AUDIOLOGY: SCIENCE TO PRACTICE

Second Edition

Steven Kramer, PhD

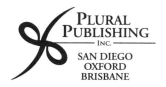
PLURAL
PUBLISHING
INC.
SAN DIEGO
OXFORD
BRISBANE

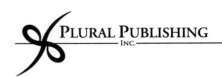

5521 Ruffin Road
San Diego, CA 92123

e-mail: info@pluralpublishing.com
Web site: http://www.pluralpublishing.com

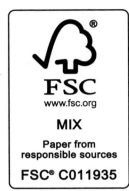

Typeset in 11/13 Garamond by Achorn International
Printed in the United States of America by McNaughton & Gunn, Inc.

For permission to use material from this text, contact us by
Telephone: (866) 758-7251
Fax: (888) 758-7255
e-mail: permissions@pluralpublishing.com

Every attempt has been made to contact the copyright holders for material originally printed in another source. If any have been inadvertently overlooked, the publishers will gladly make the necessary arrangements at the first opportunity.

Library of Congress Cataloging-in-Publication Data
Kramer, Steven J., author.
   Audiology : science to practice / Steven Kramer, author.—2E.
       p. ; cm.
   Includes bibliographical references and index.
   ISBN-13: 978-1-59756-523-3 (alk. paper)
   ISBN-10: 1-59756-523-7 (alk. paper)
   I. Title.
   [DNLM: 1. Hearing—physiology. 2. Audiology. 3. Hearing Disorders. 4. Hearing Tests—methods. WV 270]
   LC Classification not assigned
   617.8—dc23
                                                        2013000768

Contents

Preface

The second edition of this popular textbook continues its focus on providing undergraduate students, beginning audiology doctoral students, and other health care professionals the foundations for understanding the auditory system, performing and interpreting basic hearing tests as they relate to auditory disorders, and gaining an appreciation for the profession of audiology. This textbook is appropriate for students beginning a professional doctoral program in audiology, including those from traditional speech and hearing undergraduate programs or those who may not have had any background in speech, language, and hearing sciences. It is expected that the knowledge obtained in this textbook will be applicable to the readers' future education or clinical practices. For some, it may help them decide to go into the profession of audiology. To facilitate learning, the principles and procedures described in this textbook are further enhanced through the use of a companion workbook, *Audiology Workbook*, by Steven Kramer and Lesli Guthrie, in which there are extensive sets of related questions and activities, along with a complete answer set, for most of the chapters in this textbook.

Although this textbook is intended for readers with little or no background in audiology, it is not a cursory overview. Instead, it presents a comprehensive and challenging coverage of hearing science and clinical audiology, but written in a style that tries to make new and/or difficult concepts relatively easy to understand. The approach to this book is to keep it readable and to punctuate the text with useful figures and tables. Each chapter has a list of key objectives, and throughout the chapter key words or phrases are italicized and included in a glossary at the end of the textbook. In addition, most of the chapters have strategically placed reviews (synopses) that can serve as quick refreshers before moving on, or that can provide a "quick read" of the entire text. Having taught undergraduates in speech, language, and hearing sciences, as well as beginning audiology doctoral students for a number of years, I have learned a lot about how students learn and what keeps them motivated. In my classes and in this textbook, I

first gain their attention and interest with a fascinating look at the structure of the ear, rather than the more traditional approach of beginning with physics of sound. After getting them interested in the ear and audiology, I cover some information about acoustics so that they have the tools to understand how the ear works and how hearing loss is assessed (which is what they really want to know). Of course, the order of the chapters can be changed to suit any instructor.

As with other introductory audiology textbooks, this textbook provides comprehensive descriptions of basic audiological test equipment, standards, audiograms, pure-tone tests (including masking), speech tests, and immittance measures. Where appropriate, variations in procedures for pediatrics are presented. This textbook includes many examples on how to interpret and describe audiograms and immittance data. The reader is also introduced to some specialized tests like auditory brainstem response (ABR), otoacoustic emissions (OAE), wide-band middle ear power (WMEP), and tests for functional hearing losses. Beginning students also have a lot of interest in knowing about some common hearing disorders, and this book provides concise descriptions of selected auditory pathologies from different parts of the auditory system, with typical audiological findings for many of the more commonly found ear diseases and hearing disorders. As a special addition, James Jerger, a legend in audiology, and Cheryl DeConde Johnson have contributed a very interesting chapter on the historical highlights of audiology over the past 70 plus years—a must-read for anyone involved with audiology. In addition, Gus Mueller and Earl Johnson have contributed an excellent chapter that introduces the student to hearing aids and cochlear implants.

Features and Additions to this Edition

This edition of the textbook includes many additions and updates from the previous edition, and there has been some reorganization throughout the book. The easy-to-read style and clearly explained concepts popular with the first edition have been retained and improved throughout this edition. Two new chapters have been added, one on clinical pure-tone masking, and one on hearing screening. Much of the supplemental material from the first edition is now incorporated into the main content of the chapters. Some additional details and figures have been added on vestibular anatomy and physiology, acoustic resonance, speech acoustics, wide-band middle ear power (WMEP) measures, and masking for speech testing. In addition, James Jerger has revised his contributed chapter on the historical pathways in audiology, including the addition of an educational audiology path, thanks to the contribution of Cheryl DeConde Johnson. Gus Mueller and Earl Johnson have also revised their chapter on hearing aids to reflect many updates that have taken place in amplification options over the past five years. And finally, most of the updates and additions to this textbook have also been added to the second edition of the companion workbook, *Audiology Workbook, 2nd edition*, by Steven Kramer and Lesli Guthrie.

Contributors

Cheryl DeConde Johnson, EdD
Speech, Language, and Hearing Sciences
University of Colorado
Boulder, Colorado
Chapter 13

James Jerger, PhD
Distinguished Scholar-in-Residence
School of Behavioral and Brain Sciences
The University of Texas at Dallas
Dallas, Texas
Chapter 13

Earl E. Johnson, PhD
Coordinator, Auditory and Vestibular Dysfunction
Research Enhancement Award Program
James H. Quillen VA Medical Center, Mountain
    Home, TN
East Tennessee State University
Johnson City, Tennessee
Chapter 11

Steven J. Kramer, PhD
School of Speech, Language, and Hearing Sciences
San Diego State University
San Diego, California
Chapters 1, 2, 3, 4, 5, 6, 7, 8, 9, 10, and 12

H. Gustav Mueller, PhD
Professor
Department of Hearing and Speech Sciences
Vanderbilt University
Nashville, Tennessee
Chapter 11

To the hearing impaired children on my school bus route many years ago, who inspired me to pursue an education in audiology;

To my students then, now, and the future, who make my work enjoyable, challenging, and rewarding;

To my colleagues who provide me an exciting place to work and lasting friendships.

PART I

FUNDAMENTALS OF HEARING SCIENCE

Part I of this textbook focuses on anatomy and physiology of the auditory and vestibular systems, as well as fundamental concepts in acoustics traditionally covered in hearing science courses. The first three chapters are ordered in somewhat of a nontraditional way. Chapter 1 provides a detailed look at the auditory and vestibular structures, their relationships to each other, and their orientations in the skull. You will find yourself eager to learn how these sensory organs function, but will have to be a little patient and wait for Chapter 3. In Chapter 2, you will learn some important concepts regarding basic properties of sound, including frequency, amplitude, phase, and the physical properties of speech sounds. An understanding of the material in Chapter 2 will provide you with the important concepts and tools needed to learn and appreciate the physiology of the hearing and balance systems covered in Chapter 3. The objective of Part I of this textbook is to provide you with a solid foundation in hearing science that is important for understanding the clinical concepts presented in Part II of the textbook. Finally, you are encouraged to use the newly updated Audiology Workbook (2014) to maximize your learning and enjoyment of the material covered in this textbook.

1

Anatomy of the Auditory and Vestibular Systems

After reading this chapter, you should be able to:

1. Visualize the location of the auditory and vestibular organs in your own head and be able to describe the locations of these structures within the temporal bone.
2. Divide the ear into its five major divisions based on anatomy, and identify the primary parts within each division.
3. Identify the parts of the outer ear and middle ear, and the major landmarks observed in an otoscopic view of a normal tympanic membrane.
4. Describe the relationship of the bony and membranous labyrinths within the inner ear and their different fluids.
5. Sequence different anatomical views as they progress from a more general view to detailed views of the cells and neurons within the organ of Corti, the semicircular canals, and the otolith organs.
6. Identify the sensory and support cells within the organ of Corti.
7. Describe several differences between the inner hair cells (IHCs) and the outer hair cells (OHCs) within the organ of Corti.
8. Define and describe the afferent and efferent neural systems within the auditory system as they relate to the hair cells, brainstem auditory nuclei, and primary auditory cortex.
9. Identify and locate the sensory structures of the vestibular organs and their primary nuclei within the brainstem.

The ear is a fascinating structure! Relatively few people come to appreciate the intricacies of the sensory structures and neural connections responsible for hearing (auditory system) and balance (vestibular system). You are in for an enjoyable journey through these sensory structures no matter what your background or where your career interests lie. For some, this glimpse into the anatomy of the auditory and vestibular systems becomes a pivotal moment that propels them to pursue audiology as a career. This chapter will give you a detailed look at the different parts of the ear, their orientations to each other, and how they are interconnected. The approach taken in this chapter is to present the anatomy with very little discussion on the function of the different structures. The functions of the auditory and vestibular systems are covered in Chapter 3.

This chapter is filled with diagrams and photos. As the adage goes, "a picture is worth a thousand words." The text in this chapter is meant primarily to orient you to the figures, with the expectation that you will navigate through the figures to learn the anatomy and the unique vocabulary associated with these sensory systems. As you progress through this anatomy chapter, keep looking back at previous figures to establish their relationships to each other. Eventually, you will come to mentally visualize these structures in your own head. So for now, sit back and enjoy a pictorial presentation and description of the anatomy of the auditory and vestibular systems.

General Orientation to the Parts of the Auditory and Vestibular Systems

Figure 1–1A provides a general orientation of the auditory and vestibular structures as they would appear within the skull when looking from the front of the head. Although this figure only shows the details for the right ear, the same structures occur on both sides. As you can see, there are structures that run from the side of the skull (lateral direction) to a location toward the middle of the skull (medial direction). Figure 1–1B is a closer view of these structures in a coronal view or section, which is derived by an imaginary plane that results in a front/back view of the human body. Anatomical planes of reference and their commonly used anatomical directions are described in Table 1–1.

Each ear is divided into five general divisions based on their location. The five general divisions of the ear are the outer ear, middle ear, inner ear, 8th cranial nerve, and the central auditory nervous system. Table 1–2 lists the five general divisions of the ear along with some of the primary structures that are identified in Figure 1–1. Although these divisions are convenient, they are connected and work together to receive and process sounds. Obviously, we have two ears and each has the same anatomical and neural components; therefore, in this textbook most of the anatomical descriptions are given only for one ear. The term *central auditory* (or *vestibular*) *system* is used to refer to the neural pathways in the brainstem and cortical areas; the term *peripheral auditory* (or *vestibular*) *system* is used to refer to auditory or vestibular structures that are outside the central nervous system. The peripheral sensory organ for hearing is called the *cochlea*. The peripheral sensory organs for the vestibular system include three *semicircular canals*, a *saccule*, and a *utricle*. The utricle and saccule are often collectively referred to as the *otolith organs*.

The auditory and vestibular structures are attached or embedded into the part of the skull that is called the *temporal bone*, which is shown in Figure 1–2. Most people are only familiar with the part of the ear that is visible on the side of their head, called the *auricle*. If you wiggle your ear or put your finger into your ear, you will notice that these parts of the ear are somewhat compliant because they are composed primarily of cartilage. These cartilaginous parts of the outer ear are attached to the lateral side of the temporal bone (and removed in Figure 1–2).

Figure 1–3 shows the details of the temporal bone from two directions. In the top part of Figure 1–3, you can see the opening of the bony part of the *external auditory canal* (also called the *external acoustic meatus*). This bony part of the ear canal is a continuation of the cartilaginous

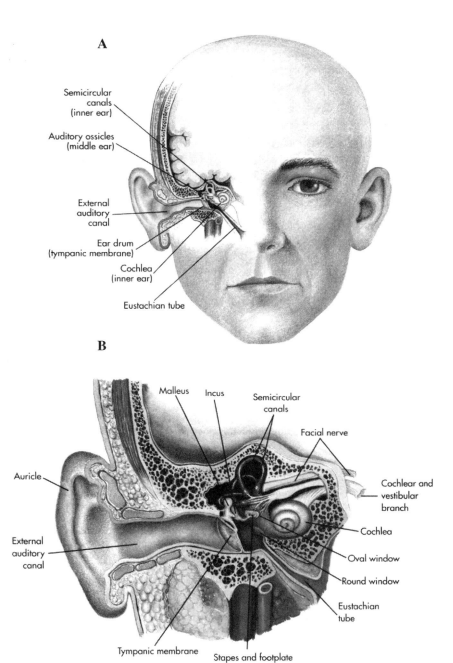

A

Semicircular canals (inner ear)

Auditory ossicles (middle ear)

External auditory canal

Ear drum (tympanic membrane)

Cochlea (inner ear)

Eustachian tube

B

Malleus   Incus   Semicircular canals

Facial nerve

Auricle

Cochlear and vestibular branch

External auditory canal

Cochlea

Oval window

Round window

Eustachian tube

Tympanic membrane   Stapes and footplate

Figure 1–1. A. Orientation of auditory and vestibular structures in the human skull. **B.** Coronal view of the auditory and vestibular structures. See Table 1–2 in order to relate the various structures seen here to the general divisions of the auditory and vestibular systems. From Seidel, Ball, Dains, & Benedict, 2003, p. 314. Copyright 2003 by Mosby, Inc.

Table 1-1. Commonly Used Terms for Anatomic Planes of Reference and Related Directions Used in Reference to Humans and Four-Legged Animals

Planes of Reference	Result in Humans	Related Directions in Humans	Result in Four-Legged Animals	Related Directions in Four-Legged Animals
Coronal	Front/back	Anterior/posterior	Head/tail	Rostral/caudal
Sagittal	Left/right	Lateral/medial	Left/right	Lateral/medial
Transverse	Top/bottom	Superior/inferior	Top/bottom	Superior/inferior

Table 1-2. Five Major Divisions of the Auditory/Vestibular Systems with Primary Structures that Correspond to Those Shown in Figure 1-1B

Outer Ear	Middle Ear	Inner Ear	Cranial Nerve (CN)	Central Nervous System
Auricle	Tympanic membrane	Cochlea (with oval and round windows)	Cochlear nerve (8th CN)	Brainstem
External auditory canal	Ossicles (malleus, incus, stapes)	Semicircular canals	Vestibular nerve (8th CN)	Cortices
	Eustachian tube	Saccule, utricle (not shown)	Facial nerve (7th CN)	

Note: More detailed structures for each division are listed in later sections.

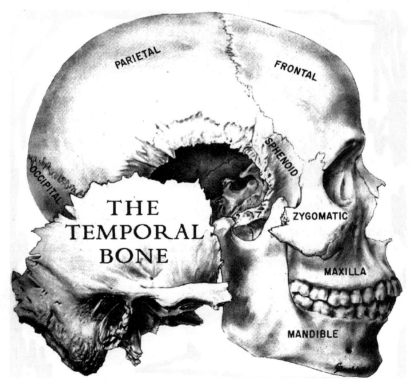

Figure 1-2. The temporal bone and its relation to the other parts of the human skull. From Anson & Donaldson, 1967, p. 1. Copyright 1967 by W. B. Saunders.

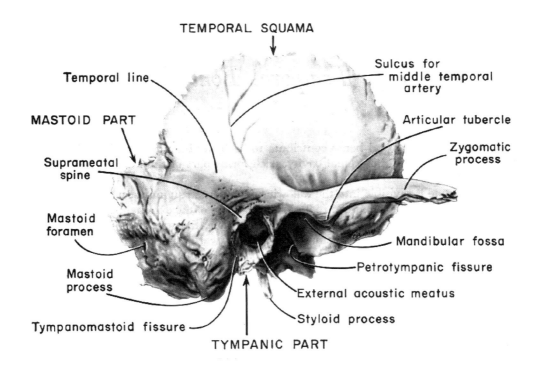

TEMPORAL SQUAMA

Temporal line

MASTOID PART

Suprameatal
spine

Mastoid
foramen

Mastoid
process

Tympanomastoid fissure

TYMPANIC PART

Sulcus for
middle temporal
artery

Articular tubercle

Zygomatic
process

Mandibular fossa

Petrotympanic fissure

External acoustic meatus

Styloid process

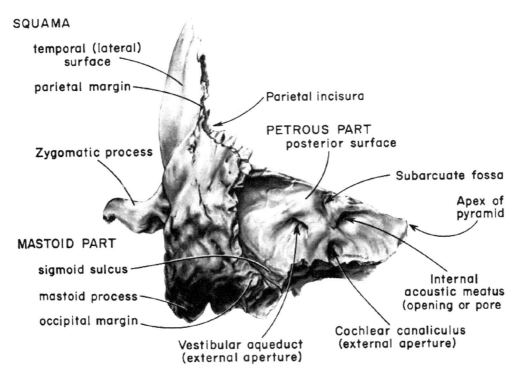

SQUAMA

temporal (lateral)
surface

parietal margin

Parietal incisura

PETROUS PART
posterior surface

Zygomatic process

Subarcuate fossa

Apex of
pyramid

MASTOID PART

sigmoid sulcus

mastoid process

occipital margin

Internal
acoustic meatus
(opening or pore)

Cochlear canaliculus
(external aperture)

Vestibular aqueduct
(external aperture)

Figure 1–3. Anatomic details of the temporal bone. The *top part of the figure* shows the lateral surface of the temporal bone as viewed from the side of the head. The *bottom part of the figure* shows the temporal bone as viewed from the top of the head, and reveals the petrous portion of the temporal bone. From Anson & Donaldson, 1967, p. 4. Copyright 1967 by W.B. Saunders.

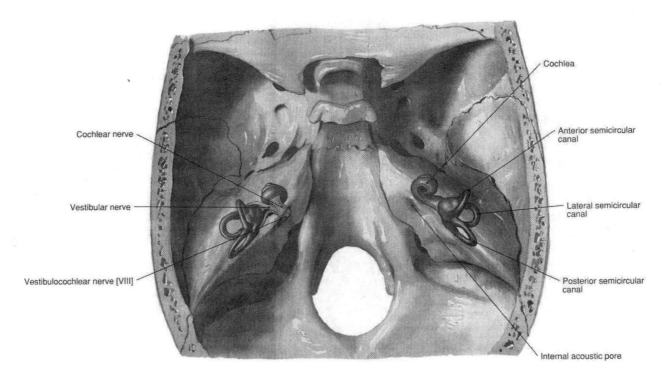

Cochlea

Anterior semicircular canal

Cochlear nerve

Lateral semicircular canal

Vestibular nerve

Posterior semicircular canal

Vestibulocochlear nerve [VIII]

Internal acoustic pore

Figure 1–4. Transverse section of the human skull at the level of the petrous bone with an artist's rendition showing the relative locations of the cochlea, vestibular organs, and cranial nerves on both sides of the head as if the petrous bone were transparent. From "Atlas of Human Anatomy" (14th ed., p. 778), by Sobotta, 2008, in R. Putz & R. Pabst (Eds.). Copyright 2008 by Elsevier GmbH, Urban & Fisher Verlag.

part of the ear canal that has been removed. The temporal bone is divided into four main parts, tympanic, mastoid, squamous, and petrous. The temporal bone also has two small processes, the *styloid process* and the *zygomatic process*, which interface with other non-auditory structures. The ear canal runs through the tympanic part of the temporal bone, whereas the middle ear and inner ear structures are housed in the *petrous* part of the temporal bone. As seen in the bottom part of Figure 1-3, the petrous part of the temporal bone is directed medially into the skull; this allows the inner ear structures to be located away from the lateral surface of the skull for greater protection.

Besides being internally located in the skull, the protective nature of the petrous part of the temporal bone is also enhanced by its pyramidal shape and hardness. Figure 1-4 is a transverse section through the skull showing the location of the inner ear's cochlea and semicircular canals. In Figure 1-4, the top of the petrous portion of the temporal bone has been removed in order to expose the sensory organs, which are actually a series of canals within the petrous part of the temporal bone. Notice in Figure 1-4 that the cochlea is more anterior and medial to the semicircular canals, and that the top of the coiled cochlea "points" horizontally in an anterior-lateral direction. Can you visualize these structures in your own head? In the following sections, the anatomical details of the auditory system are described first; then the anatomical details of the vestibular system are presented.

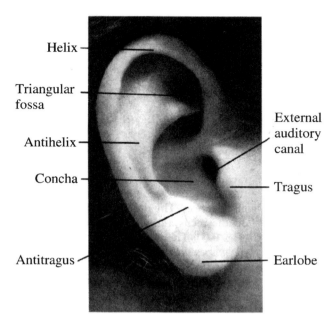

Helix

Triangular fossa

Antihelix

Concha

Antitragus

External auditory canal

Tragus

Earlobe

Figure 1–5. A picture of an auricle with key landmarks identified. Adapted from Seidel, Ball, Dains, & Benedict, 2003, p. 315. Copyright 2003 by Mosby, Inc.

Outer Ear

The outer ear is the most visible, but least important, of the auditory structures. This visible portion of the outer ear that is attached to the lateral surface of the temporal bone is called the *auricle*. There are several ridges and indentations in the auricle formed by cartilage. Although there are some variations among individuals, the primary features of the auricle are labeled in Figure 1–5. To get a better sense of the auricle's anatomy, use your own auricle as the example. Begin by touching your earlobe with your finger. The *earlobe* is the lower portion of the auricle where earrings are often attached; it is primarily fatty tissue and is not cartilaginous as is the rest of the auricle. Immediately superior and anterior to the earlobe you can place your finger in an indentation that separates the *tragus* anteriorly and the *antitragus* posteriorly. Do you feel those landmarks? The tragus is the flap of cartilage that you have, undoubtedly, used when

you close off your ear by pushing this flap in with your finger. Now run your finger superiorly from the antitragus along the ridge of cartilage called the *antihelix*, which ends at an indentation called the *triangular fossa*. If you move your finger to the outer rim of the ear, you can trace the ridge of cartilage that is called the *helix* that runs around the outer border of the auricle. The relatively large bowl-shaped indentation just before the entrance (meatus) to the external auditory canal is called the *concha*.

The *external auditory canal* is the other part of the outer ear. The external auditory canal is the canal that leads from the auricle to the middle ear. Figure 1–6 shows a coronal section of the external auditory canal. The external auditory canal is approximately 2.5 cm in length and has a somewhat curved route. The lateral half of the external auditory canal is formed by cartilage, and the medial half is formed by bone of the tympanic portion of the temporal bone. The external auditory canal can be straightened by pulling up and back on the auricle (as is done during a clinical examination of the outer ear), which lifts the cartilaginous portion of the external auditory canal. Along the cartilaginous portion of the ear canal are small hairs, as well as glands that produce earwax, called *cerumen*. The hairs and cerumen help protect and clean the external auditory canal. The bony portion of the external ear canal is covered tightly by the thin lining of skin tissue.

Middle Ear

The middle ear is a small air-filled cavity that begins at the *tympanic membrane* (ear drum). The tympanic membrane forms the boundary between the external auditory canal and the middle ear (see Figure 1–1B). Figure 1–7 shows photos of the right and left tympanic membranes, surrounded by the external auditory canal wall, as they would appear when viewed through an *otoscope*, an instrument used to look into the ear canal. The tympanic membrane is semitranslucent, slightly cone shaped, and pearl gray in color. The primary components of the middle ear are the tympanic

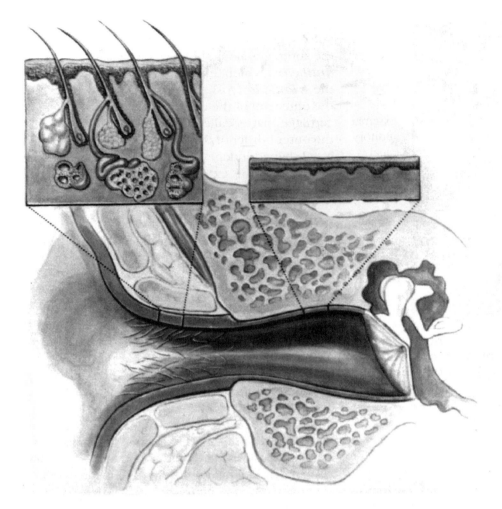

Figure 1–6. A drawing of the external auditory canal. The *insets* illustrate how the various parts differ in the presence or absence of hair follicles and cerumen glands. From Office of Visual Media, Indiana University School of Medicine, 1994. Copyright, 1994, Indiana University School of Medicine.

Right Ear

Left Ear

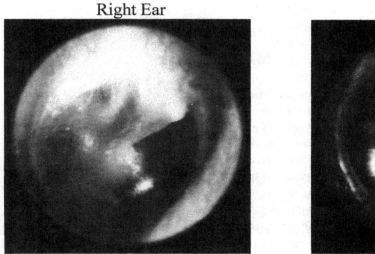
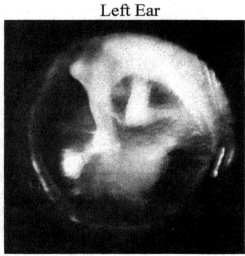

Figure 1–7. Photos of the tympanic membranes for the right and left ears as they would appear when viewed through an otoscope. From Touma & Touma, 2006, pp. 2 & 7. Copyright 2006 by Plural Publishing.

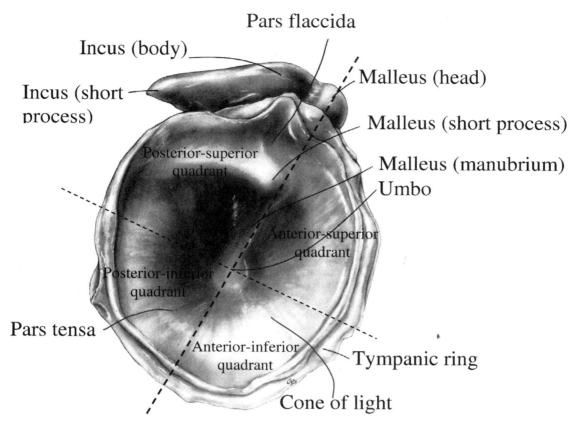

Figure 1–8. Drawing of a tympanic membrane and related middle ear structures. The superimposed *dotted lines* divide the tympanic membrane into four quadrants. Adapted from Anson & Donaldson, 1967, p. 54. Copyright 1967 by W. B. Saunders.

membrane, the ossicles (bones) with two small muscles attached, and the eustachian tube.

Figure 1–8 is a drawing of the tympanic membrane with some landmarks and structures labeled. The more easily seen landmark visible through the tympanic membrane is the *manubrium* (handle) of the *malleus* (one of the ossicles). This bony landmark is clearly visible through the tympanic membrane along the upper half, where the manubrium is attached to the tympanic membrane. The *umbo* is a term used to describe the location where the tip of the manubrium attaches to the center of the tympanic membrane. There is often a *light reflex* or *cone of light* seen on the tympanic membrane that is a characteristic reflection of the light from the otoscope due to the curved

shape of the tympanic membrane (seen better in Figure 1–7).

Notice also that the upper portions of the ossicles lie above the superior border of the tympanic membrane and would not be visible with an otoscope. Most of the tympanic membrane has a fibrous tissue layer, the *pars tensa*, that lies between the skin lining the external ear canal wall and the mucous tissue lining the middle ear space. This fibrous tissue layer within the tympanic membrane provides strength to the membrane. In the anterior part of the tympanic membrane, however, there is a small area that does not have the fibrous tissue layer; this thinner area of the tympanic membrane is called the *pars flaccida* or *Shrapnell's membrane*. The outer rim of the tympanic membrane is called the *tympanic ring* (or *tympanic annulus*). The tympanic ring is embedded into an indentation in the tympanic portion of the temporal bone, and this indentation is called the *tympanic sulcus*, which serves to hold the tympanic membrane in place. As seen in Figure 1-8, the tympanic membrane can be described by quadrants as visualized by an imaginary line running along the manubrium and a bisecting perpendicular line. These quadrants allow one to describe where different structures or pathologies are located. For example, the cone of light in a normal ear is typically found in the anterior–inferior quadrant.

The middle ear *ossicles* are a series of three bones, the *malleus, incus,* and *stapes,* which are connected to each other and form the *ossicular chain.* Details of the ossicular chain are shown in Figure 1-9, as viewed from inside the middle ear cavity looking toward the inner surface of the tympanic membrane (not shown). The manubrium of the malleus attaches to the tympanic membrane (see Figure 1-7). The top part of the manubrium is readily visible through the tempanic membrane and is called the *lateral process.* In addition to the manubrium, the malleus is composed of a neck, an anterior process, and a head. The head of the malleus *articulates* (united by joints) with the body of the incus. In addition to its body, the incus has a short process and a long process. At the end of the long process of the incus is the *lenticular process,* which articulates with the head of the stapes. In addition to the head, the stapes has an anterior crus, posterior crus (plural is crura), and a footplate. The *footplate of the stapes* is connected to the inner ear through the *oval window.* You should look back and forth between Figure 1-1, Figure 1-8, and Figure 1-9 in order to get a sense of how the tympanic membrane and ossicular chain are oriented to each other and how they are oriented within the middle ear.

The middle ear also has a *eustachian tube* that connects the middle ear to an opening into the *nasopharynx,* an area above the tonsils in the upper part of the oral cavity/throat. Figure 1-10 shows the anatomy of the eustachian tube and its relationship to the nasopharynx. The eustachian tube is composed of a bony (osseous) portion

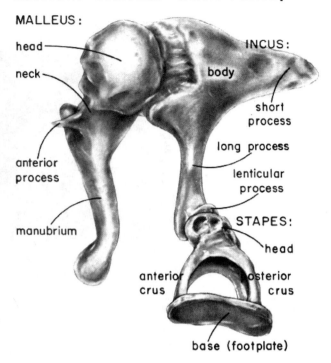

AUDITORY OSSICLES – Normal Anatomy

MALLEUS:

head

neck

anterior process

manubrium

INCUS:

body

short process

long process

lenticular process

STAPES:

head

anterior crus

posterior crus

base (footplate)

Figure 1-9. Drawing of an ossicular chain, composed of the three bones, malleus, incus, and stapes. Adapted from Anson & Donaldson, 1967, p. 76. Copyright 1967 by W. B. Saunders.

that originates in the middle ear cavity and a cartilaginous portion that extends to the back of the nasopharynx. The cartilaginous portion of the eustachian tube is normally closed but is opened by action of the *tensor veli palatini* muscle during chewing or swallowing. The periodic opening of the eustachian tube allows the middle ear to maintain its air-filled environment at atmospheric pressure, since it connects to the outside world through its opening in the nasopharynx. As shown in Figure 1-10C, the adult eustachian tube is longer than in a young child, and is oriented at about a 45° angle from the middle ear to the nasopharynx compared with a shallower angle in the young child (Bluestone, 1991). These developmental differences in the eustachian tube make it more difficult for the infant to maintain a normal air-filled environment of the middle ear, and this

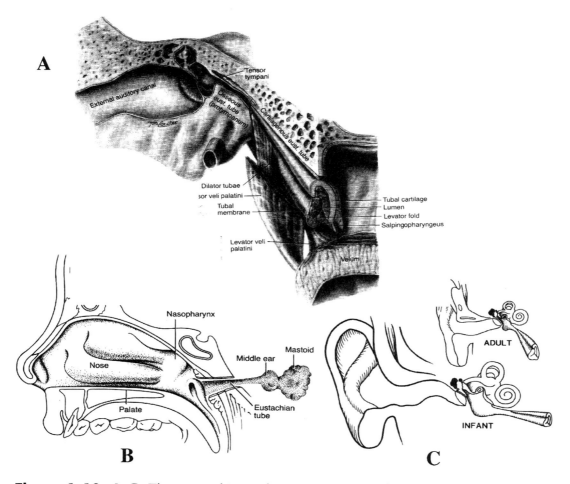

Figure 1–10. A–C. The eustachian tube. **A.** Anatomy of the eustachian tube with its bony and cartilaginous parts. The eustachian tube is normally closed, and is opened briefly by the tensor veli palatini muscle during chewing or swallowing. **B.** Illustration showing the eustachian tube from the middle ear to an opening in the nasopharynx. **C.** Illustration showing the differences in the angle of the eustachian tube between adults and infants. Adapted from Bluestone & Klein, 1988, pp. 5–7. Copyright 1988 by W.B. Saunders.

is a primary reason why infants and toddlers have more middle ear problems than adults.

The middle ear also has two small muscles, the *stapedius muscle* and the *tensor tympani muscle*, which attach to the ossicular chain by their corresponding tendons. The stapedius muscle arises from the posterior wall of the middle ear cavity and attaches to the head of the stapes. The stapedius muscle is innervated by the stapedial branch of the facial nerve (7th cranial nerve). The tensor tympani muscle arises from the bony wall above the eustachian tube and attaches to the upper part of the manubrium of the malleus. The tensor tympani muscle is innervated by a branch of the trigeminal nerve (5th cranial nerve). These middle ear muscles are involved in a reflexive response to loud sounds, called the acoustic reflex. Evaluation of the acoustic reflex is one of the basic audiological clinical procedures that will be described in more detail in later chapters.

Synopsis 1–1

- Each ear is divided into five general divisions:
  - Outer ear
  - Middle ear
  - Inner ear
  - 8th cranial nerve
  - Central auditory nervous system
- The peripheral auditory and vestibular structures are located in the temporal bone of the skull. The parts of the temporal bone include the tympanic, mastoid, squamous, and petrous, as well as two processes, the zygomatic and styloid.
- The organs for hearing and balance are within the petrous portion of the temporal bone, which affords them good protection due to the more medial location, dense composition, and pyramidal shape.
- The cochlea is anterior and medial to the semicircular canals, and the tip of the cochlea points horizontally in an anterior–lateral direction.
- The main components of the outer ear are:
  - Auricle
    - Helix
    - Antihelix
    - Tragus
    - Antitragus
    - Earlobe
    - Triangular fossa
    - Concha
  - The external ear canal, which is irregularly shaped with cartilaginous and bony parts, has an adult length of about 2.5 cm. There are cerumen and hair glands in the cartilaginous part.
- The middle ear is a small air-filled cavity that begins with the tympanic membrane at the end of the external ear canal. The main components and their parts are:
  - Tympanic membrane (pars tensa, pars flaccida, umbo, tympanic ring): semitranslucent and pearl gray in color. Notable landmarks of a normal tympanic membrane, when viewed with an otoscope, include the manubrium of malleus, lateral process of malleus, umbo, and a light reflex (from the otoscope).
  - Ossicular chain: malleus (manubrium, neck, lateral process, anterior process, head), incus (body, short process, long process, lenticular process), and stapes (head, anterior and posterior crura, footplate). The footplate is attached to the inner ear at the oval window.

- Two small muscles: stapedius muscle connects to the stapes; the tensor tympani muscle connects to the malleus. The stapedius muscle is innervated by a branch of the 7th cranial nerve; the tensor tympani muscle is innervated by a branch of the 5th cranial nerve. The stapedius muscle is involved in the human acoustic reflex as described in Chapter 3.
- Eustachian tube: a cartilaginous tube from the middle ear space to the nasopharynx to maintain atmospheric pressure in the middle ear. It is normally closed but opens (by tensor veli palatini muscle) with chewing and swallowing. Infants and young children have developmental differences in shape and function, which is a primary reason for ear infections in young children.

Inner Ear

The inner ear is a series of canals and cavities within the petrous portion of the temporal bone, called the *bony labyrinth*. A cast made of the bony labyrinth would look something like that shown in Figure 1–11. Keep in mind that the entire inner ear is smaller than the end of your little finger. The coiled structure on the right of Figure 1–11 is the cochlea, which houses the sensory organ for hearing. The cochlea spirals about 2 ¾ turns, and if uncoiled is about 35 mm long (Yost, 2000). The wider part of the cochlea is called the base, and the tip of the cochlea is called the apex. The height of the cochlea from base to apex is only about 5 mm. On the left side of Figure 1–11 you can see the three semicircular canals (anterior, posterior, and lateral or horizontal) of the vestibular system. These three semicircular canals are oriented in three orthogonal planes and respond

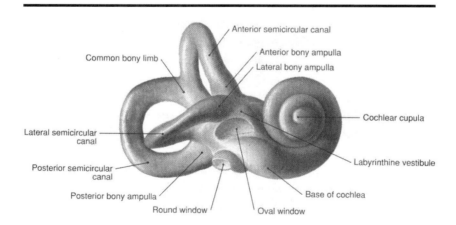

Figure 1–11. The bony labyrinth of the right inner ear as it appears in a cast taken from the system of canals and cavities within the petrous portion of the temporal bone. From "Atlas of Human Anatomy" (14th ed., p. 778), by Sobotta, 2008, in R. Putz & R. Pabst (Eds.). Copyright 2008 by Elsevier GmbH, Urban & Fisher Verlag.

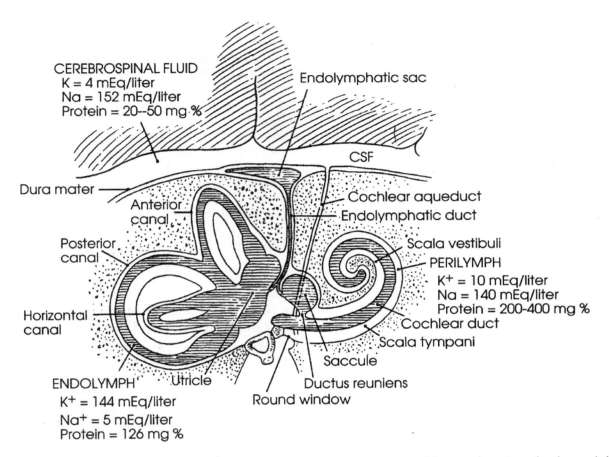

Figure 1–12. Cross-section of the petrous portion of the temporal bone showing the bony labyrinth (*unfilled areas*) and the membranous labyrinth (*filled areas*). The membranous labyrinth is suspended within the bony labyrinth and is filled with endolymph, whereas the bony labyrinth is filled with perilymph. From Baloh & Honrubia, 2001, p. 29. Copyright 2001 by Oxford University Press, Inc.

primarily to angular accelerations of the head. The *vestibule* is the area of the bony labyrinth that lies between the cochlea and the semicircular canals. Inside the vestibule is where the saccule and utricle organs of the vestibular system are located. The saccule and utricle are often referred to as the *otolith organs*, and respond primarily to linear accelerations of the head. The vestibule is also the location of the *oval window*, through which the stapes footplate of the ossicular chain connects to the cochlea. The *round window* is another membrane-covered small opening in the cochlear portion of the bony labyrinth between the middle ear cavity and the cochlea. As you will

learn in Chapter 3, because the inner ear is filled with fluid, vibrations can occur within the cochlea through reciprocal movements (in and out) of the stapes in the oval window with movements (out and in) of the round window membrane.

Suspended within the bony labyrinth of the inner ear is a *membranous labyrinth*. The membranous labyrinth has the same general shape of the bony labyrinth. The membranous labyrinth is where the auditory and vestibular sensory cells are located. Figure 1–12 shows a cross-section drawing of the bony labyrinth and membranous labyrinth. The entire inner ear is filled with fluids; however, the fluid within the membranous labyrinth is different from the fluid within the bony labyrinth (surrounding the membranous labyrinth). The bony labyrinth is filled with fluid called *perilymph*, which is similar to cerebral spinal fluid. Perilymph has a high sodium (Na⁺) concentration and low potassium (K⁺) concentration. The membranous labyrinth is filled with fluid called *endolymph*. Endolymph has high potassium (K⁺) concentration and low sodium (N⁺) concentration. Endolymph is similar to fluids found inside cells (intracellular) and, therefore, in the cochlea is unique in that this type of fluid is found as an extracellular fluid. Notice, in Figure 1-12, that the membranous labyrinth (and its endolymph) is continuous between the cochlea and the vestibular organs by way of a small channel called the *ductus reuniens*. The membranous labyrinth also has an extension to the dural area of the brain through the *endolymphatic duct*, which ends in the *endolymphatic sac*. The perilymph of the bony labyrinth connects to the cerebral spinal fluid through a narrow bony canal called the *cochlear aqueduct*. In the following sections, a more detailed look at the anatomy will be presented separately for the sensory organs of hearing and the sensory organs for balance.

The Sensory Organ of Hearing

Now let's take a more detailed look at the fine structure of the cochlea. Figure 1-13 shows another drawing of the bony labyrinth of the inner ear, but with a transverse section that runs through the center of the cochlea so we can see inside the cochlea (top half of cochlea removed). The central bony core of the cochlea is called the *modiolus*, which is a porous area of bone that forms the inner wall of the cochlea. The modiolus is where the nerve fibers from the sensory cells of the cochlea come together and form the

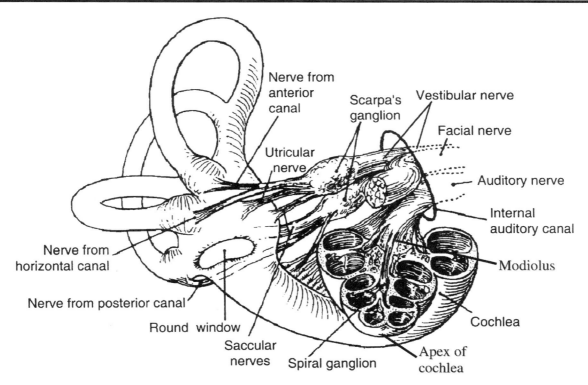

Figure 1–13. A drawing of the bony labyrinth with a transverse section through the cochlea (mid-modiolar view) revealing the modiolus and cochlear chambers (scalae). From Baloh & Honrubia, 2001, p. 11. Copyright 2001 by Oxford University Press, Inc.

auditory portion of the 8th cranial nerve. Because the top half of the cochlea has been removed in Figure 1–13, we can see circular-looking cross-sections of the coiled cochlea at different locations. Figure 1–14 shows actual photomicrographs of a cochlea. Figure 1–14A shows the modiolus after a portion of the bony wall was chipped away and the membranous labyrinth removed. As you can see, the modiolus (inner core of the cochlea) resembles a screw in which the modiolus has a bony thread, the *osseous spiral lamina*, spiraling around the bony shaft. Figure 1–14B shows the cochlea as a cross-section through the middle of the cochlea (and resembles the cut cochlea seen in Figure 1–13) with the membranous labyrinth in place. Notice that the osseous spiral lamina partially divides the bony labyrinth into different sections (called scalae). Actually, coming off of the osseous spiral lamina is a small triangular-shaped part of the membranous labyrinth, called the *scala media*, that attaches to the outer wall of the bony labyrinth. Thus, the scala media separates the bony labyrinth into two other sections, one called *scala tympani* and one called *scala vestibuli*. As we will see in more detail soon, the sensory organ of hearing, called *organ of Corti*, lies within scala media along one side of its membranous surface, the *basilar membrane*. The basilar membrane is the portion of the membranous labyrinth that is attached from the osseous spiral lamina to the outer wall of the bony labyrinth. The other surface of the membranous labyrinth is called *Reissner's membrane*. Reissner's membrane is also attached from the modiolus part of the bony labyrinth to the outer wall of the bony labyrinth. You can identify each of these scala by remembering that the scala tympani is the part of the bony labyrinth next to the basilar membrane and organ of Corti. It may also help to remember that the scala tympani terminates at the round window membrane which is drum-like (hence, "tympani"), whereas scala vestibuli is the part of the bony labyrinth next to Reissner's membrane and terminates at the oval window in the vestibule (hence, "vestibuli"). The scala tympani and scala vestibuli are filled with perilymph, whereas scala media is filled with endolymph (except in portions of the organ of Corti,

as described later). The scala media does not quite go all the way to the apex of the coiled bony labyrinth, which results in a space at the apex, called the *helicotrema*. At the helicotrema, the scala tympani and scala vestibuli are continuous with each other. Keep in mind that the cochlea, including the scala media, spirals from base to apex, as shown in Figure 1–15.

We are now ready to take a look at the fine structure of the organ of Corti. Figure 1–16 is a drawing of a cross-section of the three scala from a part of the continuously spiraling cochlea. Be sure to look back at earlier figures to get a perspective on how this drawing relates to the entire cochlea. As you will see, many of the following figures will zoom further and further into this cross-section of the scala media to view the details of the organ of Corti. In Figure 1–16, you can again see how the membranous labyrinth divides the cochlea into its three scala by attaching to the osseous spiral lamina and the outer wall of the bony labyrinth. Scala tympani is next to the basilar membrane and scala vestibuli is next to Reissner's membrane. Scala media is the membranous labyrinth itself. Recall that scala tympani and scala vestibuli contain perilymph, whereas scala media contains endolymph. As can be seen in Figure 1–16, along the outer wall of the scala media is the *stria vascularis*, a highly vascularized system of cells that maintains the ionic charge of the endolymph and is very important for the biological function of the organ of Corti.

The organ of Corti is a collection of different specialized cells that are found within the scala media along the basilar membrane. You should now be even more impressed by how small the organ of Corti is when you think of where it is in relation to the entire inner ear, which itself is smaller than a dime.

The details of the organ of Corti are shown in Figure 1–17. When describing some of the structures of the organ of Corti, keep in mind that "inner" is toward the modiolus and "outer" is toward the stria vascularis along the outer wall of the cochlea. Figure 1–17 shows a two-dimensional "slice" through the organ of Corti; however, these cells are laid out, one next to the other, along the

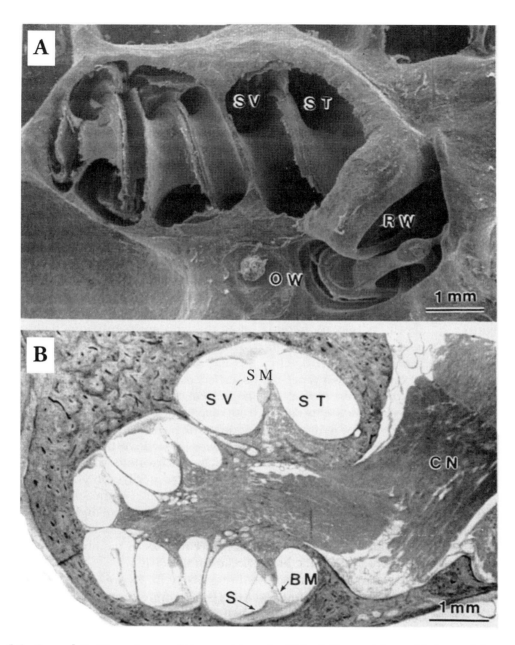

Figure 1–14. A and B. Two views of the cochlea. **A.** Chinchilla cochlea with bony labyrinth opened to show the coiled modiolus. **B.** Mid-modiolar cross-section through cochlea. **SV**, scala vestibuli; **ST**, scala vestibuli; **SM**, scala media; **BM**, basilar membrane; **S**, stria vascularis; **CN**, cochlear nerve; **OW**, oval window; **RW**, round window. From Harrison, 1988, p. 12. Copyright 1988 by Charles C. Thomas.

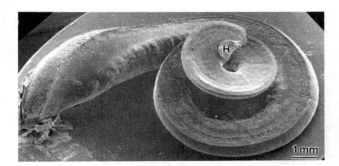

Figure 1–15. A plastic cast of the human co-chlea. **H,** helicotrema. From Harrison, 1988, p. 13. Copyright 1988 by Charles C. Thomas.

entire length of the coiled cochlea from its base to its apex. To help visualize this, imagine that all the cells in Figure 1–17 repeat as they go in and out of the page, which you can get a sense of from the organ of Corti depicted in Figure 1–16. The cells of the organ of Corti consist of two types of functionally relevant cells, the *inner hair cells* (IHCs) and the *outer hair cells* (OHCs). Spiraling from the base to the cortex are about 3,500 IHCs "lined-up" in a single row, and about 12,000 OHCs "lined-up" in three rows (Yost, 2000). The tops of the IHCs and OHCs have bundles of hairs called *stereocilia.* Above the stereocilia of the hair cells is another membrane, the *tectorial membrane.* The tectorial membrane is attached to the *spiral limbus,* a cell that curves up from the osseous spiral lamina (see Figure 1–16). Notice that the ste-reocilia of the OHCs are attached to the underside of the tectorial membrane, whereas the stereo-cilia of the IHCs are not attached to the tectorial membrane. The other cells of the organ of Corti, shown in Figure 1–17, are there to provide struc-tural support and shape for the organ of Corti. The IHCs are supported by the *inner support cells.* The OHCs and IHCs are separated by the *tun-nel of Corti,* a space in the center of the organ of Corti that is formed by the inner and outer *pillar cells.* The OHCs (unlike the IHCs) are surrounded by spaces called *spaces of Nuel.* Each OHC sits on top of a support cell, called a *Deiter cell* (also called outer phalangeal cell). Each Deiter cell has a process called a *phalangeal process* that reaches

up to the upper surface of an adjacent OHC and fills in what would have been a space between the OHCs at the upper surface. Figure 1–18 shows a closeup of the OHCs where you can see how the phalangeal processes of the Deiter cells extend to the upper surface of the organ of Corti. Fig-ure 1–19 shows a photomicrograph looking down on the top surface of the organ of Corti in its three-dimensional view, after pulling back the tectorial membrane. Here you can see the single row of IHCs and the three rows of OHCs. Notice that the stereocilia of the OHCs have a characteristic "W" appearance, whereas the stereocilia of the IHCs have a characteristic shallow "crescent" shape. Also in Figure 1–19, a section has been removed in order look inside the organ of Corti, where you can see the tunnel of Corti and some of the cell bodies of the organ of Corti. Notice that the tops of all the cells are tightly joined across the upper surface of the organ of Corti. This surface, com-prising a tight mosaic of the tops of all the cells, is called the *reticular lamina.* Can you identify the reticular lamina in Figures 1–16 and 1–17? The reticular lamina serves as the boundary between endolymph and perilymph within the scala media: Endolymph is above the surface of the reticular lamina and surrounds the stereocilia of the hair cells, whereas perilymph is below the surface of the reticular lamina in the spaces within the organ of Corti (spaces of Nuel and tunnel of Corti). The perilymph within the organ of Corti is thought to permeate the basilar membrane and surrounds the bodies of the OHCs.

As seen in Figure 1–20, the stereocilia on each hair cell are arranged in three to four rows with increasing heights, and many are joined to each other by small microfilaments called *cross-links* and *tip links.* Besides the overall number and number of rows of IHCs and OHCs, there are other differences between IHCs and OHCs as shown in Figure 1–20. The IHCs are flask shaped, have a centralized nucleus, and the cytoplasmic organ-elles are distributed throughout the cell body. The OHCs are more cylinder shaped, have a nucleus closer to the base of the cell, and the organelles are more organized along the cells' outer walls (which has important physiological relevance, as discussed in Chapter 3).

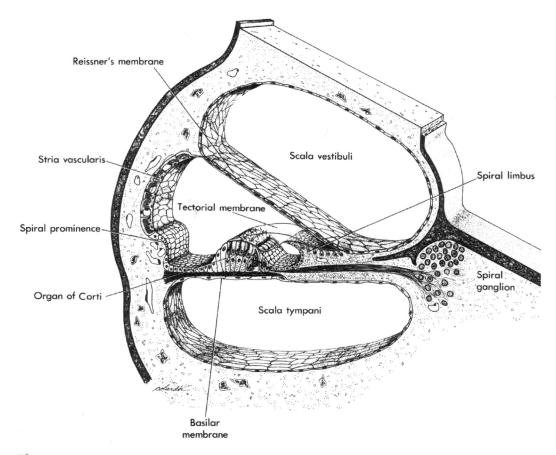

Figure 1–16. Cross-section of the cochlea showing the three scalae and the organ of Corti in scala media. From Fawcett, 1994, p. 929. Copyright 1994 by Chapman and Hall.

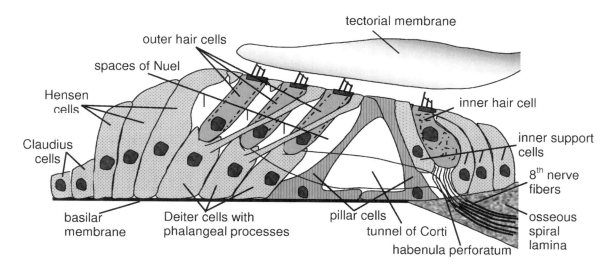

Figure 1–17. Cross-section of the organ of Corti.

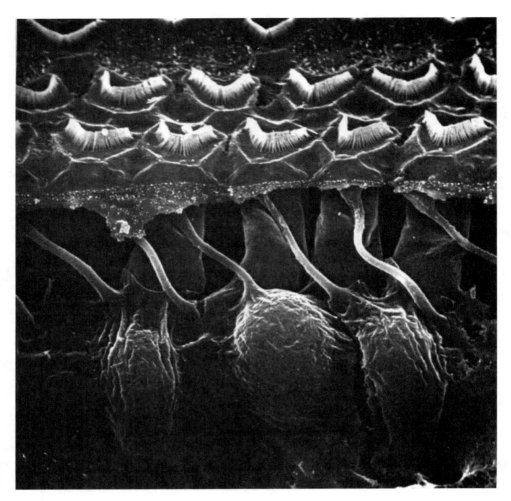

Figure 1–18. Close-up view within the organ of Corti showing the phalangeal processes of the Deiter cells and how they fill in the gaps at top surface of the adjacent outer hair cells, forming part of the reticular lamina. From Bagger-Sjöback, Anniko, & Lundquist, 1984, p.15. Copyright 1984 by Butterworths and Company Ltd.

Synopsis 1–2

- The inner ear houses the auditory organ, which is the cochlea, and the vestibular organs, which include three semicircular canals and two otoliths (saccule and utricle).

- The middle ear connects to the inner ear membranous labyrinth at the footplate of the stapes in the oval window.

- The membranous labyrinth of the cochlea, the scala media, divides the cochlea into three chambers: (a) scala media (the membranous labyrinth), (b) scala tympani (next to the basilar membrane), and (c) scala vestibuli (between Reissner's membrane and the outer wall of the cochlea).

- Because the membranous labyrinth ends just before the apex, the scala vestibuli and scala tympani are joined in this area, which is called the helicotrema.

- Along the outer wall of the membranous labyrinth is a highly vascularized network of cells, the stria vascularis, which maintains the ionic composition of the endolymph.

- The organ of Corti is found within the scala media along the basilar membrane. The cells of the organ of Corti (in order from modiolus to the outer wall) include:
  - Inner sulcus cells
  - Inner support cells
  - Inner hair cells (IHCs)
  - Inner and outer pillar cells (which form the tunnel of Corti)
  - Three rows of outer hair cells (OHCs) sitting on top of Deiter cells
  - Hensen cells
  - Claudius cells

- The organ of Corti has a membrane, the tectorial membrane, which attaches to the spiral limbus on the modiolus side and to the Hensen cells across the organ of Corti. The stereocilia of the OHCs are imbedded within the underside of the tectorial membrane, whereas the stereocilia of the IHCs are not directly in contact with the tectorial membrane.

- The OHCs are surrounded by spaces of Nuel. The Deiter cell below each OHC has a phalangeal process that reaches up to the upper surface of the organ of Corti to fill in any spaces at the surface above the spaces of Nuel. In this way, the upper surfaces of all the cells of the organ of Corti (below the tectorial membrane) are tightly butted against each other to form a mosaic of cells, the reticular lamina, with only the stereocilia sticking out above the surfaces of the hair cells. The reticular lamina serves as the boundary between endolymph above and perilymph below (in the spaces of the organ of Corti).

- Endolymph is similar to fluids typically found within cells (high K^+, low Na^+) and is unique as an extracellular fluid in the inner ear. The bony labyrinth (surrounding the membranous labyrinth) is filled with a fluid called perilymph, which is similar to cerebral spinal fluid (high Na^+, low K^+).

- Each cochlea has about 3,500 IHCs (arranged in one row) and about 12,000 OHCs (arranged in three rows). Each hair cell has small hair-like bundles of tiny hairs, called stereocilia, arranged in three to four rows with increasing height toward the outer wall of the cochlea, and are connected by cross-link and tip-link filaments. The stereocilia on each IHC appear as a shallow crescent shape. The stereocilia on each OHC appear as a W shape.

- The OHCs differ from IHCs in their overall number, arrangement, shape, and organization of their internal cellular organelles.

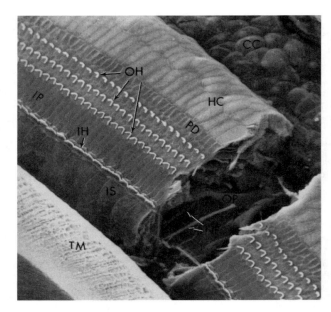

Figure 1–19. A view of the top surface of the organ of Corti with the tectorial membrane (*TM*) pulled back to reveal the reticular lamina and the stereocilia of the three rows of outer hair cells (*OH*) and the single row of inner hair cells (*IH*). The top surface of the tunnel of Corti is defined by the top plates of the inner pillar cells (*IP*) and separates the inner hair cells from the outer hair cells. A section is opened up to view below the reticular lamina. **OP**, outer pillar cells; **PD**, phalangeal processes of Deiter cells; **HC**, Hensen cells; **CC**, Claudius cells; **IP**, inner pillar cells. From Kimura, 1984, p. 102. Copyright 1984 by Butterworths and Company Ltd.

The Sensory Organs of Balance

There are five separate structures that make up the peripheral vestibular system of the inner ear: three semicircular canals (anterior, posterior, and horizontal) and the saccule and utricle. The semicircular canals are involved in rotational movements (accelerations) of the head, whereas saccule and utricle are involved in linear movements (accelerations) of the head. More details on the physiology of the vestibular organs are provided in Chapter 3. The membranous labyrinth of the vestibular portion of the inner ear is filled with endolymph and is continuous with the endolymph in the cochlea,

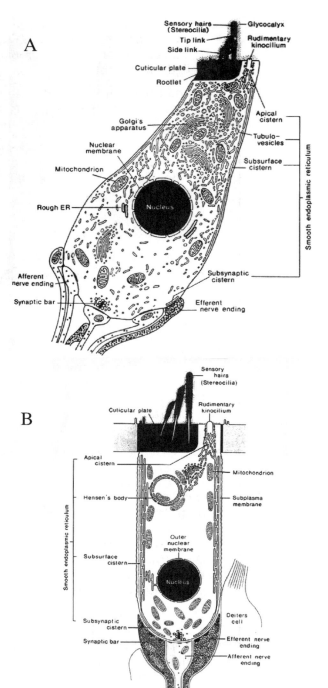

Figure 1–20. Drawings of inner hairs cells (**A**) and outer hair cells (**B**) that illustrate their different shapes, location of the nucleus, and organization of the cell's cytoplasm. Notice also that the stereocilia are connected by tip links and side links. Adapted from Lim, 1986, pp. 75 & 76. Copyright 1986 by W.B. Saunders.

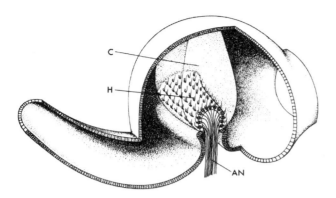

Figure 1–21. A crista within the ampulla of a semicircular canal. **C**, cupula; **H**, hair cells; **AN**, afferent nerves. From Barber & Stockwell, 1976, p. 22. Copyright 1976 by C. V. Mosby.

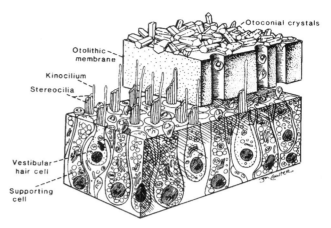

Figure 1–22. A macula of the otolith organ showing the otoconia crystals on the surface of the gelatinous otolithic membrane. From Furman & Cass, 1996, p. 6. Copyright 1996 by F. A. Davis.

through the ductus reuniens. The sensory organ of each semicircular canal is called the *crista ampullaris* and is located within the membranous labyrinth. Each crista is located in an enlargement of the membranous (and bony) labyrinth, the *ampulla,* at the anterior end of each semicircular canal near the vestibule (see Figure 1-11). The saccule and utricle each have a sensory organ, the *macula.* Unlike the cochlea, where the sensory cells continue along the entire length of the coiled cochlea, the sensory cells of the vestibular organs are localized to a patch of cells within each ampulla for the cristae rather than continue around the semicircular canal; likewise, the sensory cells are situated along one edge of the maculae of the saccule and utricle.

Figure 1-21 shows a diagram of a crista. The crista is composed of sensory hair cells that have their stereocilia embedded into a gelatinous membrane, the *cupula,* which extends above the hair cells and completely seals off the semicircular canal. Remember, there is a separate crista for each semicircular canal. Figure 1-22 shows a diagram of a macula. The maculae comprise sensory hair cells distributed along one side of the saccule or utricle. The stereocilia of the hair cells within each macula are embedded in a gelatinous otolith membrane; however, the macula also has a layer of dense calcium carbonate crystals, *otoconia,* on

the top of the otolith membrane, which adds mass to the macula.

As with the inner and outer hair cells of the organ of Corti, the vestibular organs have two types of hair cells, type I and type II. Type I hair cells are more flask shaped (similar to IHCs of the organ of Corti) and type II are more cylinder shaped (similar to OHCs of the organ of Corti). Functional relevance of having two types of hair cells within the vestibular organs is not as distinct as for the IHCs and OHCs of the organ of Corti (discussed more in Chapter 3). The stereocilia of the hair cells of the cristae are arranged in two or three rows with increasing heights, and each hair cell has a single large cilium, a *kinocilium,* adjacent to the tallest row of stereocilia. The kinocilia have functionally relevant orientations for stereocilia bending during head movements that produce distinct physiological responses (discussed more in Chapter 3). In the crista, the kinocilia are oriented away from the utricle for the anterior and posterior canals, and are oriented toward the utricle for the horizontal semicircular canal. It should be noted that in the hair cells of the organ of Corti, kinocilia are not present; however, each hair cell has a rudimentary base of a kinocilium embedded in the top surface of the hair cell adjacent to the tallest row of stereocilia, and which also provides functionally relevant orientations for stereocilia bending as part of the ear's physiological response to sound vibrations.

Auditory and Vestibular Neural Pathways

Referring to Figure 1–1 and Figure 1–13, you can see the location of the 8th cranial nerve, the *vestibulocochlear* (or *cochleovestibular*) *nerve*. As the name implies, the 8th cranial nerve is composed of the *cochlear* (or *auditory*) *nerve* that connects to the cochlea, and the *vestibular nerve* that connects to the different vestibular organs. The 8th cranial nerve exits the petrous part of the temporal bone through an opening in the posterior wall, the *internal auditory canal*. Notice that the 7th cranial nerve (facial nerve) also exits the petrous bone through the internal auditory canal. In the following sections, the auditory neural pathways are first described, followed by the vestibular neural pathways.

Auditory Nervous System Pathways

Most of the nerve fibers in the cochlear nerve are *afferent neurons* (approximately 30,000) that carry impulses from the organ of Corti to the brainstem; however, there are a small number of *efferent neurons* (about 1,200) that carry impulses from the brainstem to the organ of Corti. Figure 1–23 shows the connections of the auditory neurons (both afferent and efferent) to the hair cells in the organ of Corti. Keep in mind that the auditory neurons are distributed from/to hair cells along the entire length of the coiled organ of Corti. As you can see in Figure 1–23, most of the afferent nerve fibers (*inner radial fibers*) come from connections with the IHCs. In fact, approximately 95% of the 30,000 afferent neurons are connected to the 3,500 IHCs, i.e., many afferent neurons connect to each IHC (Spoendlin, 1978). The remaining afferent neurons (*outer spiral fibers*) come from OHCs that are located approximately 0.6 mm basally from where they cross the tunnel of Corti.

Each outer spiral fiber has collaterals coming from several OHCs distributed across their three rows.

The efferent auditory nerve fibers within the organ of Corti are much fewer in number and more difficult to trace. A greater proportion of the efferent nerve fibers connect to the OHCs than to the IHCs (Gelfand, 2004). Figure 1–24 shows that the efferent fibers have different types of connections to the IHCs and OHCs. For the OHCs, both the efferent neurons and the afferent neurons synapse directly with the body of the hair cell. This suggests that the efferent nerve fibers can have a direct influence on the OHCs. However, for the IHCs, only the afferent neurons synapse directly with the body of the hair cell, whereas the efferent neurons synapse with the afferent nerve dendrites after they leave the IHC, and do not have direct connections with IHC (Spoendlin, 1978). The functional significance of these differences in neural connections to the different hair cells is not yet fully understood.

The afferent auditory neurons coming from the cochlear hair cells enter the modiolus through tiny holes, *habenula perforata* (see Figure 1–23), in the osseous spiral lamina. The cell bodies of the afferent auditory neurons are located in the modiolus near the osseous spiral lamina within a bony canal, *Rosenthal's canal*. The afferent auditory nerve cell bodies are called *spiral ganglia* (singular = *spiral ganglion*) and are distributed along the spiraling cochlea. The cell bodies for the efferent nerve fibers are located in the pontine region of the brainstem near the *superior olivary complex* (SOC), and their axons travel as the *olivo-cochlear bundle* (OCB) in the 8th cranial nerve, following the same route to the organ of Corti as the afferent nerve fibers through the modiolus, habenula perforata, and to the corresponding hair cells. The efferent nerve fibers that connect to the OHCs originate from the area around the *medial superior olive* (MSO) on both sides of the brainstem, with the majority coming from the contralateral side. The efferent nerve fibers that connect to the IHCs originate from the area around the lateral superior olive (LSO) on both sides of the brainstem, again with the majority coming from the contralateral side.

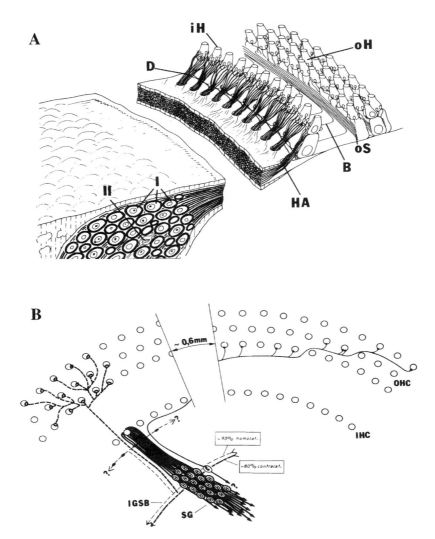

Figure 1–23. Illustration showing the afferent neurons entering the cochlea through the habenula perforata (*HA*) with multiple synapses with the inner hair cells (*iH*). The cell bodies of the cochlear neurons (**I**, type I neurons; **II**, type II neurons) are shown in Rosenthal's canal along the spiral lamina of the modiolus. **oH**, outer hair cell; **oS**, outer spiral bundle; **B**, basilar fibers; **D**, dendrites. From Spoendlin, 1984, p. 133. Copyright 1984 by Butterworths and Company Ltd. **B.** Innervation pattern of cochlear neurons in the organ of Corti. *Solid lines* indicate afferent neurons; *dashed lines* indicate efferent neurons. **SG**, spiral ganglion; **IGSB**, intraganglion spiral bundle; **IHC**, inner hair cell; **OHC**, outer hair cell. From Spoendlin, 1988, p. 204. Copyright 1988 by Raven Press.

The afferent nerve fibers of the cochlear branch of the 8th cranial nerve exit the internal auditory canal and travel a short distance to enter the brainstem at the junction of the pontine (pons) and medullary (medulla) regions of the brainstem. The term *nucleus* is used to identify a location within the brainstem where there is a collection of specialized cell bodies. This is similar to the use of ganglion to describe a collection of specialized cell bodies in the peripheral sensory systems (e.g., spiral ganglion in the cochlea). Connections and pathways in the brainstem and cortical regions of

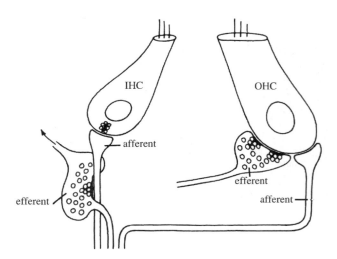

Figure 1–24. Illustration showing the different synapse of afferent and efferent neurons with an inner hair cell (*IHC*) and an outer hair cell (*OHC*). From Spoendlin, 1984, p. 144. Copyright 1984 by Butterworths and Company Ltd.

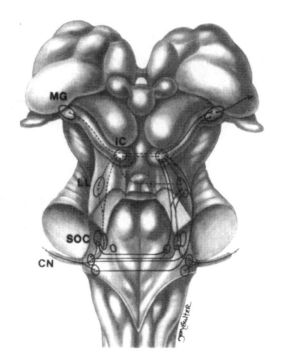

Figure 1–25. Drawing of the posterior surface of the brainstem, with superimposed pathways and nuclei of the central auditory system. Nuclei include cochlear nuclei (*CN*), superior olivary complex (*SOC*), lateral lemniscus (*LL*), inferior colliculus (*IC*), and medial geniculate body (*MG*). From Møller, 2000, p. 131. Copyright 2000 by Academic Press.

the brain are considered to be part of the central nervous system. As shown in Figure 1-25, the primary auditory nuclei, in ascending order, are the *cochlear nucleus, superior olivary complex, lateral lemniscus, inferior colliculus*, and *medial geniculate* (in the thalamus). Each of these auditory nuclei is present on both sides of the brainstem. The central auditory afferent pathway involves multiple synapses with multiple cells within multiple brainstem nuclei.

The neural connections of the central auditory system within the brainstem are relatively complex, are not easy to document, and may vary slightly among species. A complete description is beyond the scope of this introductory text. However, a relatively simplified schematic representation of the afferent auditory pathways is shown in Figure 1-26 representing input to the brainstem from the cochlea on one side of the head (the pathways would be duplicated from the other ear). The nerve fibers of the cochlear portion of the 8th cranial nerve enter the brainstem at the lateral side of the pontine region of the brainstem. All of the cochlear 8th nerve afferent neurons synapse with cells in the cochlear nucleus on the

same side (ipsilateral) as the ear. Upon entering the cochlear nucleus, each afferent auditory nerve fiber sends collaterals to different areas of the cochlear nucleus. The afferent (ascending) outputs from the cochlear nucleus take different paths depending on the location of the cells. The primary neural output of the cochlear nucleus comes from the anterior-ventral (AVCN) part of the cochlear nucleus and travels to the other side of the brainstem (contralateral); however, even these neurons can take different paths, for example, some neurons from the AVCN cross the midline and synapse with cells in the contralateral lateral lemniscus or inferior colliculus, while others synapse in cells of either the ipsilateral or contralateral superior olivary complex. The primary afferent pathways consist of connections to the contralateral side of

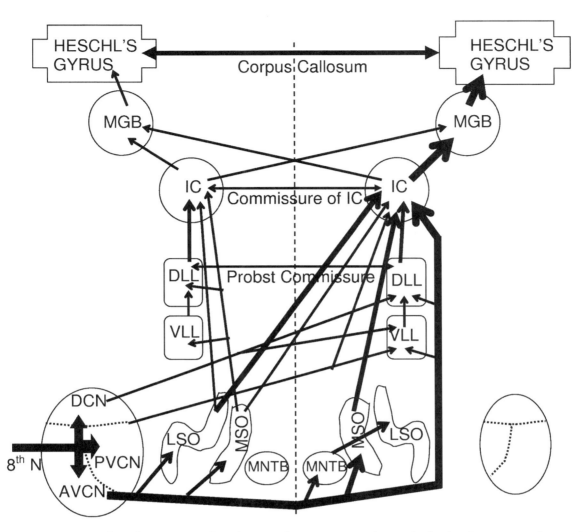

Figure 1–26. Central auditory neural pathways from one ear through the brainstem to the auditory cortex as gleaned from several references. The *dotted line* represents the midline of the brainstem. There are multiple pathways coursing along an ipsilateral route and a more dominant contralateral route. **8th N** 8th cranial nerve; **AVCN** anterior–ventral cochlear nucleus; **PVCN** posterior–ventral cochlear nucleus; **DCN** dorsal cochlear nucleus; **LSO** lateral superior olivary complex; **MSO** medial superior olivary complex; **MNTB** medial nucleus of trapezoid body; **VLL** ventral lateral lemniscus; **DLL** dorsal lateral lemniscus; **IC** inferior colliculus; **MGB** medial geniculate body.

the brainstem; however, there is also an ipsilateral ascending representation from the superior olivary complex. Notice that the first location where there would be connections from both ears is at the superior olivary complexes. To add to the complexity, there are *commissures* (interconnections) across the brainstem between the lateral lemnisci and between the inferior colliculi. From the me-

dial geniculate on each side of the brainstem, the neurons travel to the ipsilateral primary auditory reception area of the cortex. The primary auditory reception area of the cortex is located along the upper surface of the *temporal lobe* in *Heschl's gyrus* (Figure 1–27). The two hemispheres of the cortex, including the temporal lobes, are interconnected through the *corpus callosum.*

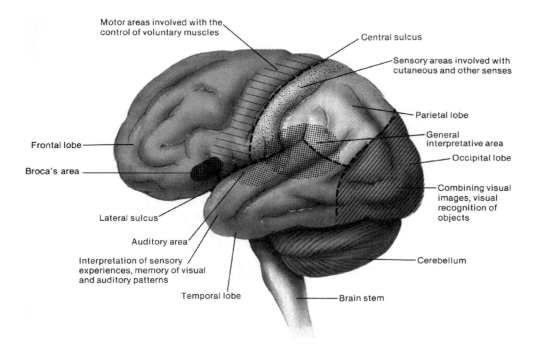

Figure 1–27. The left side of the brain with the different lobes and major landmarks identified. The primary auditory area (Heschl's gyrus) is on the upper surface of the temporal lobe. There is an auditory reception area on the temporal lobe on both sides of the brain. From Van de Graaf, 1988, p. 333. Copyright 1988 by W. C. Brown.

Vestibular Nervous System Pathways

The vestibular organs provide the central vestibular system with information about the orientation (relative to gravity) and changes in head movement (more in Chapter 3). Refer to Figure 1–1 and Figure 1–13 to see the vestibular portions of the 8th cranial nerve. As with the cochlea, there are afferent neurons and a much smaller number of efferent neurons making connections with the hair cells of the vestibular organs. As mentioned earlier, there are two types of hair cells in the vestibular organs, type I and type II. Similar to the IHCs of the cochlea, the type I hair cells have relatively large and direct afferent nerve connections with the body of the hair cell, and the efferent neurons connect to the afferent neurons after leaving the hair cell. The type II vestibular hair cells, like the OHCs of the cochlea, have both afferent and efferent connections directly with the body of the hair cell (see Figure 1–24). The proportion of type I and type II

hair cells varies among species and among the different vestibular organs. (A complete description of the vestibular neural connections to the peripheral organs is beyond the scope of this text.) The afferent pathways are involved in carrying the sensory information from the vestibular organs to the central vestibular nuclei where they are involved with a variety of reflexive actions (e.g., with eye movements and spinal reflexes). The cell bodies for the peripheral vestibular afferent neurons are gathered together in *vestibular ganglia*, also known as *Scarpa's ganglia*, located just peripherally to the internal auditory canal. The afferent neurons from the posterior semicircular canal and part of the saccule form an inferior branch of the vestibular nerve, whereas those afferent neurons from the other two semicircular canals, the utricle, and the remaining part of the saccule form the superior branch of the vestibular nerve.

The vestibular branches of the afferent vestibular portions of the 8th cranial nerve exit the

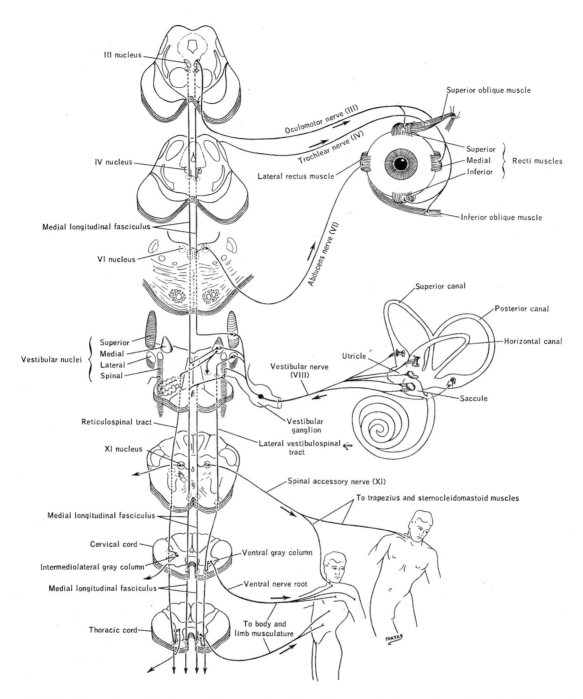

Figure 1–28. Central vestibular pathways showing the vestibulo-ocular reflex (*VOR*) on the top right, and the vestibulo-spinal reflex (*VSR*) on the bottom right. From House, Panskey, & Siegel, 1979, p. 240. Copyright 1979 by McGraw-Hill, Inc.

petrous portion of the temporal bone through the internal auditory canal, along with the cochlear branch of the 8th cranial nerve and the 7th cranial nerve. The vestibular portions of the 8th cranial nerve enter the brainstem at the same level of the pontine region of the brainstem as the cochlear portion of the 8th cranial nerve; however, the vestibular neurons synapse with cells within specialized vestibular nuclei within the brainstem and a small number go directly to the cerebellum. Figure 1–28 shows the main vestibular nuclei and pathways for the *vestibulo-spinal reflex* (VSR) and the *vestibulo-ocular reflex* (VOR). The central vestibular nuclei for these systems are in the pontine-medullary region of the brainstem (one on each side of the brainstem), but are distinct from the auditory nuclei. The vestibular neurons of the 8th cranial nerve from each side of the head synapse on the ipsilateral (same) side as the sensory organs. As with the auditory nuclei, there are interconnections between the vestibular nuclei on the left and right sides of the brainstem. The VSR has direct connections from portions of the vestibular nuclei to motor neurons in the spinal cord (vestibulo-spinal tracts) and indirect connections through the reticular formation (reticulo-spinal tract), which act to reflexively control the relevant skeletal muscles as needed. The VOR involves connections from parts of the vestibular nuclei to the oculomotor nuclei through the medial longitudinal fasciculus (MLF) or indirectly through the reticular formation. The VOR acts to reflexively control the relevant muscles of the eyes as needed. For more detailed descriptions of the vestibular organs and neural pathways, the reader is referred to Barin (2009).

Synopsis 1–3

- The 8th cranial nerve, the vestibulocochlear nerve, has branches from each semicircular canal, the saccule, the utricle, and the cochlea. The 8th cranial nerve exits the petrous portion of the temporal bone through the internal auditory canal. It is also joined in the internal auditory canal by the 7th cranial nerve.

- There are about 30,000 afferent neurons from each cochlea that send information from the cochlea to the brainstem. There are also about 1,200 efferent auditory neurons that send information from the brainstem to each organ of Corti.

- Approximately 95% of afferent auditory neurons originate from IHCs as inner radial fibers. Several inner radial fibers are attached to each IHC. The remaining 5% of afferent neurons, called outer spiral fibers, come from collaterals originating from a more basal location from multiple OHCs across all three rows, and then cross the tunnel of Corti to exit with the inner spiral fibers through the habenula perforata in the osseous spiral lamina.

- Cell bodies for the auditory afferent neurons are called spiral ganglia. The spiral ganglia are distributed from base to apex within the modiolus of the cochlea in Rosenthal's canal (near the osseous spiral lamina).

- The neurons of the efferent auditory pathway, called the olivocochlear bundle, originate in the SOC. More of the efferent neurons connect to the OHCs than the IHCs. Those neurons connecting to the OHCs originate in the MSO region of the SOC from both sides of the brainstem, but more from the contralateral side; those connecting to the IHCs originate in the LSO region of the SOC from both sides of the brainstem, also with more from the contralateral side.

- OHCs have both afferent and efferent synapses with each hair cell body allowing direct efferent control to OHCs. The IHCs have only afferent synapses with each hair cell body, but the efferent neurons synapse on the afferent neurons associated with the IHC.

- The cochlear and vestibular portions of the 8th cranial nerve enter the brainstem at the level of the pontine–medulla junction.

- The afferent auditory neurons send collaterals to synapse with cells in three different regions of the cochlear nucleus. From the cochlear nucleus, central auditory neurons take several paths, which include both ipsilateral and contralateral auditory brainstem nuclei. The auditory nuclei within the brainstem (one on each side of the brainstem) are (in ascending order):
  - Cochlear nucleus (CN)
  - Superior olivary complex (SOC)
  - Lateral lemniscus (LL)
  - Inferior colliculus (IC)
  - Medial geniculate body (MGB)

- From each cochlea, there is a predominance of contralateral neural pathways for the auditory system in the brainstem; however, there are also other pathways, some of which do not synapse in each of the nuclei, and there are interconnections between the nuclei on each side of the brainstem.

- From each MGB, the neurons proceed to the ipsilateral temporal lobe and terminate in the primary auditory reception area called Heschl's gyrus. The temporal lobes from each side of the brain are also connected through the corpus callosum.

- The vestibular central afferent pathway involves connections from each branch of the peripheral vestibular nerve to parts of the vestibular nuclei in the pontine-medullary region of the brainstem, as well as some connections to the cerebellum. Portions of the brainstem vestibular nuclei connect to the spinal tract to reflexively control skeletal muscles (VSR). Other portions of the vestibular nuclei connect to the oculo-motor system to reflexively control eye muscles (VOR).

References

Anson, B. J., & Donaldson, J. A. (1967). *The surgical anatomy of the temporal bone and ear*. Philadelphia, PA: W. B. Saunders.

Bagger-Sjöback, S., Anniko, M., & Lundquist, P. G. (1984). Techniques in ultrastructural anatomy. In I. Friedman, & J. Ballantyne (Eds.), *Ultrastructural atlas of the inner ear* (p. 15). Boston, MA: Butterworths and Company.

Baloh, R. W., & Honrubia, V. H. (2001). *Clinical neurophysiology of the vestibular system*. New York, NY: Oxford University Press.

Barber, H. O., & Stockwell, C. W. (1976). *Manual of electronystagmography* (p. 22). St. Louis, MO: Mosby.

Barin, K. (2009). Clinical neurophysiology of the vestibular system. In J. Katz, L. Medwetsky, B. Burkard,

& L. Hood (Eds.), *Handbook of clinical audiology* (6th ed., pp. 431–466). Baltimore, MD: Lippincott Williams & Wilkins.

Bluestone, C. D. (1991). Physiology of the middle ear and eustachian tube. In M. M. Paparella, D. A. Shumrick, J. L. Gluckman, & W. L. Meyerhoff (Eds.), *Otolaryngology* (3rd ed., Vol. I, pp. 163–197). Philadelphia, PA: W. B. Saunders.

Bluestone, C. D., & Klein, J. O. (1988). *Otitis media in infants and children* (pp. 5–7). Philadelphia, PA: W. B. Saunders.

Fawcett, D. W. (1994). *Bloom and Fawcett: a textbook of histology* (p. 929). New York, NY: Chapman and Hall.

Furman, J. M., & Cass, S. P. (1996). *Balance disorders: a case-study approach* (p. 6). Philadelphia, PA: F. A. Davis

Gelfand, S. A. (2004). *Hearing: an introduction to psychological and physiological acoustics* (4th ed.). New York, NY: Marcel Dekker.

Harrison, R. V. (1988). *The biology of hearing and deafness*. Springfield, IL: Charles C. Thomas.

House, E. L., Panskey, B., & Siegel, A. (1979). *A systematic approach to neuroscience* (3rd ed.). New York, NY: McGraw-Hill.

Kimura, R. S. (1984). Sensory and accessory epithelia of the cochlea. In I. Friedman, & J. Ballantyne (Eds.), *Ultrastructural atlas of the inner ear* (p. 102). Boston, MA: Butterworths and Company.

Lim, D. J. (1986). Effects of noise and ototoxic drugs at the cellular level in the cochlea: a review. *American Journal of Otolaryngology, 7*, 75–76.

Møller, A. R. (2000). *Hearing: Its physiology and pathophysiology* (p. 131). San Diego, CA: Academic Press.

Office of Visual Media, Indiana University School of Medicine. (1994). Personal communication.

Seidel, H. M., Ball, J. W., Dains, J. E., & Benedict G. W. (2003). *Mosby's guide to physical examination*. St. Louis, MO: Mosby.

Sobotta. (2008). In R. Putz & R. Pabst (Eds.), *Atlas of Human Anatomy* (14th ed., p. 778). Munchen, Germany: Elsevier GmbH, Urban & Fisher Verlag.

Spoendlin, H. (Ed.). (1978). *The afferent innervation of the cochlea*. San Diego, CA: Academic Press.

Spoendlin, H. (1984). Primary neurons and synapses. In I. Friedman, & J. Ballantyne (Eds.), *Ultrastructural atlas of the inner ear* (p. 133). Boston, MA: Butterworths and Company.

Spoendlin, H. (1988). Neural anatomy of the inner ear. In A. F. Jahn & J. Santos-Sacchi (Eds.), *Physiology of the ear* (p. 204). New York, NY: Raven Press.

Touma, J. B., & Touma, B. J. (2006). *Atlas of Otoscopy*. San Diego, CA: Plural Publishing.

Van de Graaf, K. M. (1988). *Human anatomy* (p. 333). Dubuque, IA: W. C. Brown.

Yost, W. (2000). *Fundamentals of hearing* (4th ed.). San Diego, CA: Academic Press.

2

Properties of Sound

After reading this chapter, you should be able to:

1. Describe how sound waves are produced, how they propagate, how fast they travel through air, and how they change with distance.
2. Define frequency, period, amplitude, starting phase, and wavelength; graph the time-domain waveform of pure tones with different frequencies, amplitudes, and starting phases.
3. Define how intensity and pressure are related to each other; specify the minimum reference levels for intensity and pressure; specify the range of audibility for intensity (in watts/m^2) and pressure (in μPa).
4. Understand why and how to use decibels to quantify intensity and pressure; describe the range of audibility of intensity and pressure using decibels; define dB IL and dB SPL; describe the threshold of audibility across frequency.
5. Perform simple decibel calculations to compare the intensity and/or pressure of two sounds or to illustrate how intensity or pressure changes with distance.
6. Describe periodic and aperiodic complex vibrations; interpret time-domain and spectral graphs of complex vibrations; describe the importance of Fourier analyses.
7. Describe the basic acoustic characteristics of speech and understand how to read spectrograms.
8. Understand how filtering can be used to shape the spectrum of noise; recognize commonly used filter shapes.
9. Discuss and interpret graphs related to the psychoacoustic (perceptual) properties of loudness, pitch, temporal integration, and localization.

We live in a world of sounds, some of which are meaningful and some of which are just part of our noisy environment. We often take for granted the remarkable ability of the auditory system to extract meaningful sounds from the less meaningful so that we can sense danger, localize the source of a sound, communicate, learn, and even be entertained. Even when asleep you learn to tune out familiar sounds, but may wake up at an unfamiliar sound. At a noisy party, you are able to focus on a conversation with one person while ignoring the background conversations, but you readily become aware when someone calls your name from across the room or your favorite song begins. When you listen to an orchestra or band you may find yourself listening to the whole song or picking out the various instruments. Our ability to hear in our everyday world requires the auditory system to process the complex sounds from our environment. The process of hearing involves the generation of sounds, their travels and interactions within the environment, physiological processing by the ear, neural processing in the nervous system, and psychological/cognitive processing by the brain. The sounds we hear have basic physical properties that are processed by the auditory system into meaningful information.

Acoustics is the study of the physical properties of sounds in the environment, how they travel through air, and how they are affected by objects in their environment. As you will see in this chapter, any simple vibration can be uniquely described by its frequency, amplitude, and starting phase. Complex vibrations can be described as combinations of simple vibrations. However, not all sounds generated in the environment are audible and the audible range may be different across species; for example, dogs and cats are more responsive to higher pitched sounds than are humans. The human ear is capable of hearing a wide range of frequencies over an extensive range of amplitudes. But how does frequency relate to our perception of pitch? How does amplitude relate to our perception of loudness? How do we compare the loudness of sounds across frequencies? How do we use our two ears to localize the source of sounds? These types of questions come under the area of *psychoacoustics*, which is the study of how

we perceive sound. The psychoacoustic aspects of sound covered in this chapter include some basic perceptions of pitch, loudness, temporal integration, and localization. After reading this chapter, perhaps you will be able to answer the age-old philosophical question that goes something like, "If a tree falls in the woods and there are no living creatures around, does it make a sound?"

The definitions and terminology reviewed in this chapter are necessary in order to be able to better understand topics that are covered in the following chapters, including the physiology of the auditory system, the clinical procedures used to evaluate hearing loss, and the function of hearing aids. A thorough understanding of acoustics requires knowledge of some mathematical concepts and formulas; however, in this introductory text only the basic concepts are presented, and every attempt is made to keep the mathematics to a minimum. The interested reader is referred to other textbooks (Gelfand, 2004; Mullin, Gerace, Mestre, & Velleman, 2003; Speaks, 1999; Villchur, 2000) for a more thorough treatment of acoustics and psychoacoustics.

Simple Vibrations and Sound Transmission

Sounds are produced as a result of an object being set into vibration. Some familiar examples include vibrations of guitar strings, tuning forks, stereo speakers, engines, other musical instruments, thunder, and the vocal cords while speaking. Almost any object can be made to vibrate, but some objects vibrate more easily than other objects depending on their mass and elasticity. Although most sounds in our environment are complex vibrations, we begin by looking at very simple vibrations called *pure tones*. Pure tones are used by audiologists as part of the basic hearing evaluation. In addition, an understanding of pure tones is useful because all complex vibrations can be described as combinations of different pure tones, which was mathematically proven by a man named Fourier. Today, we have electronic instruments that can perform *fast Fourier transforms* (FFTs) to determine the different pure tones that comprise any complex vibration.

The vibrating sound source sets up sound waves that travel, called *propagation (propagate)*, through some elastic medium, such as air, water, and most solids. Propagation of sound through air occurs as a result of the back and forth movement of air molecules around their position of equilibrium in response to the back and forth vibration of an object. The air molecules closest to the vibrating object move back and forth first. Because of the inertial and elastic properties of the air molecules, the air molecules only move within a localized region, but as they push against adjacent air molecules the process repeats itself, which causes the pressure variations to propogate through the medium. When the vibrating object moves outward, the air molecules are pushed together causing an increase in the density of air molecules (more molecules per volume), called *condensation*, and this corresponds to an increase in sound pressure. When the vibrating object moves in the opposite direction, there is a decrease in the density of air molecules, called *rarefaction*, and this corresponds to a decrease in sound pressure. Figure 2–1 illustrates how these increases and decreases in the density of air molecules occur in response to a simple vibrating object such as tuning fork. When the vibration repeats itself over and over, as depicted in Figure 2–1, there are continuing cycles of condensation and rarefaction that produce a continuous sound, which can be measured at different points in the surrounding area. In Figure 2–1, you can see the areas in which the air molecules are more densely packed (condensations) and where the air molecules are less densely packed (rarefactions). The condensations and rarefactions reflect a repetitive pattern of increasing and decreasing air pressure. For unobstructed sound waves in air, the air molecules move outward in a spherical direction and the actual size of the air pressure peak (amplitude) diminishes with distance because of friction, as well as because the pressure is being radiated in an increasing spherical pattern; and at some distance the pressure will no longer be measurable because the energy is spread out over a large enough spherical area. The

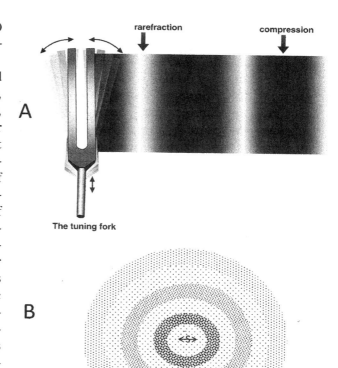

Figure 2–1. A. A vibrating tuning fork illustrates alternating areas of increased density of air molecules (condensation) and decreased density of air molecules (rarefaction) that is propagated across the air. **B.** Propagation of spherical sound wave with condensation and rarefaction phases. Notice that as the distance from the sound source increases, the force is distributed over a wider area.

actual amplitude of a sound at any point in space obviously depends on the original intensity of the sound, that is, louder sounds will travel greater distances than softer sounds.

Sound propagation can also be influenced by how the waves are reflected or interfered with by objects or walls. Much of our real-world listening situations are in closed environments, whereby much of the sound energy does not penetrate the walls but instead bounces off the walls. The angle at which a sound will bounce off a wall is similar to a ball bouncing off the wall. The angle of reflection will depend on the angle of incidence relative to the perpendicular. This becomes even more complicated when the encountered object is curved (convex or concave), or in a room with four walls, where the sound may bounce back and forth among the walls. We also need to appreciate how sound waves might interact with an object in its environment. Some sounds will bounce off an object, whereas other sounds easily go around the object, which is primarily dependent on the sound's wavelength (see section on wavelength). As you will learn in the following sections, there are also areas in which the condensation phase of a wave meets up with another wave's rarefaction phase, resulting in wave cancellation points (where no sound is present), also known as *standing waves*. In addition, materials have certain absorption characteristics that come into play in determining how sounds act in the real world. Understanding acoustics in these types of environments is especially important when designing theater or music venues (something acoustic engineers are trained to do, but it is well beyond the scope of this textbook).

Another characteristic of sound waves is the speed or velocity with which they are propagated through the medium. Sound travels faster in water and most solids than it does in air. The *speed of sound* in air is about 343 m/s or 1,126 feet/s,[1] which is much slower than the 186,282 miles/s that light travels. You probably use this knowledge, maybe unknowingly, when you estimate how many miles away you are from a storm by counting the seconds between when you see the lightning (seen instantaneously) and when you hear the thunder (heard later). Your estimate of how far away the storm is will be more accurate if you divide the number of counted seconds by five in order to take into account that the speed of sound is about one fifth of a mile per second.

When the increases and decreases in pressure occur in the direction of the vibrating object, as for sound waves, the sound is called a *longitudinal wave*. The process of localized back and forth movement of air molecules results in the propagation of a longitudinal sound wave through the air. When this sound wave reaches the ear, the corresponding increases (condensation) and decreases (rarefaction) in air pressure cause the tympanic membrane to move in and out, thus beginning the process of hearing. You will see in the later chapters how vibrations are received by the ear and how the ear transforms vibrations into auditory information. Before that, however, we need to turn our attention to understanding the basic physical parameters of sound, frequency, amplitude, and starting phase.

Frequency

Pure tones are characterized by regular repetitive movements. Imagine holding a pencil in your hand and moving it up and down on a piece of paper at a consistent height and speed. As you are moving your hand up and down, move the paper from right to left: You should see a pattern that looks something like those shown in Figure 2–2. The actual separation of the peaks that are produced will depend on the speed at which you move the paper (the slower the paper, the closer the peaks). In order to be able to quantify the pattern of vibratory movement, the motion is typically displayed as a function of time along the *x*-axis. The *y*-axis represents a measure of magnitude or amplitude of the vibrations (e.g., how far up and down you moved your hand). When the pattern of movement is displayed with amplitude as a function of time, it is called a *time-domain waveform* or simply a *waveform*.

A *cycle* of vibration describes the pattern of movement as the object goes through its full range of motion one time. In other words, one cycle represents the movement of an object from its starting point to its maximum peak, then to its negative peak, then back to its starting point. Figure 2–3 shows one cycle of a pure tone.

---

[1]The speed of sound in air is dependent upon both the temperature and the density. The values given in the text are approximations for 68° Fahrenheit. The speed of sound in air slows down as temperature decreases, for example, it is about 341 m/s or 1,086 feet/s at 32° Fahrenheit.

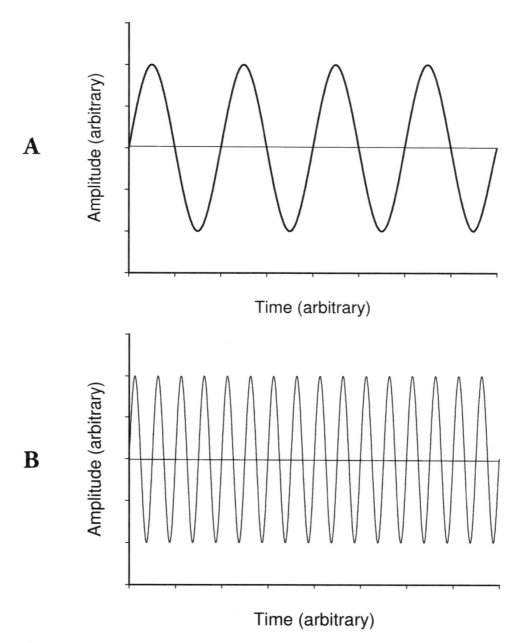

Figure 2–2. A and B. Representations of two different pure-tone vibrations as a function of time. The vibration in (**A**) is slower than the vibration in (**B**) when the time scales are equal.

Most vibrations repeat themselves; therefore, pure tones are usually described by how many cycles occur in one second, called the *frequency* of vibration. However, instead of using cycles per second as the unit of measure for frequency, the term *hertz* (Hz) is used to mean the same thing. For example, a vibration that repeats itself 100 cycles per second is called a 100 Hz pure tone. Conversely, a 100 Hz pure tone is one that completes 100 cycles in one second. An 8000 Hz pure tone is one

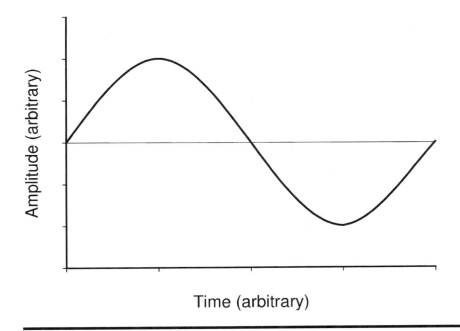

Figure 2–3. A waveform showing one cycle of vibration. The vibration moves from its starting point to its maximum peak, then to its negative peak, then back to its starting point.

that completes 8000 cycles in one second. The *frequency range of audibility for humans* is 20 to 20,000 Hz. Figure 2–4 gives some examples of different frequencies as they would appear with a one second time scale. As you can notice, it is difficult to visually count the number of cycles as the frequency increases, and counting would be extremely difficult for much of the audible frequency range. However, another way to graphically represent the different frequencies of pure tones is to change the time scale along the *x*-axis. In other words, only a few cycles (or even a single cycle) are plotted over a specified time scale. The actual frequency is calculated from knowing how long it takes to complete one cycle. The time that it takes to complete one cycle is called the *period* of the vibration. Figure 2–5 shows some examples of how the period is related to frequency. For the top example in Figure 2–5, you can see that the time it takes to complete one cycle is equal to 0.01 s (one hundredth of a second), which means it would be able to complete 100 cycles in 1.0 s (100 Hz). For the middle example in Figure 2–5, the time it takes to complete one cycle is 0.001 s, which means this vibration would be able to complete 1,000 cycles in one second (1000 Hz). For the bottom example of Figure 2–5, the time it takes to complete one cycle is 0.0001 s, which

means this vibration would be able to complete 10000 cycles in one second (10000 Hz). You can see that there is a reciprocal trade-off between the period and the frequency. The following equation shows how you can calculate the period (T) if you know the frequency, or how you can calculate the frequency (f) if you know the period:

$$T \text{ (in seconds)} = 1/f \text{ (in hertz)}$$

$$f \text{ (in hertz)} = 1/T \text{ (in seconds)}$$

This inverse relation means that as the frequency increases the period decreases. It is also important to keep in mind that when frequency is described in cycles *per second* (Hz), the period would be calculated as *seconds* (s). However, other units are often used, and one must be sure that the conversions between frequency and period are using the appropriate units. For example, frequency is often measured in units of *kiloHertz* (kHz) (*kilo* means 1,000), such that 1 kHz = 1000 Hz, 2 kHz = 2000 Hz, and so forth. The period is often measured in units of *milliseconds* (ms) (milli means 1/1,000), such that 1 ms = .001 s, 2 ms = .002 s, and so forth. Table 2–1 shows the relation between period and frequency for pure tones commonly used in studies of hearing and hearing tests. As the pattern in

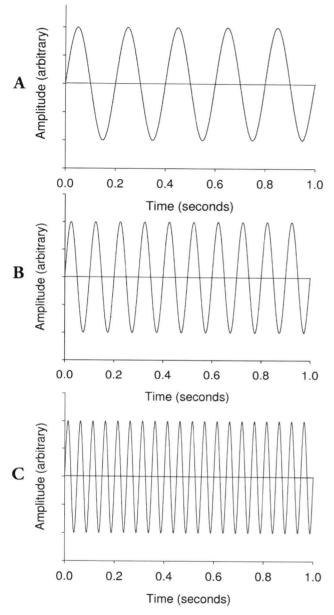

Figure 2–4. A–C. Examples of three different frequencies as they would appear with a one second time scale. The number of cycles per second determines the frequency of vibration. The more cycles per second, the higher the frequency.

Table 2-1 shows, for each doubling of frequency, the period decreases by half, or for each halving of frequency, the period doubles. In order to help understand the relations in Table 2-1, try covering one column at a time and see if you can fill in

Table 2–1. Relationship Between Frequency and Period (In Seconds and Milliseconds) for Commonly Used Frequencies

Frequency (Hz)	Period (s)	Period (ms)
250	0.004	4.0
500	0.002	2.0
1000	0.001	1.0
2000	0.0005	0.5
4000	0.00025	0.25
8000	0.000125	0.125

the correct information by using the information in the other columns. Fortunately, there is an electronic instrument, a *frequency counter*, which can be used to determine the frequency of pure tones.

Phase

Pure tones are also called *sine waves* or *sinusoids* because of their relationship to a sine function. As illustrated in Figure 2-6, one cycle of a pure tone is the equivalent of making a full revolution around a circle, where each point on the waveform can be described by its sine function relative to its phase angle (sin θ). You can think of a vibration starting at the object's resting (non-vibratory) state, which is designated as zero degrees [sin (0) = 0], then reaching its maximum positive peak at 90° [sin (90°) = 1)], returning to its initial point at 180° [sin (180°) = 0], reaching its maximum negative peak at 270° [sin (270°) = −1], and finally returning to its starting point at 360° [sin (360°) = 0]. As Figure 2-6 shows, any point on the waveform can be found using the relationship sin θ = x/r. For example, if θ = 45°, then:

$$x = r \ [sin \ (45°)],$$
$$x = r \ (0.707).$$

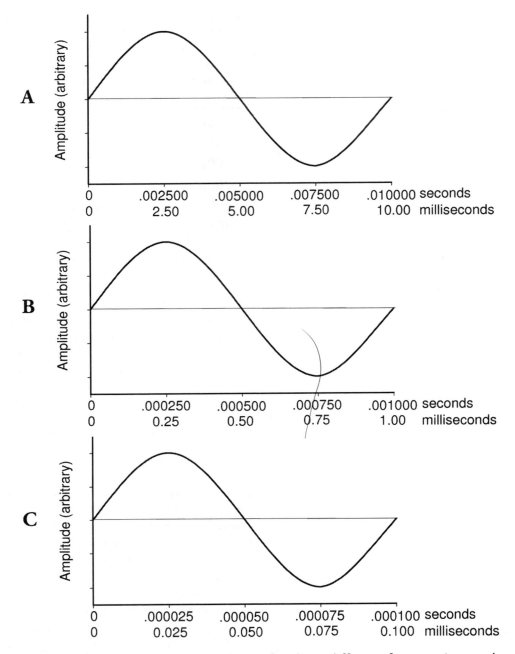

Figure 2–5. A–C. One cycle is shown for three different frequencies, each plotted with a different time scale. The time it takes to complete one cycle is the period. In (**A**) the period is equal to 0.01 s (one-hundredth of a second), which means the vibrating object would be able to complete 100 cycles in 1.0 s (100 Hz). In (**B**) the period is 0.001 s, which means this vibration would be able to complete 1000 cycles in one second (1000 Hz). In (**C**) the period is equal to .0001 second, which means this vibration would be able to complete 10,000 cycles in one second (10,000 Hz).

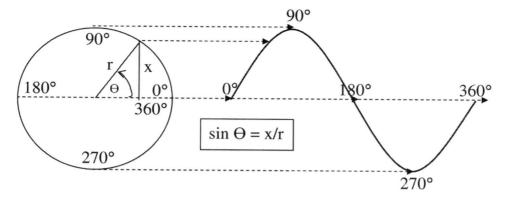

Figure 2–6. The projection of one cycle of a pure tone as it would appear relative to its position on a circle. One cycle of a waveform is the equivalent of making a full revolution around a circle. For example, the peak condensation point is equivalent to a 90° angle relative to the beginning point. The peak rarefaction point is equivalent to 270° (three-quarters around the circle). Equilibrium points are at 0°, 180°, and 360°. These simple vibrations are often called sine waves because each point on the waveform can be expressed as a sine function ($\sin \theta = x/r$) relative to its angle (θ).

Starting phase refers to the point along the waveform's cycle where the vibration begins, and is expressed in degrees relative to the angle around the circle. In other words, does the vibration first begin to move in the condensation direction or the rarefaction direction, and from what point does it begin? The waveforms shown in the previous figures have been plotted with a 0° starting phase, which means that the vibration begins from its equilibrium point and first moves toward the condensation phase, conventionally plotted as positive amplitude in the upward direction. Waveforms can begin at any point in their range of movement and go in the direction of more condensation or more rarefaction. Figure 2–7 shows an example of a sinusoid with a 180° starting phase. In this case, the vibration begins at its equilibrium point, but first moves toward the rarefaction phase and continues its cycle until it ends up back in equilibrium at the 180° starting point. Figure 2–8 shows an example of two waveforms with the same frequency, but with different starting phases, one with a 90° starting phase and one with a 270° starting phase. A 90° starting phase means that the vibration begins from its point of maximum condensation, and then

moves to its equilibrium point (amplitude = 0), continues to its point of maximum rarefaction, then back to its equilibrium point, and finally ends its cycle at the point of maximum condensation.

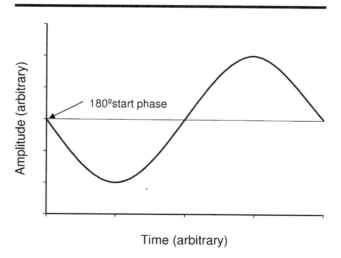

Figure 2–7. One cycle of a pure tone beginning at 180° starting phase. In this example, the movement begins with the rarefaction phase of vibration.

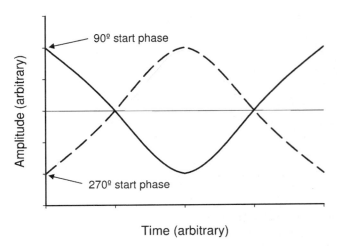

Figure 2–8. Two pure tones at the same frequency, but with different starting phases. In this example, the two waveforms are 180° out of phase with each other.

A 270° starting phase means that the vibration begins from its point of maximum rarefaction, and then moves to its equilibrium point, continues to its point of maximum condensation, then back to its equilibrium point, and finally ends its cycle back at the point of maximum rarefaction.

Our ears are not sensitive, per se, to the starting phase; a pure tone with a starting phase of 0° will sound the same as with a starting phase of 270°. However, starting phase, or phase in general, has more relevance when two or more sounds interact with each other acoustically, before reaching the ear. For the example in Figure 2–8, can you predict what the resulting sound would be? If you answered "no sound" you would have been correct, since in this example the two waveforms would cancel each other out due to the exact opposite amount of condensation in one wave

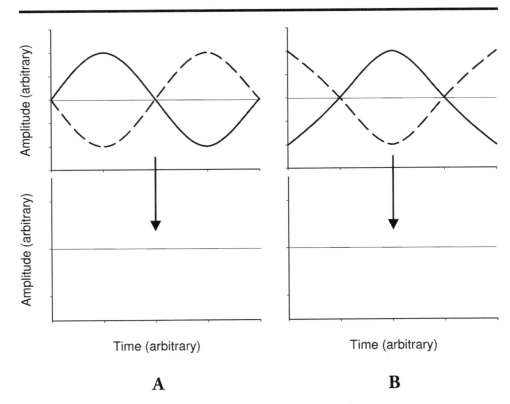

Figure 2–9. A and B. An illustration of how two pure tones of the same frequency, but which are 180° out of phase to each other, will cancel each other out. In (**A**) the *solid curve* represents a sound with a 0° starting phase and the *dashed curve* represents a sound with a 180° starting phase. In (**B**) the *solid curve* represents a sound with a 270° starting phase and the *dashed curve* represents a sound with a 90° starting phase.

with the amount of rarefaction in the other wave. Figure 2–9 again demonstrates this phase interaction with two relatively simple examples, in which two tones of the same frequency, but with opposite starting phases, are combined. For the two examples in Figure 2–9, the two tones are 180° out of phase with each other. Notice that the 180° out-of-phase relation between these (or any) two pure tones of the same frequency is maintained at all points in the waveform. Again, for these examples there would be no resulting sound pressure (and no sound) generated because each condensation point would be cancelled out by an equal rarefaction point, and the net displacement would be zero. Figure 2–10 shows two examples with two tones of the same frequency that are not 180° out of phase. In these examples, the phase relations between the two waves are more complicated and can produce places of cancellation when the points are in opposite phase directions or produce places of enhancement when the points are in the same phase direction. The combinations of the pairs of pure tones can result in more complicated waveforms. The interaction of two pure tones becomes even more complicated when they are of different frequencies as shown in Figure 2–11. In these relatively simple examples, the pairs of pure tones have the same 0° starting phase, but because they are different frequencies the phase relation between the two pure tones changes at different points in time. The phase of an individual pure tone or resultant combination of pure tones at any point in time is called the *instantaneous phase*. When a sound is made up of more than one pure tone, the resultant waveform no longer matches the pattern of a sine wave (i.e., simple wave) and is considered to be a complex vibration. As more pure tones are combined, with or without the same starting phases, the less the waveform resembles a sinusoid (complex vibrations are discussed more in a later section of the chapter).

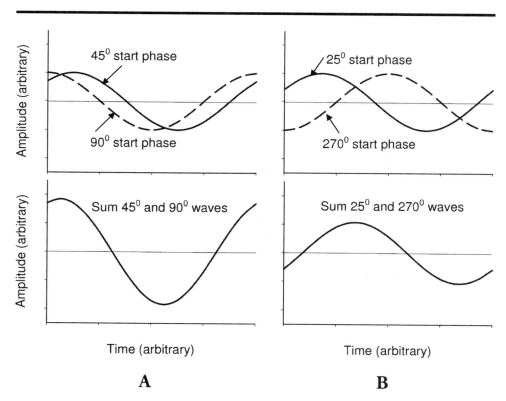

Figure 2–10. A and B. Examples of how two pure tones of the same frequency, but with different starting phases, can result in different patterns of vibration resulting from the summation of the two original waveforms.

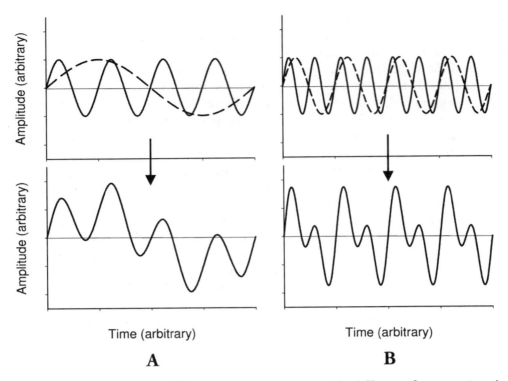

Figure 2–11. A and B. Examples of how two pure tones with different frequencies, but with the same starting phases, can result in different patterns of vibration resulting from the summation of the two original waveforms.

Amplitude

Amplitude is a general term to describe the magnitude of a sound; the larger the magnitude, the higher the amplitude. Figure 2–12 shows the waveforms of pure tones with the same frequency and starting phase, but with different maximum amplitudes along the *y*-axis.[2] For a vibrating object, maximum amplitude is related to how far the object moves back and forth. For sounds propagated through air, larger amplitudes create greater amounts of condensation and rarefaction of the air molecules. The amplitude scale along the *y*-axis is often expressed in units of displacement, intensity, or pressure.

Amplitude varies across the waveform; therefore, we need to have a way to specify the overall amplitude of a waveform. Because pure tones have equal positive and negative amplitudes, taking an average of the amplitudes at all points would result in zero amplitude and would not be useful at all. Instead, it is common to use the *root-mean-square* (RMS) *amplitude* (A_{rms}) to obtain an average amplitude for the waveform. As shown in Figure 2–13, to obtain the RMS amplitude: (a) square each of the instantaneous amplitudes to eliminate any negative values, (b) average the squared values, and

---

[2]One can describe any sinusoidal vibration by the following equation: $a(t) = A \sin(2\pi ft + \theta)$ where $a(t)$ is the instantaneous amplitude as a function of time, A is the maximum amplitude, $2\pi f$ (also called angular velocity, ω) is a measure of revolutions around a circle, and θ is the starting phase in radians.

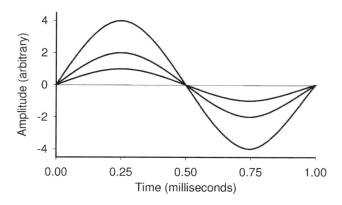

Figure 2–12. Illustration of pure tones of the same frequency with different amplitudes. Notice how the period of the vibration is the same for all three waveforms and only the height of the waveforms is different.

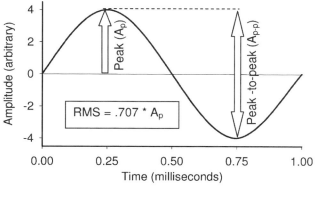

Figure 2–14. Illustration of how amplitude can be described based on its peak (*Ap*) and peak-to-peak (*Ap-p*) values. The RMS amplitude is equal to $0.707 \times Ap$.

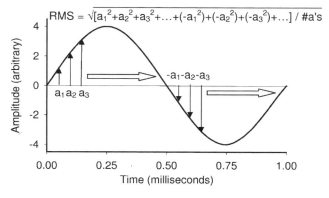

Figure 2–13. Quantification of amplitude by the method of root mean square (*RMS*). The instantaneous amplitudes across the waveform are squared to remove the negative numbers, and then averaged to find the mean, and then the square root of the number is obtained in order to get the total RMS value.

(c) take the square root of the average. The RMS amplitude is used in many applications and, fortunately, there are electronic instruments available that directly measure RMS amplitudes of pure tones and other sounds. Figure 2–14 illustrates two other ways to describe the overall amplitude of pure tones. One way is to take the amplitude change that occurs between the positive peak and the negative peak, which is called *peak-to-peak amplitude* (A_{p-p}). Another way is to measure the amplitude from baseline (zero) to one of the peaks, which is called *peak amplitude* (A_p). The RMS amplitude for a pure tone is equal to 0.707 times the peak amplitude; however, this is not the case for more complex sounds.

Synopsis 2–1

- The back and forth vibration of a sound source sets up alternating areas where the air molecules are pushed together, called condensation, and areas where the air molecules are pulled apart, called rarefaction. The air molecules move only within a small localized area, but the condensation and rarefaction areas are passed to adjacent air molecules, which cause the waveform's pressure variations to move through the medium. Sound waves travel in air at a speed of about 343 m/s (1,126 feet/s).

- Simple vibrations, called pure tones, sine waves, or sinusoids, are characterized by their physical (acoustic) dimensions of frequency, amplitude, and starting phase.

- The frequency of a sound refers to the number of vibrations that occur in one second and has units of hertz (Hz) or kiloHertz (kHz) (1 kHz = 1000 Hz). The reciprocal of frequency is the period (T), which is the time it takes to complete one cycle of vibration and has units of seconds (s) or milliseconds (ms) (1 ms = 1/1,000 s). If either the frequency or period is known, the other can be calculated ($f = 1/T$).

- The frequency range for human hearing is about 20 to 20,000 Hz. Other species may be sensitive to other ranges of frequencies.

- The starting phase of a sound refers to where in the cycle a vibration begins its cycle, and is expressed in units of degrees around a circle (0 to 360°). For example, a vibration that begins at its equilibrium and moves toward its area of maximum condensation has a starting phase of 0°; a vibration that begins at the point of maximum rarefaction and moves toward equilibrium has a starting phase of 270°. For a single pure tone, humans cannot tell the difference between starting phases. When two or more pure tones of the same frequency but with different starting phases are combined, the phase relation at different points in time (instantaneous phase) produces a complex waveform that is the sum of the two waveforms. Combining waveforms of different frequencies with or without the same starting phase will produce more complex waveforms. Two pure tones of the same frequency that are 180° out of phase will cancel each other out and not produce any sound.

- The amplitude of a sound refers to how far an object moves back and forth and/or the amount of maximum and minimum air pressure created. The larger the movement or pressure variation, the greater the amplitude for any given frequency. A simple way to describe amplitude of a visually displayed waveform is to measure the distance or pressure between the highest point of condensation peak and the lowest point of rarefaction peak, called peak-to-peak amplitude (A_{p-p}). Measures can also be made between the condensation or rarefaction peak to the equilibrium point, called peak amplitude (A_p). A more practical measure is called root-mean-square (RMS) amplitude, which is the way that most measurement instruments measure a sound's overall amplitude. The RMS method averages the amplitudes across the entire waveform by squaring each value (to remove all negative values), then averaging these squared values, and finally taking the square root to bring it back into scale.

Intensity and Pressure

The overall amplitude of a sound wave is typically quantified and measured in units of sound pressure or sound intensity to describe how the sound energy is distributed over some area of the propagating wave. For any given sound wave, there is a corresponding sound intensity and sound pressure. If you know either the intensity or the pressure, the other quantity can be derived. Intensity and RMS pressure are related to each other by the following formulas:

$$I = p^2$$
$$p = \sqrt{I}.$$

It should be intuitive that the farther away you are from a sound's source, the softer it will become. As the energy gets further away from the sound source (assuming there are no obstructions), it is distributed over a greater spherical area. The decrease in a sound's intensity with distance is known as the *inverse square law*. The inverse square law states that the intensity (I) decreases by the square of the distance between any two points (d) and is expressed by the following formula:

$$I = 1/d^2.$$

For example, if the distance is doubled, the intensity decreases by one fourth (I = 2^2). Now let's see how pressure changes with distance. Because of the previously discussed relation between intensity and pressure for any given sound wave, the

inverse square law for pressure is obtained by substituting p^2 for I in the above formula, which results in the following formula to describe how pressure changes with distance:

$$p^2 = 1/d^2$$
$$p = 1/d.$$

This formula says that the sound pressure is inversely related to the distance between two points (rather than the distance squared that was used for intensity).

Sound *intensity* is actually a measure of power that is distributed over an area, and has units of watts/cm^2 or watts/m^2 depending on the system of measurement being used (MKS or CGS). Sound *pressure* is a measure of force distributed over an area and has units of dynes/cm^2, newton/m^2, or microPascals (µPa) depending on the system of measurement being used. For this text, we will only use units of watts/m^2 for intensity and µPa for pressure. For our purposes, we are most interested in the range of sound intensities or pressures that are audible, that is, from the smallest amount needed to barely hear a sound, up to the largest amount that the ear can tolerate. Table 2–2 summarizes the intensity and pressure ranges for the human ear. Based on accepted standards derived from the lowest average levels (thresholds) obtained from young adults, the lowest average intensity needed to hear a sound, called the *reference level for intensity*, is 0.000000000001 w/m^2 (or 1.0×10^{-12} w/m^2). The lowest average pressure needed to hear a sound, called the *reference level for pressure*, is 20 µPa (or 2.0×10^1 µPa).

Table 2–2. Intensity and Pressure Ranges From the Least Audible (Reference Level) to the Upper Limit that Is Tolerated (Pain Threshold)

	Intensity (w/m²)[a]		Pressure (µPa)[b]	
Upper limit (pain)	100	or 1×10^2	200,000,000	or 20×10^7 (or 2.0×10^8)
Lowest audible (reference level)	0.0000000000001	or 1×10^{-12}	20	or 20×10^0 (or 2.0×10^1)

[a]Watts per square meter.
[b]MicroPascals.

Remarkably, these lower levels of audition correspond roughly to a vibration about the size of a hydrogen molecule (Gelfand, 2004). The highest intensity (also called the threshold of pain) that can be tolerated is approximately 100 w/m^2 (or 1.0×10^2 w/m^2). The highest pressure that can be tolerated is approximately 200,000,000 μPa (or 2.0×10^8 μPa). As you can see, the upper tolerated limit of sound intensity is 100,000,000,000,000 (or 10^{14}) times greater than the least audible sound (from 1.0×10^2 w/m^2 to 1.0×10^{-12} w/m^2). For pressure, the upper tolerated limit is 10,000,000 (or 10^7) times greater than for the least audible sound (from 2.0×10^1 μPa to 2.0×10^8 μPa). Recall that intensity and pressure are related by p = $\sqrt{I}$; therefore, it follows that the range of pressures (10^7) would be equal to the square root of the range of intensities ($\sqrt{10^{14}} = 10^7$). It may have struck you by now that these amplitude ranges are quite large, and it would be quite cumbersome if you were trying to graph them on a linear scale. Fortunately, linear scales can be transformed into ratio scales, as described in the next section on decibels, and makes working with intensity and pressure ranges much more manageable.

Decibels

In order to avoid linear scales of intensity or pressure ranges that would require working with large numbers or scientific notation, we transform these scales into a more manageable scale called the *decibel scale*. Any decibel scale is a ratio scale in which a measured value is related to a specified reference value. For example, as was mentioned above, the most intense sound that can be tolerated is 10^{14} times greater than the lowest sound intensity that can be heard. If we consider the lowest audible sound intensity as the reference, this least audible sound could be expressed as 1 or 10^0; then the range of sound intensity can be written as

a ratio of $10^{14}/10^0$. The next step in the transformation to a decibel scale is to take the logarithm[3] (or log) of that ratio, the *Bel*. The logarithm is the difference in the exponents of the terms in the ratio. Stated another way, the log is the power to which 10 must be raised to produce the number defined by the ratio. In our example, the difference in exponents is 14, which means that the range for intensity, in Bels, would be from 0 (least intense) to 14 (most intense). The upper limit would be the same as saying that 10 must be raised to the 14th power (10^{14}). Because the range for Bels only goes from 0 to 14, it is considered too restrictive to effectively describe the range of audible sounds; thus, to expand the range, the Bel is multiplied by a factor of 10 and is called the *decibel* (dB). The decibel can be written as:

$$dB = 10 \; log \; (X_{meas}/X_{ref}),$$

where X_{meas} equals the sound that is being measured and X_{ref} equals the reference sound to which X_{meas} is to be compared.

It is important to see that when the measured value is the same as the reference value, that is, $X_{meas} / X_{ref} = 1$, it would be equal to 0 dB because the log of 1 (or log 10^0) equals 0. Applying a decibel conversion to describe the range of sound intensity, the upper limit of intensity would be 140 dB greater than the least audible intensity, as determined by the following calculation:

dB intensity (at upper limit)

$= 10 \; log \; (10^{14}/10^0)$

$= 10 \; log \; (10^{14})$

$= 10 \; (14)$, *where log of 10^{14} equals 14*

$= 140 \; dB$.

Let's look at another example and calculate how many dB some arbitrary measured intensity, say 1×10^{-6} w/m^2, is above the lowest intensity needed

---

[3]A logarithm (log) of a number is the power to which 10 must be raised to obtain that number. Some simple examples are for powers of 10, in which the exponent is the log; for example, the log of 1,000 or $10^3 = 3$. It is also important to remember that the log (1) = 0. Another useful example that you may want to memorize is log (2) = 0.3. Calculators can be used to find logs of other less obvious numbers. Other sources should be consulted for a review of logarithms.

to hear. In other words, how much more intense is this higher intensity level of sound above the least audible intensity? The calculation would be:

dB intensity = 10 log (10⁻⁶ / 10⁻¹² w/m²)

When the standard reference value for intensity (10^{-12} w/m²) is used or implied in the denominator of the decibel formula, the result is called decibel *of intensity level* (dB IL). The equation for dB IL would be:

dB IL = 10 log (I$_{meas}$ w/m² / 10⁻¹² w/m²).

When the measured intensity is the same as the reference level for intensity, this would be the same as taking the log of (1), which would become 0 dB IL. By using a decibel scale, we have now defined the range of human hearing for intensity that goes from 0 to 140 dB IL. It is important to realize that 0 dB IL does not mean the absence of sound; it only means that the measured sound intensity is the same as the standard reference intensity (the least intensity needed to hear a sound for normal listeners, 1.0×10^{-12} w/m²). However, as we will see later, the lowest audible intensity can change depending on frequency, type of earphones, and other specified listening conditions, but these variations are always referenced to the universally accepted standard reference intensity of 1.0×10^{-12} w/m².

Now let's look at some other examples. Suppose you made a sound measurement and found it to be 10^{-5} w/m² (0.00001 w/m²). How many dB IL is this sound? The calculation would be as follows:

dB IL = 10 log (10⁻⁵ w/m² / 10⁻¹² w/m²)

= 10 log (10⁷)

= 10 (7), where log of 10⁷ equals 7

= 70 dB.

The decibel can be used to describe the ratio of any two numbers as long as the proper reference value is specified in the denominator. Suppose you were interested in expressing, in dB, how the intensity of one sound compares with the intensity of another sound. For example, assume one sound has an intensity that is 10,000 times more intense than another sound. In this case, the less intense sound can be considered the reference and written as 1 in the denominator; the ratio of these two sounds would be 10,000/1 (i.e., without needing to use the 10^{-12} w/m²). The dB of the louder sound, as referenced to the softer sound, would be calculated as follows:

dB intensity of louder sound
  = 10 log (10,000/1)

  = 10 log (10⁴)

  = 10 (4), where log of 10⁴ equals 4

  = 40 dB.

As another example, if the intensity of a sound is doubled, how many dB has that sound increased? In this example, the increase in intensity can be thought of as a ratio of 2/1 (the louder sound is twice as intense as the softer sound) and, therefore, would show an increase of 3 dB. The calculation would be as follows:

dB intensity increase

  = 10 log (2/1)

  = 10 (0.3), where the log of 2 equals 0.3

  = 3 dB.

The formula for converting to decibels can be applied to anything that can be expressed as a ratio as long as the reference value is known. For example, we could calculate the decibel difference between a larger bag of oranges (X$_{meas}$) as compared with a smaller bag of oranges (X$_{ref}$). If there are twice as many oranges in the larger bag than the smaller bag, there would be 3 dB more oranges in the larger bag than the smaller bag.

The decibel scale that is used most in audiology is *decibels (dB) of sound pressure*. In order to derive the decibel scale for sound pressure, it is important to go back to the previous relation between pressure and intensity ($I = p^2$). This relation requires that pressure squared (p^2) be substituted for intensity (I) in the general equation for decibels. The derivation is as follows:

dB sound pressure

$$= 10 \log (p^2_{meas} / p^2_{ref})$$

$$= 10 \log (p_{meas} / p_{ref})^2$$

$$= 20 \log (p_{meas} / p_{ref}),$$
where $\log (x)^2$ *equals* $2 \log (x)$.

Notice that for dB of sound pressure, the log of the pressure ratio is multiplied by 20 instead of by 10 as was used for dB of sound intensity. Using the formula for dB of sound pressure, any pressure ratio can be expressed in decibels. The decibel scale for sound pressure would also range from 0 to 140 dB, because the upper limit for pressure is 10^7 times greater than the lowest pressure. The calculation would be expressed as follows:

dB sound pressure upper limit

$$= 20 \log (10^7 / 10^0)$$

$$= 20 \log (10^7)$$

$$= 20 \ (7), \textit{where} \log \textit{of} \ 10^7 \ \textit{equals} \ 7$$

$$= 140 \ dB.$$

Following examples similar to those we used for intensity, let's relate any measured pressure to the lowest pressure needed to hear (20 µPa). When the specific reference value for sound pressure is used or implied in the denominator of the dB sound pressure formula, it is called *dB of sound pressure level* (dB SPL). The formula for dB SPL would be:

$$dB \ SPL = 20 \log (P_{meas} \ \mu Pa / 20 \ \mu Pa).$$

Whenever the measured sound pressure is equal to the standard reference level for sound pressure (20 µPa) it would be equal to 0 dB SPL (i.e., 20 log [1] = 0). In decibels of sound pressure, we have now defined the range of human hearing which also goes from 0 to 140 dB. It is important to realize that 0 dB of sound pressure does not mean the absence of sound pressure; it only means that the measured sound pressure is the same as the standard reference sound pressure. A sound that is 0 dB SPL has the same pressure as the standard reference pressure of 20 µPa. However, as with intensity, the lowest audible pressure can depend on frequency, type of earphones, and other specified listening conditions, but these are always referenced to the universally accepted standard reference value of 20 µPa.

Let's look at some other decibel examples using pressure. Suppose you made a sound measurement and found it to be 200,000 µPa. What is the dB SPL of this sound? The calculation would be as follows:

$$dB \ SPL = 20 \log (200,000/20 \ \mu Pa)$$

$$= 20 \log (10^4)$$

$$= 20 \ (4), \textit{where} \log \textit{of} \ 10^4 \ \textit{equals} \ 4$$

$$= 80 \ dB \ SPL.$$

What if you wanted to compare one sound to another sound? For example, suppose the pressure of one sound is 1,000 times more than the pressure of another sound. This defines the pressure ratio of these two sounds, that is, 1,000/1. In dB pressure, this would be expressed using the following equation:

dB pressure of louder sound

$$= 20 \log (1,000/1)$$

$$= 20 \log (10^3)$$

$$= 20 \ (3), \textit{where} \log \textit{of} \ 10^3 \ \textit{equals} \ 3$$

$$= 60 \ dB.$$

How about the situation in which we double the pressure of a sound. How many dB greater is the louder sound? The calculation would be as follows:

dB pressure increase

$$= 20 \log (2/1)$$

$$= 20 \ (0.3), \textit{where the} \log \textit{of} \ 2 \ \textit{equals} \ 0.3$$

$$= 6 \ dB.$$

Table 2-3. Illustration of Intensity and Pressure Ranges

Intensity					Pressure				
w/m^2	Ratio (I_{meas} / I_{ref})	Scientific Notation	log_{10}	dB IL[a]	μPa	Ratio (P_{meas} / P_{ref})	Sci Not.	log_{10}	dB SPL[b]
1×10^2	100,000,000,000,000:1	10^{14}	14.0	140	20×10^7	$\sqrt{100,000,000,000,000}$:1	$\sqrt{10^{14}}$	7.0	140
1×10^1	10,000,000,000,000:1	10^{13}	13.0	130	$20 \times 10^{6.5}$	$\sqrt{10,000,000,000,000}$:1	$\sqrt{10^{13}}$	6.5	130
1×10^{-0}	1,000,000,000,000:1	10^{12}	12.0	120	20×10^6	$\sqrt{1,000,000,000,000}$:1	$\sqrt{10^{12}}$	6.0	120
1×10^{-1}	100,000,000,000:1	10^{11}	11.0	110	$20 \times 10^{5.5}$	$\sqrt{100,000,000,000}$:1	$\sqrt{10^{11}}$	5.5	110
1×10^{-2}	10,000,000,000:1	10^{10}	10.0	100	20×10^5	$\sqrt{10,000,000,000}$:1	$\sqrt{10^{10}}$	5.0	100
1×10^{-3}	1,000,000,000:1	10^9	9.0	90	$20 \times 10^{4.5}$	$\sqrt{1,000,000,000}$:1	$\sqrt{10^9}$	4.5	90
1×10^{-4}	100,000,000:1	10^8	8.0	80	20×10^4	$\sqrt{100,000,000}$:1	$\sqrt{10^8}$	4.0	80
1×10^{-5}	10,000,000:1	10^7	7.0	70	$20 \times 10^{3.5}$	$\sqrt{10,000,000}$:1	$\sqrt{10^7}$	3.5	70
1×10^{-6}	1,000,000:1	10^6	6.0	60	20×10^3	$\sqrt{1,000,000}$:1	$\sqrt{10^6}$	3.0	60
1×10^{-7}	100,000:1	10^5	5.0	50	$20 \times 10^{2.5}$	$\sqrt{100,000}$:1	$\sqrt{10^5}$	2.5	50
1×10^{-8}	10,000:1	10^4	4.0	40	20×10^2	$\sqrt{10,000}$:1	$\sqrt{10^4}$	2.0	40
1×10^{-9}	1,000:1	10^3	3.0	30	$20 \times 10^{1.5}$	$\sqrt{1,000}$:1	$\sqrt{10^3}$	1.5	30
1×10^{-10}	100:1	10^2	2.0	20	20×10^1	$\sqrt{100}$:1	$\sqrt{10^2}$	1.0	20
1×10^{-11}	10:1	10^1	1.0	10	$20 \times 10^{0.5}$	$\sqrt{10}$:1	$\sqrt{10^1}$	0.5	10
1×10^{-12}	1:1	10^0	0.0	0	20×10^0	$\sqrt{1}$:1	$\sqrt{10^0}$	0.0	0

[a]dB IL = 10 log (I_{meas}/I_{ref})
[b]dB SPL = 20 log ($P_{meas}/P_{reference}$)

Notice that if the pressure of a sound is doubled, it increases by 6 dB, whereas if the intensity of a sound is doubled, it increases by 3 dB. However, it is important to realize that for a specific sound, the intensity and pressure must vary together $(I = p^2)$, that is, one cannot double the sound's pressure and double the sound's intensity. For example, if we double the intensity of a sound, the decibel level increases by 3 dB and the pressure also increases by 3 dB because the sound's pressure would increase by the square root of two. On the other hand, if we double the pressure of a sound, the decibel level increases by 6 dB and the intensity of that sound also increases by 6 dB because the sound's intensity is squared. These comparisons can be illustrated by the following calculations (keeping in mind that $I = p^2$), for (a) the pressure of a sound was doubled, and (b) the pressure of a sound was increased by a factor of 10:

(a) dB pressure increase
$$= 20 \log (2/1)$$
$$= 20 \log (2)$$
$$= 20 (0.3)$$
$$= 6 \, dB;$$

dB intensity increase
$$= 10 \log (2^2/1)$$
$$= 10 \log (4)$$
$$= 10 (0.6)$$
$$= 6 \, dB;$$

(b) dB pressure increase
$$= 20 \log (10/1)$$
$$= 20 \log (10)$$
$$= 20 (1)$$
$$= 20 \, dB.$$

dB intensity increase
$$= 10 \log (10^2/1)$$
$$= 10 \log (100)$$
$$= 10 (2)$$
$$= 20 \, dB.$$

Table 2–3 summarizes how the ranges of pressure and intensity for human hearing are related and how the linear scales are transformed into their respective decibel (ratio) scales. The decibel is defined as 10 times the log of an intensity ratio and 20 times the log of a pressure ratio. The decibel range between the least audible sound and the upper limit (threshold of pain) is 140 dB for either intensity or pressure. However, a tenfold increase in intensity results in a 10 dB increase, whereas a tenfold increase in pressure results in a 20 dB increase because of the relation between intensity and pressure $(p = \sqrt{I})$. One more thing to keep in mind is that decibels cannot be simply added or subtracted, that is, adding a sound of 40 dB to another sound of 40 dB does not equal 80 dB. The decibels must be converted back to pressure or intensity before being combined. For more information and practice on combining sounds, see the problems in the workbook by Kramer and Guthrie (2013) or the text by Speaks (1999).

Synopsis 2–2

- Intensity (w/m^2) and pressure (µPa) are related to each other by the equation $p = \sqrt{I}$ (or $I = p^2$). In audiology, pressure is usually used to quantify the level (amplitude) of sounds. The minimum mean sound pressure for audibility, called the reference level for pressure, is 20 µPa. The mean upper limit of pressure that can be tolerated is 20×10^7 µPa. For intensity, the reference level is 10^{12} w/m^2 and the mean upper limit is 10^2 w/m^2. The range of hearing from the lowest to the highest is 10^7 for pressure and 10^{14} for intensity (notice the relation $10^7 = \sqrt{10^{14}}$). In either case, the range on a linear scale is too cumbersome to be very useful, so the ranges are converted to decibel (dB) scales.

- Decibel scales are based on a logarithmic (log) scale. The log of a number (x) is defined as the power to which 10 must be raised to be equal to the number (x). Stated another way, the exponent of a number is the log of that number. Most calculators can easily calculate the log of any number. Some simple examples to keep in mind are:

log (10¹⁴) = 14

log (10⁷) = 7

log (10²) = 2

log (1) = 0

log (2) = 0.3

log (4) = log (2) + log (2) = 0.6

- A decibel (dB) is defined as 10 times the log of the ratio of two numbers [10 log (X_{meas} / X_{ref})]. This formula is directly applicable to the ratio scale for intensity level [10 log (I_{meas} / I_{ref})]; however, because I = p², the conversion to decibels for sound pressure follows basic rules of logs and becomes defined as 20 times the log of the ratio of two pressures [20 log (P_{meas} / P_{ref})]. When the reference (denominator) for the ratio is 20 µPa it is called dB of sound pressure level (dB SPL). When the reference for the ratio is 10^{-12} w/m² it is called dB of intensity level (dB IL).

- When the measured sound pressure or sound intensity is equal to its respective reference level (giving a ratio of 1/1), it would be equal to 0 dB because the log of 1 = 0. The range of hearing in decibels is 140 dB for either pressure or intensity as calculated for dB pressure = 20 log (10⁷) or dB intensity = 10 log (10¹⁴).

- Sound pressure increases by 6 dB when the pressure is doubled [20 log (2/1)]. Sound intensity increases by 3 dB when the intensity is doubled [10 log 2/1]. However, since one cannot double the intensity and the pressure independently within the same sound (recall that I = p²), the number of decibel change would be the same for pressure and intensity, that is, if one doubles the pressure of a sound, the formula for pressure would be 20 log (2/1) and for intensity converted to 10 log (4/1), resulting in a 6 dB increase in intensity and pressure. If one doubles the intensity of a sound, the increase would be 3 dB for both intensity and pressure, that is, for intensity the formula would be 10 log (2/1), and for pressure the formula would become 20 log (√2). A sound that is 100 times greater in pressure than another sound would be 40 dB greater; a sound that is 100 times greater in intensity than another sound would be 20 dB greater.

Audibility by Frequency

As mentioned earlier, the human ear is responsive to frequencies from 20 to 20,000 Hz; however, the ear is not equally sensitive across the frequency range (Robinson & Dadson, 1956). Figure 2-15 shows the lowest average dB SPL for threshold in normal hearing human listeners, and is typical of what is called the *threshold of audibility curve*. As this figure illustrates, auditory threshold changes with frequency. The threshold of audibility, even at 1000 Hz, can vary slightly from the data shown in Figure 2-15 under different listening

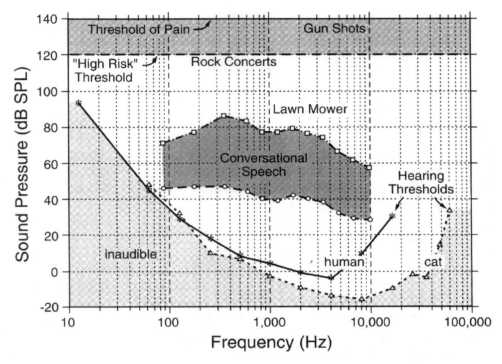

Figure 2–15. Thresholds and upper ranges of audibility as a function of frequency. The *lower line* shows the minimum levels of audibility as a function of frequency, and is typically referred to as the threshold of audibility curve. Higher dB SPL is needed in the low and high frequencies to reach threshold. The *upper line* is an estimate of the upper range of hearing, although most listeners do not tolerate levels above 100 dB SPL. Some types of sounds are included in the figure to provide some relevance of the scale. From Geisler, 1998, p. 21. Copyright 1998 by Oxford University Press.

conditions and with different types of earphones; for example, listening to sounds from speakers (called sound-field testing) with both ears may have slightly different values. From Figure 2-15, it is apparent that humans are most sensitive to frequencies between 500 and 6000 Hz, and the fluctuations in this region are less than 10 dB. As we will see later, the frequency range between 500 Hz and 6000 Hz is important for perceiving most speech sounds. On the other hand, at lower and higher frequencies, more sound pressure (or intensity) is needed for the frequencies to be just audible. Also shown in Figure 2-15 is an estimate of the upper limit for hearing, called the threshold of pain. Notice that the upper limit does not vary much as a function of frequency, probably because it involves the threshold of feeling within

the tympanic membrane, which is relatively constant across frequency (Durrant & Lovrinic, 1995). The area between the threshold curve and the upper limit curve defines the useable range for human hearing. However, most listeners find sounds above 100 dB SPL uncomfortably loud.

Wavelength

An additional acoustic parameter of pure tones is the distance that they travel in one cycle, the *wavelength*. The symbol for wavelength is the Greek symbol λ (lambda). The wavelength has units of length (e.g., feet, meters) rather than units of time, which was used to define the period. Wavelength is a measure of the distance between one point on the waveform to the same point on the next cycle, most easily seen as the distance between adjacent points of condensation (or rarefaction) in Figure 2-1. You should be able to envision that higher frequencies will have shorter wavelengths than lower frequencies because the cycles are closer together. Since the speed of sound is determined by the properties of the air and is the same for all frequencies, the wavelength can be defined by the following equation:

$$\lambda = c/f,$$

where c is the speed of sound and f is the frequency.

This equation shows that the higher the frequency, the shorter the wavelength. For example, a 2000 Hz sinusoid traveling in air (c = 343 m/s) has a wavelength of 0.17 m (or about 0.56 feet), whereas a 250 Hz sinusoid traveling in the same air would have a wavelength of 1.32 m (or about 4.5 feet). The same sinusoids traveling in water would have wavelengths that are approximately four times longer because the speed of sound in water is about four times faster than in air. Conversely, if one knows the wavelength of a sound, the frequency can be calculated by the equation:

$$f = c/\lambda.$$

The wavelength, to some extent, determines how sounds are affected as they travel past objects in their path. In a simple sense, the longer the wavelength is relative to the size of the object encountered, the less likely the object will have an effect on the amplitude of the sound. However, if the wavelength is short (as for higher frequencies) relative to the size of an object, then the object will tend to block (and reflect) the sound. You may have noticed that it is much easier to hear drums over a greater distance than the higher frequency band instruments; this is partly due to the higher frequencies being blocked by objects along the way, whereas the lower frequencies more easily go around the objects. As we will also see later in this chapter, part of our ability to localize sounds is related to the different amplitudes that occur between the two ears for higher frequencies, which

tend to be blocked by the head because of their shorter wavelengths.

Complex Sounds

As mentioned earlier, most sounds we listen to are complex sounds, which means that they are the result of combining two or more individual pure tones. Any complex vibration can be created or described by knowing the frequencies, amplitudes, and starting phases of the individual pure-tone components. The number of pure tones, along with their relative amplitudes and starting phases, will determine the type of sound we hear. A *spectrum* (plural = spectra) is a way to describe complex vibrations by plotting a graph that shows the amplitudes as a function of frequency (frequency spectrum), and/or the starting phases as a function of frequency (phase spectrum). Figure 2-16 shows an example of a complex vibration that is composed of two different pure tones with amplitudes and phases shown in the corresponding spectra.

Vibrations are generally classified as periodic or aperiodic. A *periodic vibration* is one in which the vibratory pattern repeats at regular intervals. A pure tone is an example of a *simple periodic vibration*. However, when two or more pure tones are combined into a nonsinusoidal pattern they may also be considered periodic if the wave pattern repeats itself as a function of time. These nonsinusoidal periodic vibrations are called *complex periodic vibrations* (or complex periodic tones). Complex periodic vibrations typically have a tonal or buzzing quality. The example shown in Figure 2-16 would be a complex periodic vibration because the pattern repeats itself, and the pattern would continue to repeat itself if the time scale continued. The amplitude spectrum of a complex periodic vibration (as shown on the right side of Figure 2-16) shows vertical lines at the discrete frequencies present in the vibration, and this type of spectrum is called a *line spectrum*. On the other hand, an *aperiodic vibration* is one in which the pattern of vibration does not regularly repeat itself over time, that is, there is no periodicity in

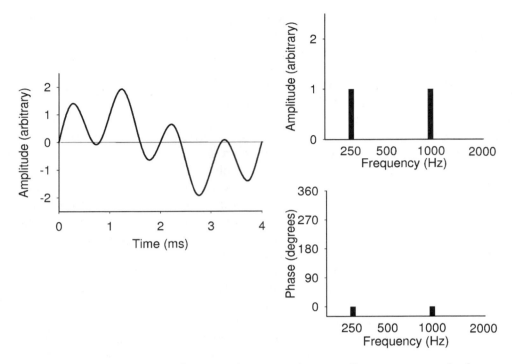

Figure 2–16. Example of a complex periodic waveform composed of two frequencies (*left*), which are described by their corresponding amplitude spectrum (*top right*) and starting phase spectrum (*bottom right*). These types of spectra are called line spectra.

the wave pattern. Aperiodic vibrations generally produce *noise*. Noise is produced by a combination of many pure tones with random starting phases. The waveform shown in Figure 2–17 is an example of an aperiodic-noise-type vibration. The spectrum shown in Figure 2–17 is a continuous horizontal line, rather than discrete vertical bars, to indicate that there are infinite frequencies present over the indicated range, and this type of spectrum is called a *continuous spectrum*. When there are an infinite number of frequencies with random phases and equal amplitudes over the entire frequency range it is called *white noise* (analogous to white light).

Aperiodic noise-type vibrations are encountered frequently in our environment, including many speech sounds (e.g., "s," "sh," "f," "th"), as well as sounds produced by things such as running water, rustling leaves, or engines. Many sounds we listen to may have components that give it tonal

(periodic) perceptions as well as a noise (aperiodic) quality, such as the speech sounds ("v," "z," "j") or the different pitches associated with the buzzing of different types of motors. In some of these latter cases, the underlying periodicity or the frequency range of aperiodic combinations will determine the overall perceptions. If we know the frequencies, amplitudes, and starting phases of all the individual components of a complex periodic or aperiodic vibration, we can construct the predictable vibration pattern that would result from their combination. Instruments are available that can perform a fast Fourier transform (FFT) on complex vibrations to determine the frequencies, amplitudes, and starting phases of the individual components.

The lowest frequency component in a complex periodic vibration is called the *fundamental frequency* (f_0). Integer multiples of the fundamental frequency are called *harmonics*, such as $1f_0$,

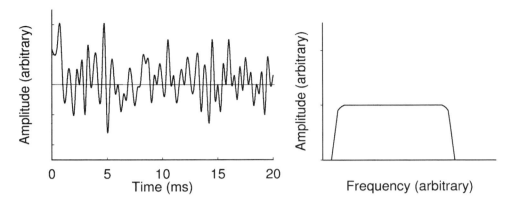

Figure 2–17. Example of an aperiodic noise vibration (*left*) and its corresponding amplitude spectrum (*right*). This type of spectrum is called a continuous spectrum.

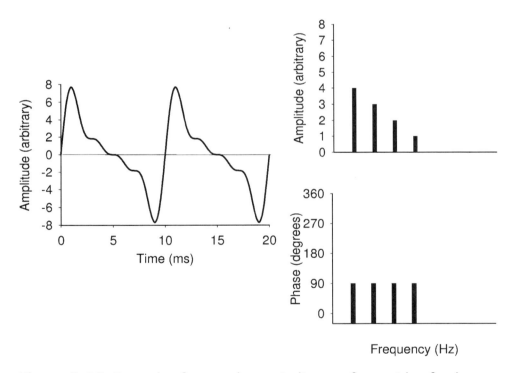

Figure 2–18. Example of a complex periodic waveform with a fundamental frequency of 100 Hz and its harmonics, 200 Hz, 300 Hz, and 400 Hz. With additional sequential harmonics added, the resulting waveform would be a sawtooth waveform.

$2f_0$, $3f_0$, and so forth. Generally, complex periodic vibrations occur when harmonically related pure tones are combined. For example, combining 100 Hz, 200 Hz, 300 Hz, and 400 Hz will produce the complex periodic waveform shown in Figure 2-18. If additional sequential harmonics were added to those shown in Figure 2-18, the resulting waveform would smooth out the smaller bumps and, with enough harmonics, would produce what is called a *sawtooth waveform*. A sawtooth waveform is a complex periodic waveform that has more of a buzzing sound quality rather than a tonal quality. You can see, in Figure 2-18, that the longest period of this complex periodic waveform is the same as the lowest frequency component (100 Hz). The fundamental frequency usually determines the primary pitch of the sound, but the other components can also be heard and will contribute to the perception of the complex periodic vibration. Adding different combinations of pure tones and using different amplitudes or phases can affect the overall shape of complex periodic waveforms. Figure 2-19 shows some additional examples of complex vibrations with their corresponding amplitude spectra.

Resonance

The frequencies to which objects vibrate most easily are called *resonant* (or *resonance*) *frequencies*. You are undoubtedly familiar with this concept when you think about musical instruments, such that strings of different length vibrate best at certain frequencies, or the smaller violin's

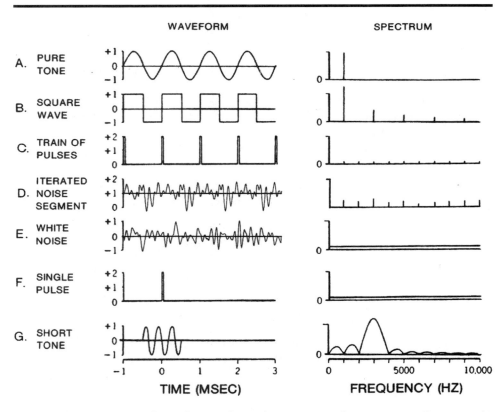

Figure 2–19. Examples of complex vibrations with corresponding amplitude and phase spectra. From *Auditory Perception: A New Analysis and Synthesis* (p. 2), by R. M. Warren, 1999, New York, NY: Cambridge University Press. Copyright 1999 by Cambridge University Press. Reprinted with permission.

sounding board emphasizes higher frequencies compared with the much larger bass which emphasizes the lower frequencies. In the case of a guitar string that is attached at both ends, when plucked, there are waves that move toward the ends of the strings and are then reflected back. This interaction of the two waves sets up characteristic interactions of the two waves into places where the displacements cancel each other, called *nodes*, and places where they combine with each other, called *antinodes*. For the guitar string, there are nodes at both ends (where the string cannot move) and an antinode at the center of the string that produces the string's musical note. The pattern of vibration between nodes at the ends of the string and an antinode in the middle is half of a cycle, as shown in Figure 2-20. These patterns of displacement as a function of distance are related to the frequency's wavelength (λ). The longest wavelength determines the string's primary resonant frequency (a.k.a. first mode or fundamental frequency) and is equal to half of a wavelength ($\lambda/2$). For a given length of string, the fundamental frequency can be calculated as:

$$f_0 = c/2L,$$

where c = speed of sound; L = length of string.

The string analogy and other vibrating objects have additional modes (e.g., harmonics) of vibrations that create other possible nodes and antinodes, as shown in Figure 2-20B corresponding to f_2, f_3, f_4, etc. Those resonance conditions whereby the fundamental frequency is equal to half a

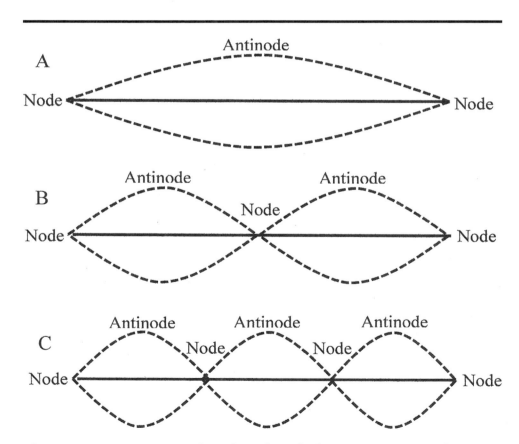

Figure 2–20. A–D. Examples of modes of vibration in a string that is attached at both ends showing the first mode or fundamental frequency (**A**), the second mode or second harmonic (**B**), and the third mode or third harmonic (**C**). Additional modes can occur at integer multiples of the first mode. At the nodes, the displacement is zero and creates standing waves.

wavelength are called *half-wave resonators*, and generate a fundamental frequency and harmonics at integer multiples of the fundamental frequency.

Resonance also occurs in tubes of different dimensions whereby the air molecules within the tube interact and produce regions of nodes and antinodes within the tube depending on the length of the tube. For example, blowing across a small tube produces a higher pitched tone compared with a lower pitched tone from a longer tube. The relationship of nodes and antinodes will depend also on whether the tube is open on both ends or only on one end, as illustrated in Figure 2–21. For the same-length tube, being open on both ends produces a higher-pitch tone than one open on only one end because of the different relationships of nodes to antinodes. As with the string example, a tube open at both ends involves half of a wavelength, and the resonant frequency is also obtained by the formula $f_0 = c/2L$. This would be a

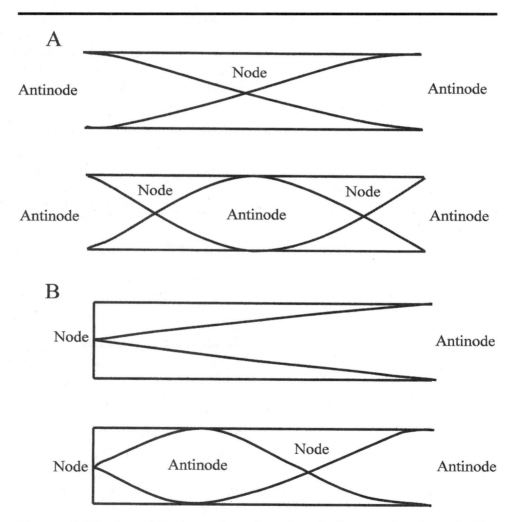

Figure 2–21. A and B. Examples of modes of vibration in tubes. **A.** The wave patterns in a tube open on both ends, called a half-wave resonator. A half-wave resonator can produce harmonics at integer multiples of the fundamental mode. **B.** The wave patterns in a tube open only on one end, called a quarter-wave resonator. A quarter-wave resonator can produce harmonics at odd multiples of the fundamental mode.

half-wave resonator with a fundamental frequency and harmonics at integer multiples of the fundamental frequency. Let's now look at a tube that is open only on one end (thinking ahead to our vocal tract, which acts much like a tube open at one end). As shown in Figure 2–21B, there must be a node at the closed end and an antinode at the open end. For the tube that is open only on one end, there is a one-quarter wavelength that can fit with the tube (between nodes and antinodes); hence, the resonant frequency can be calculated as:

$$f_0 = c/4L,$$

where c = speed of sound; L = length of tube.

These types of resonators are called *quarter-wave resonators*, and generate a fundamental frequency, along with harmonics only at odd multiples of the fundamental frequency.

Acoustics of Speech

The primary means of producing speech is through air flow supplied from the lungs, which passes through the vocal structures of the larynx and the oral and nasal cavities. The positioning and movements of the *articulators* (tongue, lips, velum, and jaws) alter the shape of the vocal path which results in specific resonance patterns of frequencies, amplitudes, and timing. The speech sounds are propagated into the environment, and received, and ideally perceived, by a listener. For example, what acoustic parameters are necessary for the listener to decide that they heard the sound /d/in the word *day*; or how does one perceive the word *day* differently than the words *die* or *bay*? Also, in today's world, human speech can be synthesized and generated through digital processing by a computer, largely based on what is known about the meaningful acoustic characteristics of the speech. Although the acoustic parameters of speech are important, keep in mind that communication involves much more than the simple production, recognition, and perception of the acoustic properties of speech.

Speech sounds can be classified into different types. On the most basic level, there are *vowels*, which are mostly complex periodic sounds, and *consonants*, which can be either complex periodic or aperiodic vibrations. Table 2–4 lists the labels used to describe different types of sounds. When the vocal folds vibrate, there is a complex

Table 2–4. Labels Used to Describe Different Types of Sounds Related to the Place of Articulation

Manner of Articulation	Voicing[a]	Bilabial	Labio-dental	Lingua-dental	Alveolar	Palatal	Velar	Glottal
Plosives or	−	p(_p_ea)			t(_t_ea)		k(_k_it)	
Stops	+	b(_b_ee)			d(_d_id)		g(_g_o)	
Fricatives	−		f(_f_in)	θ(_th_in)	s (_s_o)	ʃ (_sh_e)		h (_h_e)
	+		v(_v_ine)	ð (_th_e)	z(_z_oo)	ʒ (lu_ge_)		
Affricates	−					tʃ (_ch_in)		
	+					dʒ (_j_ot)		
Nasals	−							
	+	m (_m_e)			n (_n_o)		ŋ(ba_ng_)	
Liquids	−				l (_l_et)			
	+					r(_r_ed)		
Glides	−				ʌ(_wh_et)			
	+	w(_w_e)				j(_y_et)		

[a]Some consonants are produced without voicing (–), and some are produced with voicing (+).

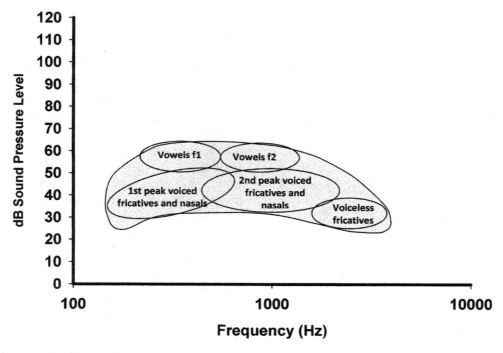

Figure 2–22. General distribution of speech sounds during normal conversational level of connected speech. The *outlined area* is called the speech banana.

periodicity to the sound and is called a *voiced sound*. When the vocal folds do not vibrate, the sound is aperiodic and is called a *voiceless sound*. Vowels are voiced and consonants can be either voiced or unvoiced. The normal average intensity level of ongoing connected speech is about 65 dB SPL, and this "volume" is primarily carried by the vowel sounds. Consonants have less energy than the vowels during connected speech, and contribute the most to word intelligibility. Figure 2–22 shows how conversational level speech sounds are distributed across the frequency and intensity scales. This general distribution of speech sounds is often referred to as the "speech banana" due to its general outline encompassing the vowels and consonants during ongoing speech. As you can see in Figure 2–22, there is as much as a 30 dB SPL difference between the loudest vowels (/u/) and the softest consonants (/th/). Notice also that the vowels tend to be more in the lower frequency, whereas many of the aperiodic noise-like consonants, called *fricatives*, are in the higher frequency range.

In the following sections, only the very basics of the acoustic properties of the different types of speech sounds are given, primarily their frequency components; however, keep in mind that amplitude and timing variations are also important acoustic properties of speech. Also, in Chapter 7 of this textbook, you will learn about the clinical speech tests that are used to assess how well a patient is able to recognize words and sentences, and how a patient's speech recognition is altered by various disorders of the auditory system. For a more in-depth understanding of speech production, speech acoustics, and speech perception, the interested reader is referred to other sources, such as Kent (2002) and Borden, Harris, & Raphael (1994).

Spectrogram

Speech is composed of basic periodic and aperiodic vibrations that occur in relatively short time periods, and is interspersed with short silent pe-

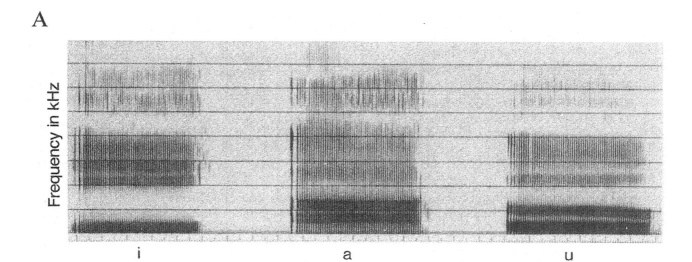

A

Frequency in kHz

i   a   u

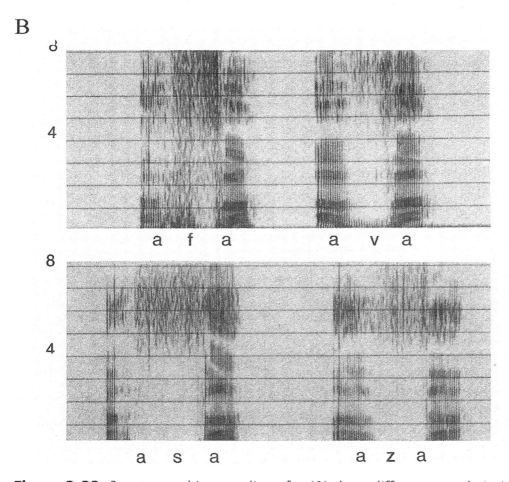

B

a f a   a v a

a s a   a z a

Figure 2–23. Spectrographic recordings for (**A**) three different vowels in isolation, and (**B**) some voiceless fricatives. Adapted from Rafael, Borden, & Harris, 2007. Pp. 111 & 124. Copyright 2007 by Lippincott, Williams & Wilkins.

riods between sounds. The frequency, amplitude, and time characteristics of speech can be analyzed with some basic equipment. One of the most important pieces of equipment used to analyze speech sounds is a *spectrograph*, which measures the spectra of speech sounds, words, or sentences (in a relatively short time window). A *spectrogram* is the display one gets from a spectrograph. A spectrogram plots frequencies (along *y*-axis) as a function of time (along *x*-axis) during some specific speech utterance that is inputted by speaking into a microphone. Amplitudes of the different frequencies are also present in a spectrogram as represented by the darkness of the frequency bands, that is, the more intense frequencies are seen as darker bands. Figure 2–23 shows examples of spectrograms for some vowels and consonants. As you can see in Figure 2–23A, the vowels show three or four darker frequency regions (bands). These darker frequency bands are called *formants*, beginning with the first formant (F1), the next higher F2, and so forth. Formants vary depending on the resonance properties associated with the positions of the articulators, and are similar to those harmonics seen with the example of the open tube, quarter-wave resonator. Vowels behave more like the complex periodic vibrations that we saw in the preceding section. Other speech sounds may be aperiodic, like the /s/ shown in Figure 2–23B, which do not have the discrete frequency bands like those seen with vowels, but instead show a wider range of frequencies as expected with a noise-type sound. The following sections give a brief overview of the acoustics properties for the various vowel-like speech sounds and the various noise-like speech sounds. Although not covered in this text, keep in mind that there are also corresponding amplitude variations associated with connected speech, as well as important temporal factors such as duration of sounds and silent intervals.

Vowels

Vowels carry most of the audible energy in speech, and generally have lower frequencies and higher intensities than consonants. Vowels are complex

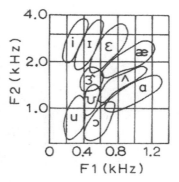
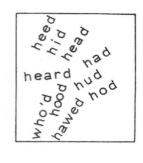

Figure 2–24. Distribution of F1 and F2 formants for English vowels for a variety of speakers. From Kent & Read, 2002, p. 107. Copyright 2002 by Thomson Learning.

periodic vibrations (voiced) that result from the vibration of the vocal folds. The frequency of vocal fold vibration is the fundamental frequency (f_0) which gives the sound its perceived pitch, and can vary depending on the vowel as well as the size of the larynx (which relates to males having a lower-sounding voice). As described earlier, vowels can be characterized by their F1 and F2. In general, the F1 varies inversely with the height of the tongue and F2 varies with the forward/backward position of the tongue. For example, /i/ is produced with the tongue in its highest position and most forward in the mouth, whereas /a/ is produced with the tongue in its lowest position and as far back as possible. Lip rounding is done for some back and center vowels and its effect is to extend the vocal tract and thus lower all formant frequencies. Keep in mind that the formant frequencies are not precise numbers, but are best considered as elliptical regions that vary depending on the speaker due to variations in size of vocal tract, articulators, and dialect. Figure 2–24 shows how the different vowels can be separated into their F1 and F2 elliptical areas, and be relatively distinct from each other.

During speech, vowels can also vary by their duration. For example, some vowels are longer in duration like those in open syllables (e.g., "see," "so"), whereas others are shorter in duration when in closed syllables (e.g., "sit" "sat"). Additionally, vowels that are produced in context with other consonants also have a dynamic shifting of their formant frequencies, called *formant transitions*, where there may be a rising or falling frequency transition depending on the their preceding and/or target consonant. Combining vowel sounds, called *semivowels* or *diphthongs* (see Table 2-4), are characterized by formant transitions, and the shifts in F2 are the most distinguishing characteristic to help recognize different semivowels and diphthongs.

Consonants

Consonants are considered the sounds that contribute most toward intelligibility as they precede and/or follow vowels to define words or parts of words. The acoustic properties of consonants are a bit more complicated than vowels, and one is not able to give as general a description as we were able to do with the formant structure of vowels. Consonants are divided into several different types (see Table 2-4). Some consonants are voiced, some have a noise quality, some only have a period of silence, and some may involve the nasal cavity. Only a brief description of these characteristics is given here, and only some selective examples are shown on a spectrogram. With some practice, you may be able to recognize the patterns of vowels and consonants in the complete sentence "The sunlight strikes raindrops in the air," shown in Figure 2-25.

Stops (or *plosives*) are produced by a brief period in which the air flow is blocked. The blockages can occur at the lips, alveolar area, or velum, and are referred to as *bilabial, alveolar,* or *velar stop.* Stops can be voiced or unvoiced depending on whether or not the vocal folds are set into vibration. During the closure, air pressure is built up and when the stop is opened, there is a burst of air flow. *Fricatives* are noise-like sounds that are produced by passing air through the oral cavity in which the articulators are positioned in a way to create turbulence in the air flow. The different fricatives are produced by the location (place) of constriction from the most forward point of the oral cavity at the lips to the rearmost position at the glottal area. Fricatives can be voiced (e.g., /v/) or unvoiced (e.g., /f/) at the same place of

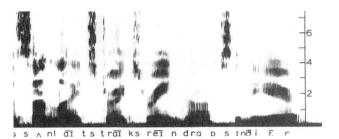

Figure 2-25. Sample spectrogram of the sentence, "The sunlight strikes raindrops in the air." From Kent & Read, 2002, p. 59. Copyright 2002 by Thomson Learning.

articulation. *Affricates* are created by the transition of a stop into a fricative. With *nasals*, the velopharyngeal port is opened so that sound energy can pass through both the nasal and oral tracts or through only the nasal tract. The formants of the nasals depend on the length of the cavity from the uvula to the nostrils, and are voiced with the vibration of the vocal folds.

Filtering

Filtering is a means by which certain frequencies are excluded and certain frequencies are allowed to pass through. Filtering can be used to generate a sound that is composed of a specified range of frequencies by filtering out some portion of a wider range of frequencies. For example, one can start with white noise and then filter out some of the frequencies so that a more restricted range of frequencies is passed.

Figure 2-26 shows the spectra for different types of commonly used filter types. The band of frequencies that is passed through to generate the sound is those represented under the curve, and those outside the curve are the frequencies that are filtered out. The high-pass, low-pass, and band-pass filters shown in Figure 2-26 each describe a range of frequencies that are "passed" and those that are excluded. The excluded frequencies are determined by the slope of the curve, called *attenuation rate* or *rejection rate*, which is usually

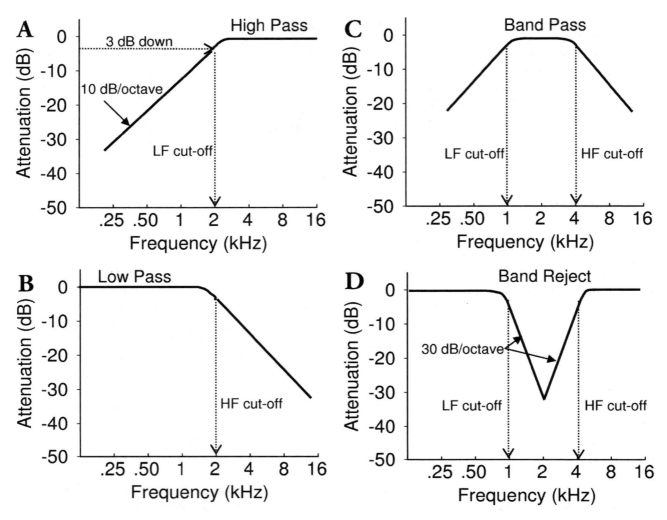

Figure 2–26. A–D. Examples of different types of filters. The *region under the curves* shows those frequencies that are heard (passed). The places where the filter begins to reject frequencies are called cutoff frequencies, which are at the 3 dB down points. The filter's rate of frequency rejection is indicated by the dB/octave. **A.** High-pass filter with 2000 Hz cutoff with 10 dB/octave rejection rate. **B.** Low-pass filter with 2000 Hz cutoff with 10 dB/octave rejection rate. **C.** Band-pass filter with 1000 Hz low frequency cutoff and 4000 Hz high frequency cutoff, with 10 dB/octave rejection rates. **D.** Band-reject filter with 1000 and 4000 Hz cutoff points, with 30 dB/octave rejection rates.

specified as a dB per octave (dB/octave). An *octave* means a doubling or halving of frequency. In the example shown in the top left panel of Figure 2–26, the filter has a slope of 10 dB/octave. The point where frequencies begin to be filtered out is called the *cutoff frequency* and is usually defined at the point which is 3 dB less than the peak (called 3 dB *down points* or *half-power point*). A high-pass filter passes all the frequencies higher than the cutoff frequency and rejects frequencies

lower than the cutoff frequency as defined by the dB/octave slope toward the lower frequencies (notice there is only one cutoff frequency). For example, the spectrum in the top left panel of Figure 2–26 would be called a high-pass filter with a 2000 Hz low frequency cutoff and an attenuation or rejection rate of 10 dB/octave. The low-pass filter passes all of the frequencies lower than the cutoff frequency and attenuates frequencies higher than the cutoff frequency as defined by the

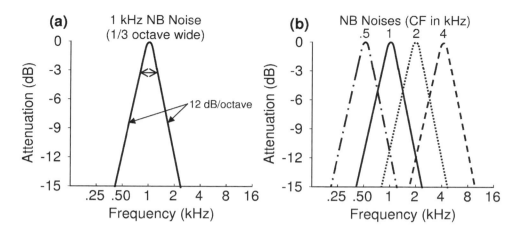

Figure 2–27. A and B. Spectra for some one-third-octave narrowband noises. **A.** The width of the filter is described by how wide the spectrum is to be at the 3 dB down points from the center frequency, with the corresponding dB/octave rejection rates. **B.** Some narrowband noises commonly used in audiology.

dB/octave slope directed toward the higher frequencies. The band-pass filter has a band of frequencies that is passed, as defined by the high and low cutoff frequencies and the dB/octave slopes in the higher and lower frequency ranges. The band-reject filter (also known as a notched filter) specifies a range of frequencies in the middle of a wider range noise that is attenuated, and those frequencies on both sides of the specified band-reject area are passed.

A special type of band-pass filtered noise is called a *narrowband noise* where there is a relatively restricted range of frequencies. These frequencies are often described by the width of the curve as measured across the 3 dB down points on both sides of the peak, called the *center frequency*. A commonly used narrowband noise is called a *one-third-octave* narrowband noise, which means the filter is one third of an octave wide at the 3 dB down points. Figure 2–27 shows the spectra for some one-third-octave narrowband noises. Narrowband noises are used frequently as noise maskers during basic hearing tests (described in Chapter 6). Filtering can also be used when analyzing or measuring a complex wave pattern in order to exclude frequencies that you are not interested in analyzing or measuring, and instead allows one to focus on those frequencies that are of interest. This type of filtering is used in many of the physiological measures from the auditory system (described in Chapter 8).

Synopsis 2–3

- Humans respond to sounds from 20 to 20,000 Hz; however, we are most sensitive to frequencies in the 500 to 6000 Hz range, which are the most important for perceiving speech.

- It takes a greater amount of sound pressure (or intensity) for lower and higher frequencies to become just audible. The variation in the just audible dB SPL as a function of frequency is called the threshold of audibility curve.

- The wavelength of a sound (λ) describes how far a pure tone travels in one cycle. The wavelength can be calculated by the equation $\lambda = c/f$, where c is the speed of sound and f is the frequency. Conversely, if you know the wavelength, the frequency can be calculated from $f = c/\lambda$.

- Complex sounds are much more typical in our environment than pure tones; however, any complex sound is the result of some combination of pure tones with specific amplitudes and starting phases. The individual sinusoidal components of complex sounds can be determined using equipment that can perform a fast Fourier transform (FFT).

- A spectrum is a graphic representation of amplitude or starting phase (along the y-axis) as a function of frequency (along the x-axis). Spectra are useful in describing complex vibrations. A line spectrum is used when discrete (and usually limited) frequencies contribute to the complex vibration. A continuous spectrum is used when a range of frequencies (all inclusive) contributes to the complex vibration.

- A periodic vibration is characterized by a waveform that repeats itself at regular time intervals. Complex vibrations are periodic if the combined waveform repeats itself over time. Periodic complex vibrations result from combinations of pure tones that are harmonically related as integer multiples of the lowest frequency, called the fundamental frequency (f_0). Different periodic complex vibrations occur depending on which harmonics are included. For example, a sawtooth waveform results when all harmonics ($1f_0 + 2f_0 + 3f_0 + 4f_0 \ldots$) are included and a square wave results when only the odd harmonics ($1f_0 + 3f_0 + 5f_0 + 7f_0 \ldots$) are included. Line spectra are usually used to describe periodic complex vibrations.

- An aperiodic complex vibration (often called a noise) does not repeat itself at regular time intervals and typically results from a range of pure tones with random starting phases. White noise (analogous to white light) has an infinite number of frequencies present with random phases.

- Most vibrating objects (except for a pure tone), including air molecules in tubes, have a fundamental frequency and additional harmonics. The vocal tract is similar to a tube that is open at one end, and is called a quarter-wave resonator. A quarter-wave resonator produces vibrations at a fundamental frequency and at odd integer harmonics. The resonance frequencies are dependent on the wavelengths associated with the length of the tube.

- Speech has specific acoustic properties generated by airflow passing through the vocal fold, oral cavity, and nasal cavity, resulting in complex periodic and aperiodic acoustic waveforms. The articulators modify the airflow depending on the targeted speech sound.

- Vowels are complex periodic vibrations with a fundamental frequency (giving rise to the pitch of the voice), and additional bands of energy called formants. The F1 and F2 are most important for vowel differentiation. Vowels are more intense than consonants in connected speech and produce the perception of voice loudness.

- Consonants can be periodic if accompanied by vocal fold vibration (voicing) or aperiodic if entirely noise-like (unvoiced). There are many types of consonants depending on the manner and place of articulation. Consonants are generally less intense than vowels and contribute most to intelligibility when in connected speech.

- Filtering is a way to exclude certain frequencies and allow other frequencies to pass through (to be heard or analyzed). Filters are used to shape the spectra of noise stimuli and/or to focus on a specific frequency range that is to be analyzed. Common types of filters include high-pass, low-pass, band-pass, and band-reject. These filters are described by their cutoff frequencies, which define where the change occurs (at 3 dB down) between those that are to be passed and those that are to be filtered out. The filtered portion is defined by the dB/octave slope (also known as the attenuation rate). Narrowband noises, used extensively in hearing testing, are filtered noises that are typically one third of an octave wide.

Psychoacoustics

The study of how humans perceive the acoustic properties of sound is called psychoacoustics. The following sections will present basic information on how frequency and intensity translate into our perception of loudness and pitch; how our thresholds change as the duration of a sound is shortened, called *temporal integration*; and, finally, how we use acoustic information to determine where sounds are coming from, called *localization*. The introductory material covered in this chapter only touches the surface of this fascinating area and only covers how normal hearing humans perceive simple sounds. For more advanced coverage of this topic for a variety of simple and complex sounds, the interested reader is referred to other texts (e.g., Durrant & Lovrinic, 1995;

Gelfand, 2004; Moore, 2003; Yost, 2000; Zwicker & Fastl, 1990).

Loudness

Loudness is generally considered the psychological correlate of intensity. Most of us have a general idea that soft and loud sounds are related to low and high intensities of sounds. As discussed earlier, the ear responds to a wide range of intensities; the minimum level is perceived as threshold and the upper limit is perceived as being uncomfortably loud. As we learned from the threshold of audibility curve, it takes a different amount of intensity to reach threshold for different frequencies. So, an obvious question is what intensities are needed to maintain equal loudness across frequencies? To answer this question, a

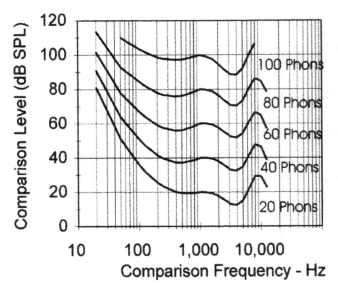

Figure 2–28. Phon scales of loudness (or equal loudness contours). Each line represents frequencies that sound equally loud for the given phon level. A phon is defined as the loudness associated with a 1000 Hz reference tone. From Yost, 2000, p. 194. Copyright 2000 by Academic Press.

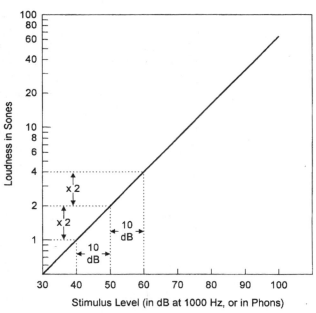

Figure 2–29. Sone scale of loudness for 1000 Hz. One sone equals the loudness associated with a 1000 Hz tone at 40 dB SPL. A doubling of loudness occurs for tenfold increases in stimulus level. From Gelfand, 2009, p. 93. Copyright 2009 by Thieme.

loudness-matching procedure is typically used in which the intensity level for different frequencies is adjusted until they sound equally loud to a 1000 Hz reference tone (Fletcher & Munson, 1933; Robinson & Dadson, 1956). The scaling unit used to compare loudness across frequencies is called a *phon*, where the phon level is equal to the SPL value of the 1000 Hz reference tone. For example, a loudness level of 30 phons is equal to a 1000 Hz tone presented at 30 dB SPL, and a loudness level of 60 phons is equal to a 1000 Hz tone presented at 60 dB SPL. The intensity levels that are needed for other frequencies to sound equally loud to the 1000 Hz reference tone, at a specified phon level, are measured to establish the corresponding phon curve across the frequency range. Different phon curves are established for different levels of the 1000 Hz reference tone. Figure 2–28 shows a series of phon curves. These phon curves are also called *equal loudness contours*. Each phon curve shows the different SPLs that are needed across

the frequency range that would be judged equal in loudness. In other words, all tones at the same phon level are judged to be equally loud even though their SPLs are different. As you can see from Figure 2–28, the general shape of the phon curves follows the threshold of audibility curve; however, they tend to flatten out across frequency as the reference level increases, especially in the lower frequencies. This means that at higher sound levels it does not take as much increase in SPL in the lower frequencies to sound equally loud to the mid frequencies.

The phon scale does not tell us much about how our perception of loudness is related to the continuum of intensity. Another question of interest is how does a scale of loudness relate to a range of sound pressures? For example, if the dB SPL is doubled, does the loudness also double? In other words, how much increase in dB SPL is needed to achieve a doubling of the perceived loudness?

The relationship of loudness to pressure (or intensity) is generally determined by using magnitude estimation or scaling method (Stevens, 1956). This type of loudness scale uses *sones* as the unit of loudness, where one sone is defined as the loudness of a 1000 Hz tone at 40 dB SPL. In these types of experiments, the subject is asked to adjust the dB SPL of the tone until the loudness is judged to be half, double, triple, and so on, of the loudness of the reference value. In other words, what dB SPL corresponds to 2 sones or 0.5 sones? The data are typically presented for a 1000 Hz tone; however, similar data can be obtained for different frequencies by making the reference value equal to the loudness in phons for the frequency being measured. Figure 2–29 shows the relationship that occurs between the loudness in sones and the dB SPL of a 1000 Hz tone (or loudness level in phons). One can see that the sone scale for loudness (on a log-log plot) shows a relatively straight line above 30 dB SPL for a 1000 Hz tone. In this region, a doubling of loudness corresponds to a 10 dB increase

in sound pressure and approximates a power function, where the slope of the line is the exponent of the power function, for example, in this case, loudness = pressure[6]. For levels between threshold and 30 dB SPL, the loudness function is much steeper and does not fit the simple power function. Notice also that the entire range of sound pressures (10^7) is compressed into a range of only around 100 sones.

Pitch

Pitch is generally considered the psychological correlate of frequency. Most of us have a sense that low- and high-pitch sounds are related to low and high frequencies. Although we are able to detect a wide range of frequencies and can attribute a general perception of pitch to these frequencies, the question of interest here is how does a scale of pitch relate to a scale of frequency, that

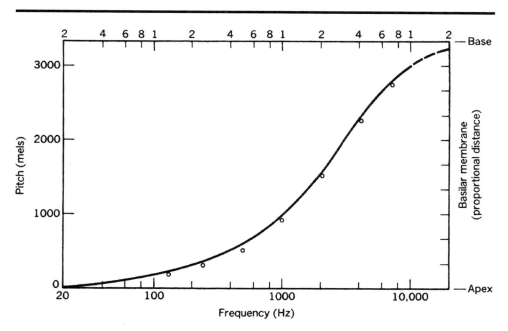

Figure 2–30. Mel scale of pitch. The pitch associated with 1000 Hz is defined as 1000 mels. The range of audible frequencies (20 to 20000 Hz) is compressed into about 3500 mels. From Gulick, Gescheider, & Frisina, 1989, p. 249. Copyright 1989 by Oxford University Press.

is, if we double the frequency of a sound, does the pitch also double? In other words, how much of a frequency increase is needed for a doubling of the perceived pitch? As we see, there is not a one-to-one correspondence between pitch and frequency. The relationship of pitch to frequency was first described by Stevens and Volkmann (1940). The pitch scale is typically presented in units called *mels*. The mel scale assigns a standard reference value of 1000 mels to the pitch associated with 1000 Hz. The subject then adjusts the frequency of a tone until the pitch is judged to be half, double, triple, and so on, of the pitch of the reference tone. In other words, what frequency best corresponds to 500, 2000, or 3000 mels?

Figure 2–30 shows the relationship that occurs between pitch in mels (linear scale) and frequency in hertz (logarithmic scale). One can see that the mel scale for pitch does not show a one-to-one relation to frequency. For example, a doubling of frequency from 1000 to 2000 Hz corresponds to a 1.5 increase in pitch (from 1000 to 1500 mels). Conversely, a doubling of pitch from 1000 to 2000 mels corresponds to about a threefold increase in frequency (from 1000 to 3000 Hz). Notice also that the entire range of frequencies (20 to 20,000 Hz) is compressed into a range of only 3500 mels, and that the data follow a curvilinear function in a semi-log plot across the frequency range.

Pitch also changes with intensity, as shown in Figure 2–31, for a variety of frequencies (Stevens, 1935). These pitch versus intensity data are called *equal pitch contours*. In general, increasing intensity results in an increased pitch for the higher frequencies and a decreased pitch for the lower frequencies (Gulick, Gescheider, & Frisina, 1989). It should be pointed out that these increases and decreases in pitch with intensity are relatively small and not generally noticeable except under controlled laboratory conditions (Cohen, 1961).

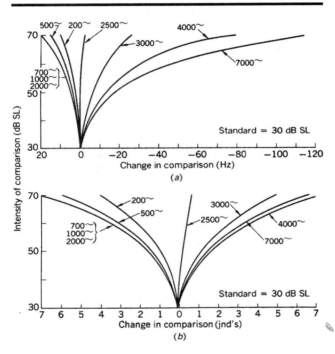

Figure 2–31. Equal pitch contours. Each line represents equal pitch as stimulus level increases. For lower frequencies, as stimulus level is increased, the frequency must be increased in order to maintain the same pitch (the pitch decreases with stimulus intensity). For higher frequencies, as stimulus level is increased, the frequency must be decreased in order to maintain the same pitch (the pitch increases with stimulus intensity). From Gulick et al., 1989, p. 251. Copyright 1989 by Oxford University

Temporal Integration

Temporal integration describes how the threshold of audibility for a sound changes with the duration of the sound. In general, as the duration of a sound is shortened to less than 200 ms, the level of the sound must be increased in order for the sound to be audible. Figure 2–32 shows how the threshold changes as a function of duration. As you can see, there is about a 10 dB increase in level (threshold shift) for a tenfold decrease in duration. In other words, as the duration is shortened from 200 to 20 ms, the sound level must be increased by 10 dB to remain audible. Similarly, as the duration is shortened from 20 to 2 ms, an additional 10 dB increase in the level of the sound is needed to remain audible. It should also be pointed out that for tones less than 10 ms in duration the quality of the sound also changes significantly, such that the tonality is lost and it is perceived as a brief click (transient) type sound. These brief transients also

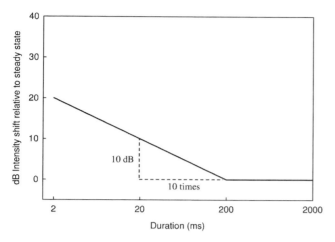

Figure 2–32. Temporal integration function. This shows how the threshold for a pure tone changes as a function of duration. As the duration is shortened by a factor of 10 (e.g., from 200 to 20 ms), the sound level must be increased by 10 dB to remain audible.

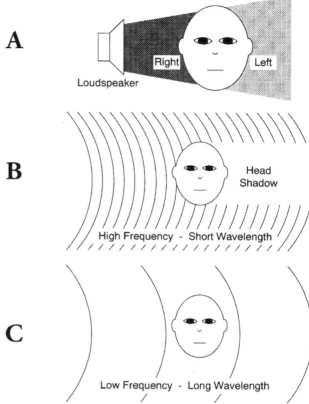

Figure 2–33. A–C. Some simplified illustrations showing factors that may be important for sound localization in the horizontal plane. **A.** Speaker is presenting sound to one side of the head. **B.** Interaural intensity differences between the two ears due to sound shadow area with reduced amplitude at the ear farther away from the sound source, which may explain some localization at high frequencies. **C.** Interaural time differences between the two ears due to distance traveled, with longer time of arrival at the ear farther away from the sound source, which may partially explain how we localize at lower frequencies. From Gelfand, 2009, p. 48.

spread their energy across a wider frequency range called *spectral splatter*. One can also see from Figure 2-32 that for sounds with durations greater than 200 ms, the threshold remains constant.

Localization

Localization refers to the ability to determine the direction from which a sound is coming. In general, our ability to localize is greatly dependent on the use of both ears, called *binaural hearing*. Most animals have a keen sense of localization, and many animals are able to move their pinnae to help them localize. Humans, on the other hand, do not move their auricles as a means of localizing. Instead, humans rely (unconsciously) on different arrival times and/or intensities of sounds at the two ears to determine from where sounds are coming. These mechanisms are referred to as *interaural time differences* or *interaural intensity differences*. These two mechanisms can explain localization of simple sounds that come from one side of the head. For localization, clearly two ears are better than one, and a typical complaint of people with hearing loss in one ear is that they have some difficulty localizing sounds.

Figure 2-33 shows how interaural time and interaural intensity mechanisms operate when listening with two ears to a sound presented to one side of the head. As shown in Figure 2-33B, higher frequencies (>1500 Hz) have shorter wavelengths when compared with the size of the head, and these frequencies tend to be blocked by the head (Fedderson, Sandel, Teas, & Jeffress, 1957).

This produces an area referred to as the *head shadow* area at the ear farther away from the sound source, making the sound less audible than at the ear closer to the sound source. As shown in Figure 2–33C, for lower frequencies, the wavelength is larger than the size of the head and wraps around the head due to diffraction and does not create interaural intensity differences; however, it does take more time for the sound to get to the ear farther away from the sound source. These interaural time differences appear to be important for lower frequency localization as long as the wavelength is larger than the distance between the two ears; however, this simple model has been shown to have some discrepancies in more recent studies (e.g., Kuhn, 1977) and these are beyond the scope of this textbook. As the direction of the sound source moves more toward the center, localization based on interaural time and intensity differences becomes more difficult. In those situations, and in vertically directed localization, spectral differences in the sound from front to back, due to the shape of the auricle, may help with localization at higher frequencies because the wavelengths are smaller than the auricle (Durrant & Lovrinic, 1995). In the real world, humans are able to move their heads and/or use visual cues to help them identify the source of a sound; and while listeners with unilateral hearing loss have some localization difficulty, they are able to localize to some degree by using these other cues.

References

Borden, G. J., Harris, K. S., & Raphael, L. J. (1994). *Speech science primer* (3rd ed.). Baltimore, MD: Williams & Wilkins.

Cohen, A. (1961). Further investigations of the effects of intensity upon the pitch of pure tones. *Journal of the Acoustical Society of America, 33,* 1363–1376.

Durrant, J. D., & Lovrinic, J. H. (1995). *Basis of hearing science* (3rd ed.). Baltimore, MD: Williams & Wilkins.

Fedderson, W. E., Sandel, T. T., Teas, D. C., & Jeffress, L. A. (1957). Localization of high-frequency tones. *Journal of the Acoustical Society of America, 29,* 988–991.

Fletcher, H., & Munson, W. A. (1933). Loudness, its definition, measurement, and calculation. *Journal of the Acoustical Society of America, 5,* 82–105.

Geisler, C. D. (1998) *Sound to synapse* (p. 21). New York, NY: Oxford University Press.

Gelfand, S. A. (2004). *Hearing: an introduction to psychological and physiological acoustics* (4th ed.). New York, NY: Marcel Dekker.

Gelfand, S. A. (2009). *Essentials of audiology* (3rd ed.). New York, NY: Thieme.

Gulick, W., Gescheider, G., & Frisina, R. (1989). *Hearing: physiological acoustics, neural coding, and psychoacoustics.* New York, NY: Oxford University Press.

Kent, R. D., & Read, C. (2002). *Acoustic analysis of speech.* Toronto, Ontario, Canada: Thomson Learning.

Kuhn, G. F. (1977). Model for the interaural time differences in azimuthal plane. *Journal of the Acoustical Society of America, 62,* 157–167.

Moore, B. (2003). *Introduction to the psychology of hearing.* San Diego, CA: Academic Press.

Mullin, W. J., Gerace, W. L., Mestre, J. P., & Velleman, S. V. (2003). *Fundamentals of sound with applications to speech and hearing.* Boston, MA: Allyn and Bacon.

Rafael L. J., Borden, G. J., & Harris, K. S. (2007). *Speech science primer: physiology, acoustic, and speech production* (5th ed., pp. 111, 124). Baltimore, MD: Lippincott Williams & Wilkins.

Robinson, D. W., & Dadson, R. S. (1956). A re-determination of the equal loudness relations for pure tones. *British Journal of Applied Physiology, 7,* 166–181.

Speaks, C. E. (1999). *Introduction to sound: Acoustics for the hearing and speech sciences* (3rd ed.). San Diego, CA: Singular.

Stevens, S. S. (1935). The relation of pitch to intensity. *Journal of the Acoustical Society of America, 6,* 150–154.

Stevens, S. S. (1956). The measurement of loudness. *Journal of the Acoustical Society of America, 27,* 815–829.

Stevens, S. S., & Volkmann, J. (1940). The relation of pitch to frequency: A revised scale. *American Journal of Psychology, 53,* 329–353.

Villchur, E. (2000). *Acoustics for audiologists.* San Diego, CA: Singular.

Warren, R. M. (1999). *Auditory perception: a new analysis and synthesis* (p. 2). New York, NY: Cambridge University Press.

Yost, W. (2000). *Fundamentals of hearing* (4th ed.). San Diego, CA: Academic Press.

Zwicker, E., & Fastl, H. (1990). *Psychoacoustics: Facts and models.* New York, NY: Springer-Verlag.

3

Functions of the Auditory and Vestibular Systems

After reading this chapter, you should be able to:

1. Understand why there is a need for the outer ear and middle ear to amplify pressures at the oval window.
2. Describe the amplifying mechanisms of the outer ear and middle ear, and how the predicted gains in pressure relate to the measured transfer functions.
3. Draw the ipsilateral and contralateral acoustic reflex pathways, and describe the functions of the acoustic reflex.
4. Understand how traveling waves occur along the basilar membrane and what is meant by basilar membrane tonotopic arrangement. Draw traveling wave envelopes for low, mid, and high frequency pure tones.
5. Discuss the different roles of the inner and outer hair cells, and describe the passive and active processes that occur in the cochlea.
6. Describe tuning curves for the passive and active cochlear processes, and discuss how damage to the active process (or outer hair cells) affects tuning curves.
7. Describe the different stages of transduction that sounds undergo from the environment through the level of the 8th nerve.
8. Discuss how frequency and intensity may be coded in the peripheral auditory system.
9. Understand the function of the vestibular organs and how they relate to visual and other sensory/motor systems.

Our sense of hearing is truly remarkable. Close your eyes for a moment and think about all those different types of vibrations in your environment that your ears are processing into useful and meaningful information: people talking, birds chirping, sound of cars in the distance, air conditioner, and/or music that may be playing. Think back to what you learned in Chapter 1 about the different parts of the auditory system, and imagine how the different components must somehow work together to allow you to hear and extract relevant information. As we will see in this chapter, the primary function of the ear is to receive vibrations from the environment and convert them into neural information that the brain can use. This change in sound energy, as it goes through the different parts of the auditory system, is referred to as the *transduction* process. The different parts of the auditory system *transduce* the sound energy from one form into another form. This chapter will detail the transduction processes through the auditory system.

Air-to-Fluid Impedance Mismatch

To begin with, the ear must somehow convert acoustic vibrations into something usable by the inner ear. If we did not have our outer and middle ear, the acoustic vibrations would impinge on the oval and round window membranes; this would be analogous to talking directly into the fluid-filled cochlea. However, when two types of media (air and water) have different properties, they have an inherent opposition to the efficient flow of energy. The total opposition to the flow of energy is called *impedance*. Energy flow is most efficient when the impedance is low or when two systems have equal impedances. When two systems have different impedances, they are said to have an *impedance mismatch*. If we were to talk directly into the cochlea, the air-to-fluid impedance mismatch would result in a loss of energy to the cochlea. You have, undoubtedly, experienced an analogous situation where you try to talk to someone who is under water and you are on the deck of the pool. In the pool analogy, about 99.9% of the sound energy would be reflected off the water's surface due to the air-to-fluid impedance mismatch, and only 0.1% would be transmitted into the water. This can also be expressed in decibels, if one considers the ratio of the reflected energy to the transmitted energy to be about equal to 1,000/1 (i.e., 99.9% / 0.1% = 999/1). In decibels, this could be expressed as:

$$dB = 10 \log (1,000/1)$$
$$dB = 10 \ (3), \text{ where log of } 1,000 = 3$$
$$= 30 \ dB.$$

In other words, we would predict that there would be about a 30 dB loss of sound energy, due to the impedance mismatch when going from air to fluid. While this analogy is useful as a basic understanding of the problem, the actual impedance mismatch would depend on knowing the precise impedance characteristics of the cochlear fluids at the oval window, something that has not yet been determined (Durrant & Lovrinic, 1995). Obviously, having a significant air-to-fluid impedance mismatch in the ear would not be an efficient way to transduce the sound energy through the ear. Therefore, one of the important functions of the outer ear and middle ear is to overcome this impedance mismatch so that there is a more efficient transfer of energy to the fluid-filled cochlea, in other words, to create a situation whereby the predicted 30 dB loss of sound energy does not occur during the transduction process. The ways in which the outer ear and middle ear overcome this impedance mismatch are discussed in the following sections.

Functions of the Outer Ear

The outer ear serves as the primary connection between the sounds in the environment and the middle ear. The auricle and external canal of the outer ear have only modest contributions to the overall processing of sound, and most pathologies of the outer ear do not cause much hearing loss. The outer ear is important, however, in protecting the more important middle and inner ear structures by allowing them to be embedded further into the skull away from potentially damaging events or foreign objects. Even the cerumen of the ear canal keeps debris and bugs away from the tympanic membrane.

The outer ear also modifies the incoming sound prior to arrival at the tympanic membrane. As mentioned in Chapter 2, many animals can move their auricles to help localize the source of a sound. Humans, on the other hand, do not have (or seem to need) the ability to move their auricles. The auricle, even without moving, can alter the spectra of sounds, especially the high frequency components, due to its shape and irregular series of depressions and ridges. These spectral variations provide some cues for sound localization, especially from the front, back, or from overhead (Gelfand, 2009). In addition, the outer ear also amplifies the sound pressure that is delivered to the tympanic membrane through the mechanism of resonance (see Chapter 2). This is the same thing that makes different-sized jars produce different pitches when struck, or when one blows air into cavities with different sizes. The size (and shape) of a cavity (or tube) will be most responsive to certain frequencies, such that smaller sizes resonate better to higher frequencies and larger sizes resonate better to lower frequencies.

The external ear canal is a tube-shaped cavity which is closed on one end. The resonant frequency of this type of tube is dependent on the relationship of the wavelength of the sound to the length of the tube. For this type of tube, enhancement of the sound pressure occurs maximally (resonant frequency) when the frequency is equal to one quarter the length of the tube. If the average adult ear canal length is 0.025 m, then the resonant frequency (f_{res}) can be calculated as:

$$f_{res} = c \, / \, 4L, \text{ where } c \text{ is the speed of sound} \text{ and } L \text{ is length of tube;}$$

$$f_{res} = 343 \, / \, 4 \times 0.025 \quad f_{res} = 3430 \text{ Hz.}$$

Remember that the ear canal is also irregular in shape and is preceded by the concha, both of which contribute to the resonance characteristics of the outer ear to enhance specific frequencies. In order to verify these theoretical advantages and determine how they are related to different frequencies, actual measurements have been made to document the changes in pressure that occur at the tympanic membrane. These types of measurements are referred to as *transfer functions*. The interested reader is referred to Shaw (1974) for more detailed data on the outer ear transfer function. In general, the outer ear provides an increase in amplitude (gain) of about 15 to 20 dB at the tympanic membrane in the frequency range 1500 to 7000 Hz (Ballachanda, 1995). This frequency range amplified by the outer ear is, somewhat remarkably, matched to those frequencies most important for understanding speech. Our auditory system is already performing some important processing at the level of the external ear that contributes to our ability to use speech for communication.

Functions of the Middle Ear

The middle ear is a mechanical system, which transduces the acoustic vibrations that strike the tympanic membrane into *mechanical vibrations* of the ossicular chain. The ossicular chain delivers the vibrations received at the tympanic membrane directly to the oval window. Without the ossicles, acoustic vibrations would strike both the oval and round window membranes at essentially the same time, and this would not allow reciprocal back-and-forth movements of these membranes that are necessary for vibrations to occur in the incompressible fluid-filled cochlea. In other words, in order for the ossicular chain to move the oval window back and forth in the incompressible fluid-filled cochlea, the round window membrane must also respond, such that an inward movement of the oval window corresponds to an outward movement of the round window membrane; and an outward movement of the oval window corresponds to an inward movement of the round window membrane. The acoustic vibrations that strike the tympanic membrane are transduced into mechanical vibrations of the ossicular chain, and then into hydromechanical vibrations within the fluid-filled cochlea. As Figure 3–1 illustrates, the back-and-forth movement of the air molecules within the ear canal results in a corresponding back-and-forth movement of

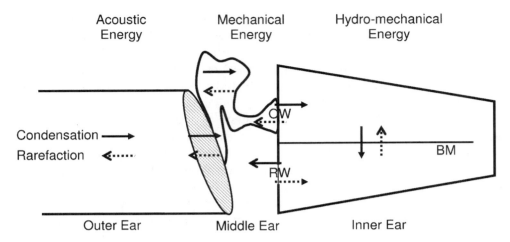

Figure 3–1. Overview of the transduction process, whereby the acoustic energy that enters the ear canal is converted into mechanical energy in the middle ear and then to hydromechanical energy in the fluid-filled inner ear. The *arrows* represent the vibration phase (rarefaction or condensation). Notice that there is a reciprocal relationship in the movement of the oval window (OW) and the round window (RW) that is necessary for the vibrational energy to occur in the incompressible fluid-filled cochlea. **BM**, basilar membrane.

the tympanic membrane, ossicular chain, and the oval and round windows (in opposite directions to each other).

Middle Ear Amplifier

As mentioned earlier, one of the primary functions of the middle ear is to overcome potential loss of energy due to the air-to-fluid impedance mismatch so that a more efficient transfer of sound to the inner ear can occur. In addition to directing the vibrations to the oval window, the middle ear is designed to function as a mechanical amplifier, whereby the sound pressures at the oval window are greater than those striking the tympanic membrane. There are three ways that the middle ear amplifies sound at the oval window. The largest amplification through the middle ear occurs as a result of the size (area) differences between the tympanic membrane and the oval window, referred to as the *area ratio advantage*. The effective area of the tympanic membrane is about 55 mm², whereas the area of the oval window is about 3.2 mm²

(Yost, 2000). Since pressure is equal to force per area (p = F/A), for a given amount of force applied to the larger area (tympanic membrane) there will be an increase in pressure on the smaller area (oval window). As an analogy, think of yourself standing on snow with snow shoes on (or standing flat-footed on sand at the beach); then think about what would happen if you took the snow shoes off (or when you stand on your toes in the sand). When the force of your body is applied over a smaller area, more pressure is applied and you sink deeper into the snow (or sand). In the middle ear, because the force that is exerted on the larger tympanic membrane is transferred by the ossicular chain to the smaller oval window, there is an increase in pressure at the oval window. If one considers the area ratio to be 17 to 1 (55 mm²/3.2 mm²), there would be about a 25 dB difference (dB = 20 log [17]). This means that the pressure at the oval window would be predicted to be about 25 dB greater than the pressure at the tympanic membrane due to the area ratio advantage.

The second mechanical amplifying mechanism of the middle ear is called the *curved membrane advantage*. This curved membrane advantage is related to the cone shape of the tympanic membrane, which tends to focus its movement in such a way that it moves the malleus with more force than if the tympanic membrane were a flat disk. The curved membrane advantage increases the pressure about twofold, which would be equivalent to about a 6 dB increase in pressure at the oval window.

The third middle ear amplifying mechanism is called the *lever advantage*. The lever advantage of the ossicular chain occurs because of the longer length of the manubrium of the malleus relative to the length of the long process of the incus. This acts like a fulcrum where the force applied to the longer arm results in more pressure being exerted at the shorter arm. For the lever advantage, the pressure at the oval window is predicted to be about 1.3 times greater than at the tympanic membrane, which would be equivalent to about a 2 dB increase (dB = 20 log [1.3]). If one combines all three of the middle ear mechanical advantages, there would be a total increase in pressure at the oval window of about 33 dB (dB = 20 log [17 × 1.3 × 2]) compared with the pressure at the tympanic membrane.

As you can see, much of the loss in sound pressure that would have occurred due to the air-to-fluid impedance mismatch has been effectively overcome by the mechanical amplifying effects of the middle ear. To better determine the range of frequencies that are enhanced by the middle ear, a transfer function can actually be measured (mostly in animals) between the tympanic membrane and the oval window as a function of frequency. The transfer function for the middle ear shows approximately a 20 to 25 dB increase in pressure (dB gain) at the oval window across a fairly wide frequency range and is especially effective in the low to middle frequencies (Békésy, 1960; Moller, 1963; Nedzelnitsky, 1980). Measures of the middle ear transfer function demonstrate that the middle ear amplifier effectively overcomes the air-to-fluid mismatch and is largely responsible for good hearing sensitivity in the middle frequencies. When the middle ear amplification is combined with the amplification from the outer ear, there is an effective transfer of pressure to the cochlea for a fairly wide frequency range, especially for those frequencies most important for the perception and recognition of speech sounds. Working together, the outer ear and middle ear avoid any loss of sound pressure that would occur due to the air-to-fluid impedance mismatch.

Acoustic Reflex

The middle ear has two small muscles, the stapedius and the tensor tympani, which attach to the ossicular chain by their corresponding tendons. The stapedial muscle is innervated by the stapedial branch of the facial nerve (7th cranial nerve), and the tensor tympani muscle is innervated by a branch of the trigeminal nerve (5th cranial nerve). These muscles are known to contract involuntarily when stimulated by loud sounds, for example, above 80 dB SPL, and this response is called the *acoustic reflex* or *middle ear reflex*. Because these muscles are oriented perpendicularly to the direction of movement of the ossicular chain, their contraction reduces the movement of the ossicular chain and lowers the sound pressure to the oval window. The acoustic reflex can reduce the pressure delivered to the oval window by as much as 10 to 20 dB SPL. A popular theory on the role of the acoustic reflex is that it affords some protection to the ear from loud sound. However, this role has been questioned, and may only be a factor in certain situations. One problem with the protection theory is that the muscles take about 20 to 100 ms to contract and fail to maintain contraction during continuous exposures; therefore, the acoustic reflex may not have much of a protective role, especially for impulsive type sounds like gunshots, explosions, or loud banging sounds. An additional problem for the protection theory is that hearing loss due to excessive continuous exposure to loud noises is quite prevalent, and if the acoustic reflex was designed for protection, it does not do a very good job in today's society. A more tenable theory for the role of the acoustic reflex is that it may reduce distortion within the movement of the ossicular chain at high intensities. This reduction in distortion may be important

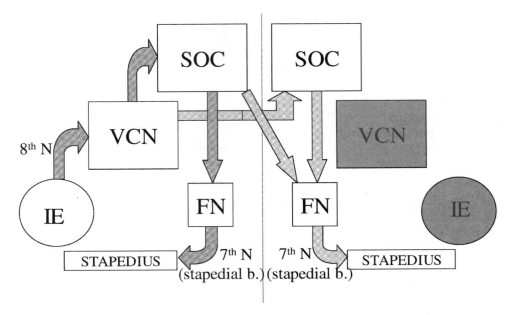

Figure 3–2. Block diagram of the acoustic reflex pathway for stimulation to one ear. The acoustic reflex is a bilateral response in which the stapedius muscles in both ears are stimulated through the ipsilateral and contralateral pathways. **IE,** inner ear; **VCN,** ventral cochlear nucleus; **SOC,** superior olivary complex; **FN,** facial nucleus; **stapedial b.,** stapedial branch of the 7th cranial nerve (facial nerve).

during your own vocalizations, especially if talking loudly in the presence of other background sounds (Borg & Counter, 1989). Although bats have a well-developed use of the acoustic reflex to protect their ears from their echo-location sounds, the precise role of the acoustic reflex in humans is still to be defined and better understood.

The acoustic reflex pathway is illustrated in Figure 3–2. In humans, most of the acoustic reflex involves the contraction of the stapedius muscles (one on each side), and the acoustic reflex is sometimes called the *stapedial reflex.* In this textbook, we will use the term acoustic reflex to refer to the stapedial reflex. The acoustic reflex involves a bilateral neural pathway in which a loud stimulus to one ear causes contraction of the stapedius muscles in both ears. The acoustic reflex pathway that is involved with the contraction of the stapedius muscle on the same side as the stimulus is called the *ipsilateral acoustic reflex* pathway. The acoustic reflex pathway that is involved with the

contraction of the stapedius muscle on the opposite side as the stimulus is called the *contralateral acoustic reflex* pathway. The ipsilateral and contralateral acoustic reflex pathways include the sensory input through the outer ear, middle ear, inner ear, 8th cranial nerve, and cochlear nucleus. From the cochlear nucleus on one side, there are connections to specialized neurons around the superior olivary complexes on both sides. The motor portion of the acoustic reflex pathway involves neurons from the areas around the superior olivary complexes to the facial nucleus and then to the stapedial branch of the 7th cranial nerve which then innervates the stapedius muscle. Figure 3–3 shows the components of the facial nerve. The facial nerve has a variety of motor and sensory functions not related to hearing; however, there is a small branch, called the *stapedial branch,* which innervates the stapedius muscle. As you will see in Chapter 8, the acoustic reflex is very useful as a diagnostic audiology test and shows characteristic

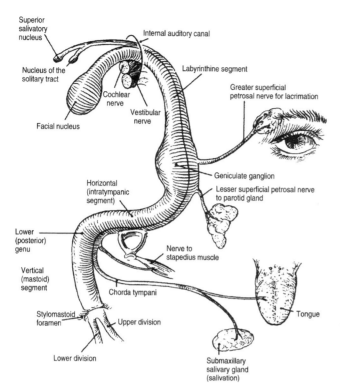

Figure 3–3. A diagram of the facial nerve that originates in the facial nucleus of the brainstem and has various motor and sensory nerve branches. The motor nerve branch that innervates the stapedius muscle is involved in the acoustic reflex. From Baloh, 1998, p. 9. Copyright 1998 by F. A. Davis.

patterns that are associated with disorders in different parts of the ear, as well as the neural integrity of the 7th and 8th cranial nerves.

Equalizing Middle Ear Pressure

The middle ear is normally an air-filled cavity. In order for the tympanic membrane and ossicles to vibrate effectively, the air pressure in the middle ear must be equal to the air pressure in the outer ear canal (impedance matched). This pressure equalization is accomplished by the eustachian tube, which connects the floor of the middle ear cavity to the nasopharynx. The eustachian tube is mostly a cartilaginous tube that is normally closed, but is periodically opened during normal physiological activities like swallowing or yawning. When the eustachian tube opens, it allows the air pressure to equalize with the environment. You have, undoubtedly, experienced this event when you "pop" your ears. The eustachian tube is opened by contraction of the *tensor veli palatini muscle* and closes when the muscle relaxes. Failure of the eustachian tube to equalize the air pressure in the middle ear can lead to middle ear infections and related hearing loss. Some of you may have experienced problems with the eustachian tubes during an airplane flight if you were unable to equalize the cabin pressure

---

Synopsis 3–1

- The inner ear is located deep within the skull where it is better protected. The outer and middle ear transduce sound energy from the environment to the inner ear where auditory processing begins.

- The tympanic membrane and ossicles transduce the acoustic vibrations into mechanical vibrations and channel them to the oval window. Because the fluid in the inner ear is incompressible, there is a reciprocal movement of the stapes footplate in the oval window and the round window membrane that allows for vibrational energy to occur in the inner ear.

- The outer and middle ear compensate for a theoretical 30 dB loss of energy that would occur due to an air-to-fluid impedance mismatch between airborne sounds and the fluid of the inner ear, thus improving our hearing sensitivity.

- The outer ear amplifies acoustic energy through resonance of its various cavities and the shape/length of the external ear canal. Measurements of the outer ear transfer function shows about a 15 to 20 dB increase in sound pressure at the tympanic membrane, especially in the middle to high frequencies.

- The mechanical amplifying effects of the middle ear include:

  - The area ratio between tympanic membrane and oval window (25 dB).

  - Curvature of the tympanic membrane, which produces more force than if it was a flat membrane (6 dB).

  - The lever ratio between the length of the manubrium and the incus (2 dB).

  - Collectively, the above three mechanical advantages produce about 33 dB increase in pressure at the oval window, which effectively overcomes the loss of energy that would occur due to the air-to-fluid impedance mismatch. Actual measures comparing pressure at the tympanic membrane to those at the oval window indicate an increase of 20 to 25 dB SPL, especially in the middle frequency range.

- The middle ear stapedius muscle contracts in response to loud sounds (greater than 80 dB SPL), called the acoustic reflex. The acoustic reflex pathway includes the 8th nerve from the cochlea, the lower brainstem auditory nuclei, the facial nucleus, and the stapedial branch of the 7th cranial nerve. The acoustic reflex pathway is bilateral, whereby input to one ear results in contraction of the stapedius muscles in both ears. The contraction of the stapedius muscles is believed to reduce distortion in the movement of the ossicular chain at high intensities. Acoustic reflex measures are very useful in assessment of a variety of auditory disorders.

- The eustachian tube of the middle ear extends to the nasopharynx to allow equalization of air pressure on the outside of the tympanic membrane with the air pressure inside the middle ear so that the proper transmission of sound vibrations can occur. The cartilaginous portion of the eustachian tube is normally closed, but is regularly opened by the tensor veli palatini during chewing, swallowing, or speaking. Young children are prone to more middle ear disorders because their eustachian tubes are not yet fully developed.

changes by opening your eustachian tubes. This happens because as the airplane takes off there is a gradual decrease in cabin air pressure and the pressure in the middle ear becomes more positive than in the cabin. During this part of the flight, the eustachian tubes can open relatively easily, even without any conscious effort because the positive pressure helps open the tubes. However, when the airplane descends and the cabin pressure is increased, the pressure in the middle ear becomes more negative than in the cabin. In this situation, the negative middle ear pressure resists opening of the eustachian tubes. More effort is needed (chewing, swallowing, popping of ears) to open the eustachian tubes during descent, and some individuals are unable to open their eustachian tubes. This may result in ear discomfort or pain, and may subsequently lead to an ear infection. As described in Chapter 1, the anatomy and function of the eustachian tube are not fully developed in young children and this is a primary reason why young children are more prone to middle ear infections than adults.

Functions of the Inner Ear

The processing of sound in the inner ear begins with the in-and-out movement of the stapes footplate in the oval window (with reciprocal movement of the round window membrane) delivering the vibrations to the fluids of the cochlea (see Figure 3–1). In other words, the mechanical pressure variations of the middle ear ossicles are transduced into pressure variations in the fluid. This is the beginning of what is called the *hydromechanical events* in the cochlea. Figure 3–4 shows how the mechanical vibrations of the stapes footplate are transduced into hydromechanical vibrations of the membranous labyrinth. You will notice in Figure 3–4 the common practice of showing the cochlea and/or basilar membrane uncoiled. The cochlea is quite small and the cochlear fluids are incompressible; therefore, the pressure vibrations are felt instantaneously throughout the entire cochlea, as if it was a solid object. It is important to realize that the fluid is not pushed through the

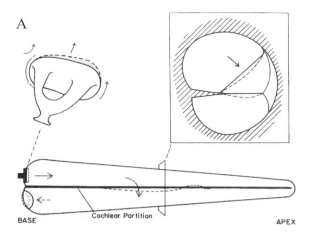

A

BASE   Cochlear Partition   APEX

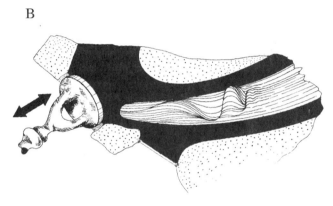

B

Figure 3–4. A. Demonstration of how movement of the stapes imparts pressure variations into the scala vestibuli, which in turn leads to displacement of the basilar membrane in the scala media. It is common to show the cochlea and/or basilar membrane uncoiled from its base to its apex for ease of illustration. From Durrant & Lovrinic, 1995, p. 150. Copyright 1995 by Williams & Wilkins. **B.** A snapshot of how a traveling wave appears on the basilar membrane in response to the pressure variations occurring in the scala media. From Dallos, 1988, p. 51. Copyright 1988 by American Speech-Language-Hearing Association.

cochlea from the oval window to the round window, but instead the vibrations are received instantaneously throughout the cochlea. Since the membranous labyrinth is suspended in the bony labyrinth, it also receives the pressure variations that are set up in the fluid. However, it is the reaction of the basilar membrane to these vibrations that is most important in the hydromechanical transduction process (see Figure 3–4B).

Traveling Waves in the Cochlea

The pressure variations in the cochlea cause the basilar membrane to react in a characteristic way, resulting in what is called the *traveling wave* (see Figure 3–4B). Much of the pioneering work in this area was done by George von Békésy in the 1950s and is summarized in Békésy (1960). Békésy's remarkable work formed the foundation of auditory theory for the next 20 years. Békésy's traveling wave occurs because of the basilar membrane's physical characteristics. As you recall from Chapter 1, and as shown in Figure 3–5, the basilar membrane is narrower at the base of the cochlea and systematically widens toward the apex of the cochlea. In addition, the basilar membrane is stiffer at the base of the cochlea and systematically becomes less stiff toward the apex of the cochlea. These physical characteristics determine how different parts of the basilar membrane respond to different frequencies. The relationship between frequency and a specific place is called a *tonotopic* arrangement. On the basilar membrane, the tonotopic arrangement is such that the higher frequencies are processed towards the base of the cochlea and the lower frequencies are processed primarily toward the apex of the cochlea. You might think of the simple analogy of a musical harp, where the shorter/tighter strings produce the higher frequencies and the longer/looser strings produce the lower frequencies.

So, how does a traveling wave occur? First of all, keep in mind that all locations along the basilar membrane receive the same vibrational input at the same time due to the incompressible nature of the fluid-filled cavity; however, because of the variations in the basilar membrane's physical characteristics, different areas of the basilar membrane move up and down at different times (phases). In other words, the narrower basal end of the basilar membrane begins to move up and down sooner

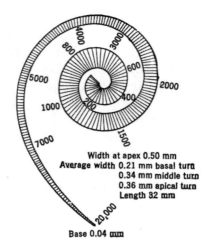

Width at apex 0.50 mm
Average width 0.21 mm basal turn
0.34 mm middle turn
0.36 mm apical turn
Length 32 mm

Base 0.04 mm

Figure 3–5. Tonotopic arrangement along the basilar membrane: high frequencies at the base and low frequencies at the apex. The tonotopic arrangement is related to the physical properties of the basilar membrane: narrow at the base and wider at the apex. From Stuhlman Jr., 1943, p. 286. Copyright 1943 by John Wiley and Sons/ Chapman & Hall.

than the more apical parts of the basilar membrane because there is less inertia to overcome (less mass) at the basal end of the membrane: The wider parts of the basilar membrane take a little longer to overcome the inertia and, therefore, begin to move a little later (phase lag) than the more basal locations. This causes one part of the membrane to move up while other areas are moving down (see Figure 3–6A). The amplitude (amount of displacement) of the traveling wave is relatively small at the base, and progressively increases until it reaches its peak amplitude at the place that responds best to the stimulating frequency; after that, the amplitude quickly decreases in more apical regions. Figure 3–6B illustrates a convenient way to show where the traveling wave stimulates different parts of the basilar membrane by showing the *envelope (outline) of the traveling wave's* motion.

In other words, because a figure cannot easily reflect a time-varying event, an artificial representation (envelope) is used to indicate the amplitudes of displacements along the basilar membrane for

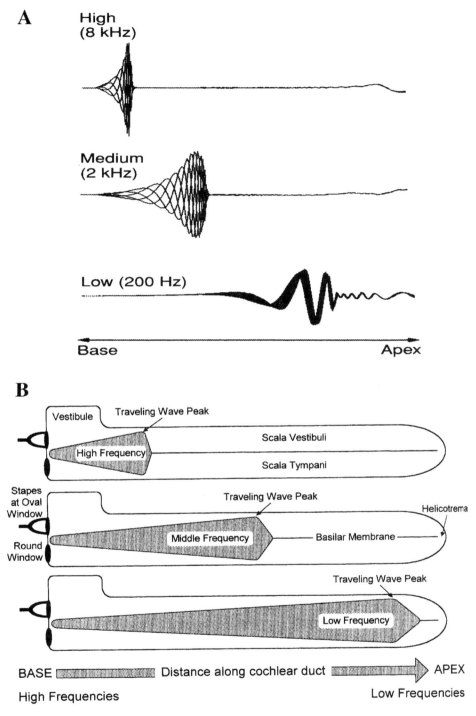

Figure 3–6. A. Displacement patterns of traveling waves showing high frequencies with peak displacements at the base, mid-frequencies further toward the apex, and low frequencies near the apex. From Salvi, McFadden, & Wang, 2000, p. 25. Copyright 2000 by Thieme. **B.** Envelopes of traveling wave activity along the basilar membrane for different frequencies. Notice that for all frequencies, the traveling wave begins at the base, reaches peak amplitude at its preferred location, and then quickly declines in amplitude. From Gelfand, 2009, p. 66. Copyright 2009 by Thieme.

different frequencies. Figure 3–6B shows examples of traveling wave envelopes for high, mid, and low frequency tones. The location where the maximum amplitude (displacement) of the basilar membrane occurs for any given pure tone is called the *traveling wave peak*. Notice in Figure 3–6 that the traveling wave for the high frequency sound only stimulates the base of the cochlea, whereas for middle and lower frequency sounds a wider part of the basilar membrane is reactive, but the displacement begins near the base and reaches its peak toward the apex. Békésy did an interesting experiment in which he introduced mechanical vibrations into the cochlea by placing a piston in a small hole at the *apex* of the cochlea, and found that the traveling wave activity still began at the base, moved in the apical direction, and reached its peak at the appropriate location dependent on the frequency of stimulation. In other words, regardless of how the vibrations enter the cochlea, there is a characteristic traveling wave that moves from the base of the cochlea and peaks at a location that is based on the tonotopic arrangement of the basilar membrane. As you will see in later chapters, one of the clinical tests of hearing involves directly sending vibrations through the skull by placing a small mechanical vibrator on the mastoid portion of the temporal bone. These bone-conducted vibrations initiate the same hydromechanical events (traveling wave) in the cochlea as those that occur when vibrations are delivered to the cochlea through the ossicular chain in the oval window.

Transduction Through the Inner Hair Cells

The next part of the hydromechanical transduction process within the cochlea is to activate the stereocilia of the inner hair cells (IHCs) and the outer hair cells (OHCs). Figure 3-7 shows how the stereocilia of the hair cells are mechanically displaced by the action of the traveling wave and contact with the tectorial membrane. When the basilar membrane moves up and down, the stereocilia of the OHCs bend back and forth due to their

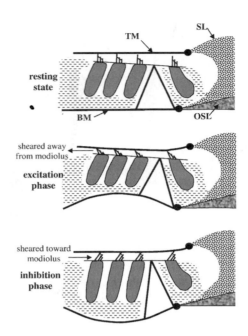

Figure 3–7. Illustration of how the stereocilia are displaced by the action of the basilar membrane and the tectorial membrane. As the basilar membrane moves up and down, the stereocilia bend back and forth due to the different pivot points of the basilar membrane and the tectorial membrane. **TM** tympanic membrane; **SL**, spiral limbus; **OSL**, osseous spiral lamina; **BM**, basilar membrane.

connections with the underside of the tectorial membrane. As the basilar membrane and the tectorial membrane move together or apart, they push (bend) the stereocilia one way or the other due to the differences in the relative pivot points of the two membranes. When the action of basilar membrane and tectorial membrane is sufficient there is enough bending of the stereocilia of the hair cells to initiate activity within the bodies of the hair cells.

Since almost all of the afferent neurons are connected to the IHCs, it is primarily the bendings of the stereocilia on the IHCs that lead to the next stage of the transduction process. When the stereocilia of the IHCs bend toward the tallest row of stereocilia (away from the modiolus) this triggers

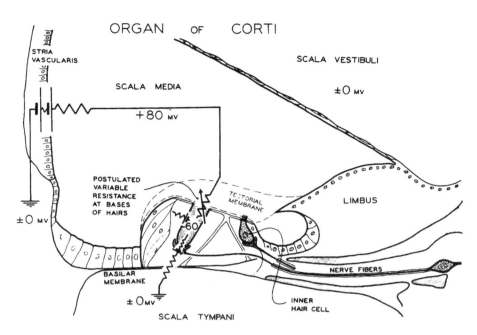

Figure 3–8. Schematic diagram illustrating the Davis Battery Theory. There is a voltage gradient of about 140 mV that drives ionic current into the hair cell, which can be varied by the amount of resistance related to the bending of the stereocilia. From Davis, 1965, p. 188. Copyright 1965 by Cold Spring Harbor Laboratory Press.

the *excitatory phase* of the IHC transduction process. As the stereocilia bend away from the tallest row of stereocilia (toward the modiolus) this triggers the *inhibitory phase* of the IHC transduction process. This stage of the transduction process involves converting the hydromechanical bending of the stereocilia into a chemical transduction process within the hair cells. Recall from Chapter 1 that the endolymph has a high K^+ content. This high K^+ concentration in the scala media, as shown in Figure 3–8, creates a +80 mV electrical potential (charge) in the endolymph, the *endocochlear potential* (EP). The EP is the highest resting electrical potential in the body and is maintained by the stria vascularis, which is often called the "biological battery" for the scala media. Inside the IHCs and OHCs there is also an *intracellular potential*, which is about −40 mV for IHCs and −60 mV for OHCs (Dallos, 1986). The EP and the intracellular potential provide a total electrical potential of

about 120 to 140 mV between the endolymph in the scala media and the inside of the hair cells. As Davis (1965) first proposed, often known as the *Davis Battery Theory*, the 120 to 140 mV electrical potential acts like the voltage of a battery, which serves as the force that drives the ionic current into the hair cell. The amount of ionic current that flows into a hair cell is modulated by changes in resistance that occur when the stereocilia bend in different directions. At the time Davis proposed his battery theory, the different roles of the IHCs and the OHCs were not yet known. From what is known today, Figure 3–8 would be more correct if the afferent neural output was shown for the IHCs and not the OHCs (are you getting curious about the role of the OHCs?).

Figure 3–9 shows how the bending of the stereocilia causes a change in the flow of ions into the hair cells. Similar intracellular ionic activity occurs for the IHCs and OHCs as the stereocilia bend

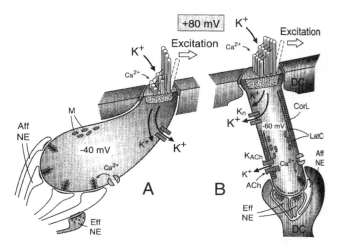

Figure 3–9. A and B. Details of how potassium ions (K$^+$) enter the hair cell by way of the stereocilia during excitation, along with the other biochemical events that occur within the hair cell to bring its intracellular potential toward equilibrium. **Aff NE**, afferent neuron; **Eff NE**, efferent neuron; **M**, mitochondria; **DC**, Deiter cell. From Geisler, 1998, p. 110. Copyright 1998 by Oxford University Press.

one way or the other. The intracellular potential becomes less negative during the influx of K$^+$ ions (excitatory phase) and more negative when the K$^+$ channels close (inhibitory phase). When the stereocilia bend in the excitatory direction (away from the modiolus), the tip links open up K$^+$ channels within the stereocilia and allow an influx (increased flow) of K$^+$ ions into the hair cell. When the stereocilia bend in the inhibitory direction (toward the modiolus), the tip links close the K$^+$ ion channels within the stereocilia and reduce the K$^+$ flow into the hair cell. During the inhibitory phase, the biochemical cell activity removes K$^+$ across the membrane. Through this series of events, the frequency of the incoming sound is now transduced from hydromechanical energy into biochemical energy. To summarize events up to this point: The incoming acoustic vibrations cause in-and-out movements of the tympanic membrane and ossicular chain, up-and-down movements of the basilar membrane (producing a traveling wave), back-and-forth bending of the stereocilia where

displacement of basilar membrane is adequate, and finally increases and decreases of ions (K$^+$) into the hair cells (both IHCs and OHCs) that result in increases and decreases of their respective intracellular potentials.

Auditory Nerve Fibers

The final stage in the transduction process of the inner ear is to convert the biochemical events within the hair cells into neural events along the 8th nerve fibers. Since at least 95% of the afferent neural information of the 8th cranial nerve comes from the IHCs, the activation of the stereocilia of the IHCs is the primary route for sensory transduction through the cochlea. For now, we will focus primarily on the activity that occurs in the IHCs. (As you are, hopefully, anticipating the activity and role of the OHCs will be discussed in a later section). The chemical-to-neural transduction process in the IHCs occurs at the chemical synapse that lies between the IHC membrane and the peripheral processes (dendrites) of the afferent auditory neurons that synapse with the IHC. Figure 3–10 illustrates the transduction process from biochemical to neural. When the intracellular potential is in its excitatory phase, there is an increase in the release of neurotransmitter substance at the synapse. When the intracellular potential is in its inhibitory phase, there is a reduction in the release of neurotransmitter substance at the synapse. The dendritic connections of the afferent nerve fibers react to the amount of available neurotransmitter substance and carry the synaptic information, called *graded potential*, to the neurons' cell bodies located in the spiral ganglion. If there is enough graded potential within a cell body to reach its criterion excitation level, then the myelinated axon of the neuron, beginning in the modiolus, sends out an all-or-none discharge, that is, the cell "fires." Once the cell fires, there is a chain reaction along the axon, through the internal auditory canal, and then to the dendrites of connecting cells in the cochlear nucleus of the brainstem.

The all-or-none discharges, called *spikes*, from an auditory nerve fiber are all of the same amplitude

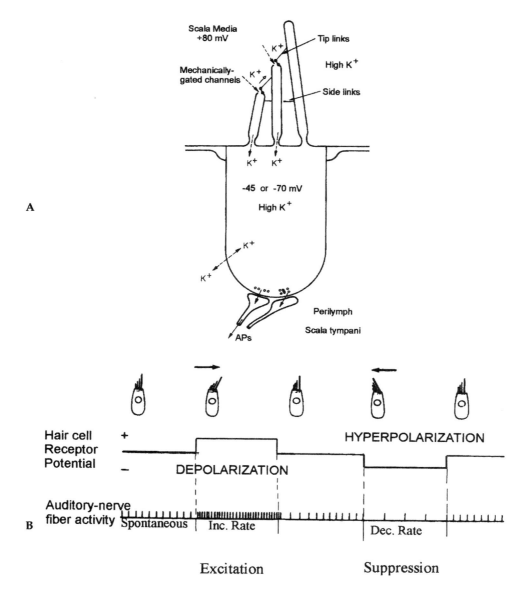

Figure 3–10. Illustration of the transduction process from hydromechanical activity of the stereocilia to neural activity in the afferent neurons attached to the hair cells. The excitation phase causes depolarization with resulting increase in the discharge rate of the neurons (relative to its spontaneous resting discharge rate). This is followed by the inhibition phase, which causes hyperpolarization resulting in a decrease in the discharge rate (relative to its spontaneous resting discharge rate). **Aps**, action potentials. From Salvi, McFadden, & Wang, 2000, p. 22. Copyright 2000 by Thieme.

and duration (see Figure 3–10B). Because there are no differences in the sizes of the discharges, the only neural information available is in the pattern of the neural spikes, for example, how many spikes occur per second or the time intervals between spikes. How the brain codes this information to determine the frequency and intensity of a sound is briefly covered later in this chapter.

Synopsis 3–2

- The transduction process through the inner ear involves hydro-mechanical events (traveling wave and bending of stereocilia on the hair cells), chemical events (changes in the hair cell potentials), and neural events (activation of the afferent nerve fibers, primarily from the IHCs.).

- The basilar membrane is narrower and stiffer at the basal end of the cochlea and becomes wider and less stiff toward the apex of the cochlea. These physical characteristics result in a tonotopic arrangement, whereby high frequencies stimulate the basal end of the membrane and low frequencies stimulate the apical end of the membrane.

- The basilar membrane and tectorial membrane move at different pivot points, which results in bending of the stereocilia away from the modiolus when the basilar membrane moves upward and toward the modiolus when the basilar membrane moves downward.

- The cochlea acts like a battery with a voltage gradient of 120 to 140 mV due to the +80 mV endocochlear potential (EP) and the −40 to −60 mV intracellular resting potential. Current flows in and out of the hair cells due to the opening and closing of K^+ channels (resistance component of the battery analogy) by the action of the tip links of the stereocilia.

- The transduction process in the inner ear involves several stages which can be summarized by the following events:

  - *In-and-out* movement of the stapes footplate creates pressure variations in the fluid that are transmitted instantaneously along the entire basilar membrane.

  - The basilar membrane reacts with a traveling wave that moves from the base of the cochlea and peaks at a location based on the tonotopic arrangement (highs toward the base, lows toward the apex)

  - *Up-and-down* movements of the basilar membrane in the vicinity of the traveling wave peak bend the stereocilia of the IHC *back and forth* by their contact with the tectorial membrane.

  - *Back-and-forth* bendings of the stereocilia *opens and closes* the ion channels by the tip links so that K^+ flow *increases or decreases* relative to the normal intracellular resting level.

  - *Increases and decreases* of K^+ into the hair cell makes the intracellular potential *less negative* (excitatory) and *more negative* (inhibitory) relative to the normal resting potential.

  - *Excitatory and inhibitory stages* of the intracellular potential cause *increases and decreases* in the neurotransmitter substances deposited in the synaptic cleft (more afferent neural activity is associated with the IHCs).

- *Excitatory and inhibitory stages* of the afferent auditory neurons connected to the IHCs cause *increases and decreases* in the all-or-none (spike) discharges, and these spikes travel to the awaiting dendrites of nerve fibers in the cochlear nucleus.

Tuning Curves

The basilar membrane acts like a series of interconnected filters. Each location along the basilar membrane responds best to a specific frequency, its *characteristic frequency* (CF). However, these filters are not precise (sharp) enough to only respond to a single frequency, as might be implied by the analogy to strings on a harp. Instead, each location on the basilar membrane can respond to a range of frequencies around its CF. The combinations of frequencies and intensities that produce a response for a particular location on the basilar membrane provide an estimate of the shape of the filter associated with that location, and this is referred to as a measure of *frequency selectivity* or *tuning*. *Tuning curves* are a useful way to describe the frequency selectivity or tuning characteristics of the auditory system. Tuning curves can be generated for a variety of physiological or psychoacoustic measures. Figure 3–11 describes typical tuning curves that are characteristic of many levels of the auditory system, including the basilar membrane, auditory neurons, and psychoacoustic measures. In essence, a tuning curve is obtained by defining the lowest intensities, over a range of frequencies, which produce a minimum criterion level of response for the measure of interest. A basilar membrane tuning curve is obtained by measuring the range of frequencies (as a function of intensity) that produce a criterion (threshold) amount of displacement for a particular location on the basilar membrane. A neural tuning curve is obtained by measuring the range of frequencies that produce a criterion increase in the discharge rate for a particular neuron. A psychoacoustic tuning curve is obtained by measuring the range of frequencies

that can interfere with (mask) the perception of a target tone near threshold. As shown in Figure 3–11, the CF of a tuning curve is defined by the frequency with the lowest intensity that produces the minimum criterion response. However, as you can see, frequencies other than the CF can also produce the criterion response when presented at higher stimulus levels. For frequencies close to the CF, the tuning curve rises fairly steeply, and this region is called the *tip of the tuning curve*. For lower frequencies, the tuning curve flattens out at a moderate intensity level for a wide range of lower frequencies, and this region is called the *low*

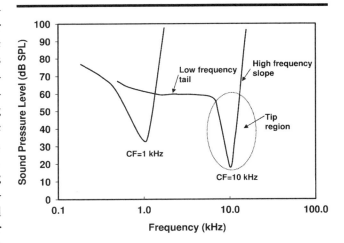

Figure 3–11. Tuning curves for a 1 kHz characteristic frequency (*CF*) and a 10 kHz CF. The most sensitive point (lowest dB SPL), called the *tip of the tuning curve*, occurs at CF. Each tuning curve shows that it is responsive to other frequencies, especially lower frequencies (but with higher dB SPLs). The lower frequencies define a *low frequency tail*. The more sensitive area around the CF is called the *tip region*.

frequency tail. For frequencies higher than the CF, there is only a continued steep slope to the tuning curve, referred to as the *high frequency slope*. A tuning curve with a relatively narrow tip region is considered to be *sharply tuned* and is the expected outcome for normal functioning ears.

Today, we know that the sharp tuning characteristics that are found in the auditory system begin at the level of the basilar membrane. However, a historical perspective needs to be interjected here. Békésy was the first to measure basilar membrane tuning curves (Békésy, 1960). Békésy's tuning curves were done in human cadavers or in physical models that he constructed. Békésy's basilar membrane tuning curves were much broader than the tuning curves we now know to occur on the basilar membrane. Békésy was well aware that the basilar membrane tuning curves he had measured were much broader than the tuning curves that others had measured from individual auditory nerve fibers of the 8th nerve, in live animal specimens, and in psychoacoustic experiments. During the 1970s to 1980s, Békésy and many others engaged in an abundance of auditory research directed at finding another filter ("second filter") that they thought must be responsible for sharpening the tuning between the basilar membrane and the auditory nerve fibers. Was it in the hair cells, the neurons, or something in the central auditory system? This issue, however, was finally resolved with advances in technology, especially laser methods, that allowed measurements of basilar membrane tuning curves to be performed in live animal specimens without compromising the integrity of the cochlea (Khanna & Leonard, 1982; Sellick, Patuzzi, & Johnstone, 1982). Figure 3–12 shows the comparison of Békésy's tuning curves with auditory nerve fiber tuning curves, as well as a later comparison using laser technology. Because the basilar membrane tuning curve in a normal live specimen is as sharp as other measures in the auditory system, there is no need of a second filter in the cochlea. Instead, as it has become clear, the sharp tuning is present in the basilar membrane and is dependent on a physiologically normal cochlea.

The relatively broad basilar membrane tuning curves found by Békésy are, as we now know, due to the physical characteristics of the basilar

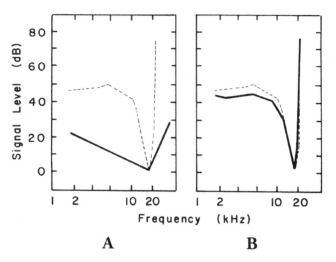

Figure 3–12. A. Comparison of the relatively broad basilar membrane tuning curve from Békésy (*solid curve*) to the sharper tuning curve of an 8th nerve fiber (*dotted curve*). **B.** Comparison of a basilar membrane tuning curve obtained with more modern laser technology (*solid curve*) to an 8th nerve fiber (*dotted curve*). Basilar membrane tuning curves from an alive and healthy specimen are as sharply tuned as 8th nerve fibers. From Dallos, 1985, p. 211. Copyright 1985 by Alan R. Liss.

membrane (width and stiffness), and this component of the traveling wave and tuning is called the *passive cochlear process*. On the other hand, the relatively sharp basilar membrane tunings seen only in healthy normal cochleae are dependent on an *active cochlear process*. The passive and active cochlear processes work together to produce the cochlear reactions to sound. Moreover, as you will see in the next section, it is the OHCs that play an important role in the active process that is responsible for the sharp frequency tuning and good sensitivity.

Role of the Outer Hair Cells

As you recall from Chapter 1, there are about three times as many OHCs as there are IHCs in each human cochlea, and less than 5% of the OHCs have afferent nerve connections (Spoendlin, 1978). This discovery suggests that the OHCs do not have the same function as the IHCs. So what is the role of the more numerous OHCs? This paradox set off another important wave of research in the late 1970s to early 1980s during which time not only was the role of the OHCs determined, but the foundation was laid for a very important physiological test called otoacoustic emissions (OAEs). The OAE test is now a routine part of the audiology test battery and is used in many newborn hearing screening programs (see Chapter 8 for more on OAEs).

About 60 years ago, even before we knew about the tuning paradox of the basilar membrane and differences between IHCs and OHCs, a mathematician named Gold (1948) concluded that some active energy process would be needed in the cochlea in order to have sharp frequency tuning. Gold suggested that this process would have to involve an active feedback loop, which would generate some vibratory energy in the cochlea. Thirty years later, a physicist named David Kemp (Kemp, 1978) gave credence to this theory by actually recording sounds that were coming out of the ear, now known as OAEs. Kemp postulated that these emissions were from some active cochlear process that generates additional mechanical activity on the basilar membrane that travels back out through the middle ear and generates very low-level acoustic sounds in the ear canal that can be measured with a very sensitive microphone. Soon after Kemp's discovery, a neuroscientist named William Brownell (Brownell, 1983) demonstrated that OHCs were able to elongate and contract in response to electrical currents. These elongations and contractions are generally referred to as the *motility* of the OHCs. The motility of the OHCs was subsequently confirmed by many investigators. Recall that OHCs have a unique organization along their outer wall consisting of structural and contractile proteins, as well as enzymes, and these elements have been shown to be partly responsible for the rigidity and motility of the OHCs. The motility of the OHCs is unique in that they can elongate and contract, rather than just contract like muscles. The stria vascularis is thought to provide the external energy source that allows the OHCs to move indefinitely and at high frequencies without

getting tired. The complete biochemistry of OHC motility is not fully understood and is beyond the scope of this textbook. The OHCs function as chemical-mechanical (motor) cells, whereas the IHCs function as chemical-neural (sensory) cells.

So, how does the OHC motility influence cochlear mechanics? Recall that the stereocilia of the IHCs are not imbedded into the underside of the tectorial membrane. We also know that, at low to moderate intensities, the traveling wave displacements of the basilar membrane that are responsible for the passive cochlear process are not sufficient to make the stereocilia of the IHCs contact the tectorial membrane to initiate bending of their stereocilia. As described earlier, it is the stimulation of the IHCs that is necessary for afferent neural transduction, therefore there must be some other mechanism needed to cause the stereocilia of the IHCs to bend. As it turns out, it is the active cochlear process of the OHCs that amplifies the displacement of the basilar membrane through the motility of the OHCs. At low to moderate intensities, the motility of the OHCs resonates with the passive process of the traveling wave motion of the basilar membrane, and this additional activity causes the displacement of the basilar membrane to be more effective. This is often explained with a swing analogy, where the amplitude of the swing's height can be increased by having someone push (adding energy) in resonance with the swing's motion (and you can imagine what happens when the push is not in resonance with the swing's motion). You can also increase the amplitude of the swing on your own by pumping your legs (adding energy) in resonance with the swing's motion. A very similar process occurs through the contraction and elongation of the OHCs. In other words, because the OHC stereocilia are firmly embedded into the tectorial membrane, the motility of the OHCs causes the basilar membrane and tectorial membrane to be pulled together and pushed apart. This active process in the cochlea amplifies the traveling wave motion of the basilar membrane enough to allow the stereocilia of the IHCs to make contact with the tectorial membrane even at low to moderate stimulus intensities. This active cochlear process is necessary for our good hearing sensitivity and frequency tuning (Kiang,

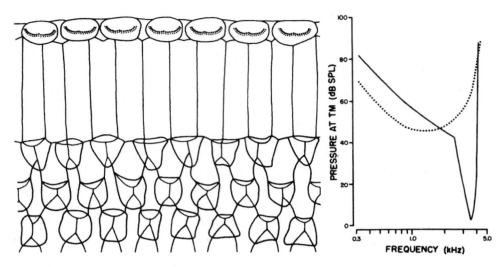

Figure 3–13. Illustration showing how the loss of outer hair cells (no stereocilia) elevates the tip region of the tuning curve and leaves only the broader tuning, which is related to the physical properties of the basilar membrane that stimulate the intact inner hair cells at higher intensities. From Liberman, Dodds, & Learson, 1986, p. 164. Copyright 1986 by Plenum Press.

Liberman, Sewell, & Guinan, 1986). At high stimulus intensities, it is believed that the displacement of the basilar membrane resulting solely from the passive cochlear process is sufficient to allow the stereocilia of the IHCs to make contact with the tectorial membrane. As Figure 3–13 illustrates, without the active process of the OHCs the basilar membrane tuning curve loses its sensitivity in the tip region and becomes broadly tuned (Liberman, Dodds, & Learson, 1985). As mentioned earlier, the broadly tuned portion of the basilar membrane tuning curve is primarily a reflection of the passive cochlear process. When damage occurs to the OHCs, the active process in the cochlear is compromised and mild-to-moderate degrees of hearing loss occur. For greater degrees of hearing loss, there is additional damage to the IHCs that also compromises the output from the passive cochlear process. An important point to realize is that when there is damage to the OHCs, the OAEs are not generated. On the other hand, if OAEs are present, it can be inferred that there is good auditory function up to at least the level of the OHCs. The absence of OAEs suggests some abnormality in auditory function, either in the OHCs, middle ear, or outer ear. As discussed in Chapter 10, OAEs are now widely used as a screening measure for newborns, and those who do not pass the OAE screen are referred for diagnostic follow-up.

As you can see, the transduction process in the cochlea includes different but related processes for the IHCs and the OHCs. The OHCs operate as a chemical-motor transduction process and the IHCs operate as a chemical-neural transduction process. Table 3–1 summarizes all of the transduction processes that we have discussed for the peripheral auditory system, including their specific mechanisms and functions.

Frequency Coding

As you might imagine, given that there is much to learn and understand about how the normal ear functions, the field is only beginning to scratch the surface on how we make use of the auditory neural information that ultimately is processed at the cortex, and how they are perceived; again, there is much more to learn through future research. At

Table 3–1. Summary of the Auditory Transduction Processes

Process	Part of Ear	Structures	Mechanism	Function
Acoustic	Outer	Auricle, ear canal	Resonance	Amplify mid to high frequencies to overcome impedance mismatch
Mechanical	Middle	Tympanic membrane, ossicles, oval window	Area, lever, and curved membrane advantages; route vibrations to oval window	Amplify low to mid frequencies to overcome impedance mismatch
Hydromechanical	Cochlea	Oval and round windows, scalae	Reciprocal in-and-out movements of oval and round windows	Instantaneous pressure variations in fluid-filled cochlea
		Basilar membrane	Passive process: traveling wave dependent on width and stiffness gradients of basilar membrane	Tonotopic place principle; highs at base and lows at apex; produces broad tuning curves
		Tectorial and basilar membranes, stereocilia	Bends stereocilia back and forth due to different pivot points of the two membranes; controls K$^+$ flow into OHCs and IHCs	Activates hair cells: toward modiolus = excitation; away from modiolus = inhibition
Chemical-motoric	Cochlea	OHCs	Active process: OHC motility, from fluctuation in K$^+$ flow, adds displacement to traveling wave to allow direct bending of IHC stereocilia	Increases sensitivity and sharpens tuning; responsible for sharp-tip region of tuning curves
Chemical-neural	Cochlea	IHCs	Increase and decrease of intracellular potential resulting from fluctuation in K$^+$ flow	Controls release of neurotransmitter substance
Neural	8th Nerve	Auditory nerve fibers	Uptake of neurotransmitter substance; if adequate, cells initiate all-or-none discharges down 8th nerve axons to cells in cochlear nucleus	Neural discharge patterns provide intensity and frequency information to central nervous system.

IHC, Inner Hair Cells; *OHC,* Outer Hair Cells.

this introductory level, only some general theories of perception are presented.

There are two general principles used to explain how we determine (code) the frequency of the incoming sound, the place theory and the frequency theory. The *place theory of hearing* refers to the tonotopic arrangement along the basilar membrane. The tonotopic arrangement of the auditory system is present at the basilar membrane, but is also a characteristic of the auditory neurons, auditory nuclei in the brainstem, and auditory reception areas of the cortex. The place theory assumes that the frequency information is first coded where the peak of the traveling wave occurs along the basilar membrane, high frequencies near the base and low frequencies near the apex, and this frequency information is preserved as the neural information goes through the auditory neural pathways. As nice as the place theory sounds, there are some limitations. One problem for the place theory comes from psychoacoustic experiments that have demonstrated that the perception of frequency does not always relate to the place predicted by the tonotopic arrangement. For example, when listening to multiple pure tones that are harmonically related the perceived pitch is determined by the lowest fundamental frequency. For example, when presented simultaneously with 1200, 1400, and 1600 Hz, the perceived pitch would be 200 Hz, even though it is not even presented to the ears. However, this 200 Hz pitch will still be perceived even when the low frequency areas are masked by a noise or have some type of damage. In other words, the place theory would predict that the 200 Hz is perceived because it generates a traveling wave at the 200 Hz location, when in fact the 200 Hz is still perceived when the apical area of the basilar membrane is unable to respond to the tone due to the noise or damage. Somehow, the pitch of this missing fundamental is still perceived because of information coming from the activity in the high frequency area of the cochlea; thus, the place theory does not explain all types of frequency coding.

An alternative theory of frequency coding, the *frequency theory*, is based on the processing of the pattern of discharges in the afferent auditory nerve fibers. However, the frequency theory also has its limitations. A simple frequency theory would be to have the number of discharges per second (*discharge rate*) in the auditory neurons correspond to the frequency of the sound. For example, we would perceive a 2000 Hz tone because neurons were discharging at 2000 times/s. However, a neuron requires a minimal period of time to recover before it can respond again, called the *absolute refractory period*, and this imposes some restrictions on the discharge rate of neurons. The absolute refractory period for an auditory neuron is about 1.0 ms; therefore, the theoretical upper limit for an auditory neuron would be 1,000 discharges per second. In fact, it is actually more typical for an auditory nerve fiber to respond up to a maximum of only 200 discharges per second, regardless of the stimulus frequency. Clearly, the discharge rate per se is not useful for coding frequency.

Let's look at some other patterns of discharges that occur in response to simple sounds to see if they could be a viable means to code frequency. One method is to measure the time intervals between the discharges, called *interspike interval* (ISI). As Figure 3–14 shows, a neuron responds with a preferred ISI; however, it also responds with other ISIs, and these can be seen to follow a specific temporal pattern. For example, the 1000 Hz tone has a preferred ISI of 1 ms, which corresponds to the period for 1000 Hz. However, notice that the other ISIs for the 1000 Hz tone occur at multiples of the period of the 1000 Hz tone. Using this strategy, a neuron does not have to discharge every cycle of the stimulus; it can skip some cycles of the stimulus due to its need for recovery time, but when it does respond it always responds at some multiple of the preferred interval. Different frequencies would have different patterns of ISIs that are related to the period of the stimulus. As you may have noticed in Figure 3–14, the relation between ISIs and the period of the stimulus holds up only for low to mid-frequencies, whereas at higher frequencies (above 2000 Hz) a preferred interval is not apparent. If, however, recordings from a neuron are displayed as a function of the period of the stimulus, called a *period histogram*,

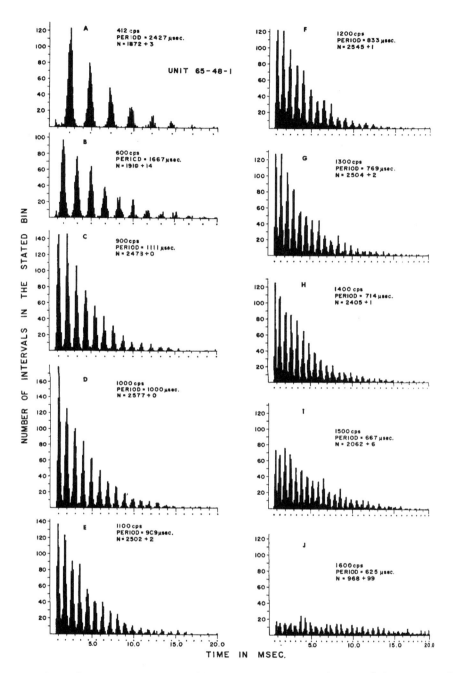

Figure 3–14. Examples of interspike interval histograms. Recordings of the intervals between discharges are plotted as a function of stimulation time. Notice how the peaks in the histograms are related to the periods of the different frequencies up to about 1500 Hz. From Rose, Hind, Anderson, & Brugge, 1967, p. 772. Copyright 1967 by The American Physiological Society.

it can be observed that the discharges always occur within the same phase of the stimulus, called *phase locking*. Figure 3–15 shows examples of phase locking. Notice that the neuron does not have to respond to every cycle of the stimulus, but when it responds it is always somewhere within the same phase of the stimulus. In other words, the neuron discharges only during the excitatory phase of the stimulus and does not respond during the inhibitory phase of the stimulus. Phase locking may be able to provide neural information for frequencies up to 4000 to 5000 Hz (Møller, 1983). The frequency theory is partially supported by the phase-locking characteristics of the auditory nerve fibers, at least for low to mid frequencies, but this theory may not be adequate to explain frequency coding in the high frequencies. Of course, it is quite plausible that the place theory and the frequency theory are used in the coding of frequency. In other words, for low to mid frequencies both

the place and neural frequency theories may explain frequency coding, whereas for high frequencies only the place theory may be involved. While we are beginning to have a more complete picture of the physiology of the different parts of the normal auditory system, there is much to learn to be able to fully understand our sense of hearing. You undoubtedly are finding yourself amazed at how we process sound and how little we understand about the mechanisms, even in normal ears, not to mention those with hearing loss. Many questions remain and make for some interesting future research.

Intensity Coding

How does the auditory system provide information that we use to code for stimulus intensity? One theory for coding intensity has to do with how much of the basilar membrane is stimulated. In other words, as intensity increases the tails of tuning curves from more basal locations are also stimulated. Figure 3–16 illustrates how a spread of activity could occur across more of the basilar membrane by crossing the tails of the tuning curves from higher frequency regions. This increase in the number of activated neurons from a wider area of the basilar membrane could code for intensity, while the activity of neurons at the tip of the tuning curve could code for the frequency.

Can a single auditory neuron code intensity? In other words, could one fiber from a single place keep increasing its discharge rate as a function of stimulus intensity? We can begin to answer this question by looking at an *input-output* (I/O) *function*, which is a measure of how the number of discharges per second changes as a function of stimulus intensity. As Figure 3–17 shows, most auditory nerves increase their discharge rates over a limited intensity range of only 20 to 40 dB above threshold (Kiang, 1965; Sachs & Abbas, 1974). This immediately suggests a problem in coding intensity over the entire 140 dB range, since neurons can only increase a maximum of 40 dB above their threshold. Liberman (1978) suggested that the range of intensity coding based on the discharge

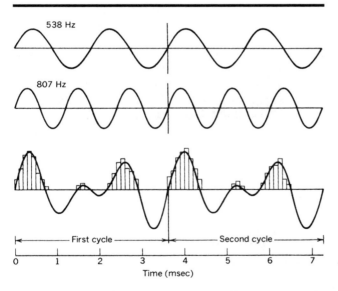

Figure 3–15. Illustration of phase locking as a means to code for frequency. In this example, two tones are played and there is a good representation of the combined tone in the preferred discharge pattern. In other words, when the nerve responded it was always in the same phase of the stimulus. From Gulick, Gescheider, & Frisina, 1989, p. 183. Copyright 1989 by Oxford University Press.

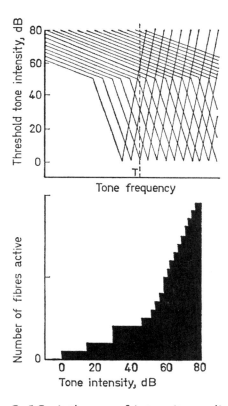

Figure 3–16. A theory of intensity coding postulated by Evans. In this theory, more nerve fibers are recruited at higher intensities because they are activated by crossing the low frequency tails of higher frequency nerve fibers. From Evans, 1975.

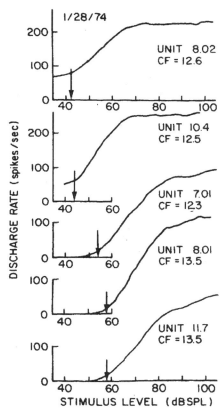

Figure 3–17. Input–output functions for some auditory nerve fibers. Most nerve fibers tend to plateau (saturate) in their discharge rates within 40 dB above threshold and, therefore, cannot use this information to code across the audible intensity range. From Sachs & Abbas, 1974, p. 1837. Copyright 1976 by American Institute of Physics.

Synopsis 3–3

- We now know that our excellent frequency selectivity (sharp tuning) and sensitivity originate along the basilar membrane only when the cochlea is physiologically healthy. Earlier measures in cadavers using compromised cochleae showed much broader tuning than had been demonstrated in the tuning of 8th nerve fibers and in psychoacoustic experiments.

- The additional mechanical energy exerted by the motility (elongations and contractions) of the OHCs at low to moderate intensities increases the displacement of the basilar membrane, much like pushing someone on a swing. The motility of the OHCs allows the stereocilia of the IHCs to be directly stimulated by the tectorial membrane in response to the basilar membrane enhanced action.

- The motility of the OHCs in a healthy, normal functioning ear is responsible for the ear's remarkable sensitivity and sharp frequency selectivity. Damage to the OHCs may lead to a mild to moderate hearing loss and a loss of frequency resolution (broader tuning curves). The OHC motility is referred to as the active cochlear process, whereas the process of traveling waves that occur along the basilar membrane due to its physical characteristics is called the passive cochlear process.

- The cochlear transduction process has both a chemical-neural mechanism involving the IHCs and a chemical-motor mechanism involving the OHCs. See Table 3–1 for a summary of the transduction process through all parts of the peripheral auditory system.

- Otoacoustic emissions, which are predictable consequences of the OHCs' motility, travel from the cochlea and back out the middle ear and are transduced into acoustic vibrations by the tympanic membrane. OAEs can be recorded with a sensitive microphone placed in the ear canal and have become a popular auditory physiological screening test.

- Because most auditory neurons respond with rates less than 200 discharges/s, the number of discharges per second is not a viable method to code for frequency. A more plausible explanation for coding frequency is by analyzing the interspike intervals or phase locking of neurons, which provide information about the period of the stimulus. Coding frequency by phase locking may be possible up to about 4000 Hz. An alternate theory for frequency coding is by the tonotopic place that is maximally activated along the basilar membrane. The place theory has limitations in explaining some psychoacoustic phenomena, especially coding low frequencies, but may be plausible for higher frequencies where the phase locking is inadequate.

- Intensity coding is also not fully understood. A single auditory nerve fiber can only increase its discharge rate over a maximum range of about 40 dB. Possible explanations for intensity coding include (a) activation of more nerve fibers at higher intensities as they cross the low frequency tails of other neurons, and/or (b) different nerve fibers may become activated at different stimulus levels.

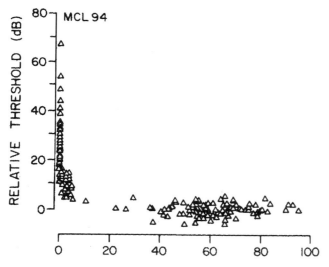

Figure 3–18. Another theory of intensity coding. Data show that different nerve fibers have different thresholds, some as high as 60–70 dB. Those fibers with low spontaneous discharge rates were the ones that had a higher range of thresholds than those with higher spontaneous discharge rates. From Liberman, 1978, p. 448. Copyright 1978 by American Institute of Physics.

rate could be expanded by staggered thresholds for different neurons attached to each IHC. As Figure 3–18 shows, neurons have been shown to have a range of thresholds, some of which do not begin to respond until 60 to 70 dB above the threshold of the most sensitive neurons attached to the IHC. Liberman showed that the thresholds of neurons were related to the spontaneous discharge rates; high-spontaneous-rate neurons had low thresholds, and low-spontaneous-rate neurons had high thresholds.

Vestibular System Function

Audiologists often see patients with balance disorders, many of whom have dizziness, and many of these disorders may be accompanied by hearing loss. A type of dizziness that originates in the vestibular organs of the inner ear is called *vertigo*, which is generally described as a sensation of "the room is spinning" or "motion sickness." Audiologists perform a variety of tests to assess different types of balance disorders. A complete description of vestibular physiology, assessment, and treatment is beyond the scope of this text. This section provides a relatively simple description of the normal physiology of the peripheral vestibular organs.

The balance system relies on sensory information from the peripheral vestibular organs, as well as from the visual and proprioceptive systems. Figure 3–19 shows how these sensory systems are integrated in the brainstem, cerebellum, and cerebral cortex, and how they affect eye movements, posture, and limb movements in certain situations (Goebel & Hanson, 1997). For example, you have probably experienced the reflexive action that occurs when you lean back in your chair just a little too far. In general, the vestibular organs provide neural information to the central nervous system that signals changes in the position of the head, as well as changes in the body's orientation relative to gravity. In other words, the vestibular organs respond to accelerations and decelerations of the head. The integration of neural activity of the vestibular, visual, and somatosensory systems is important for us to maintain an upright posture, perform coordinated complex movements, and maintain a visual target while moving. The vestibular system operates, for the most part, without conscious control, and we are not generally aware of its importance until it is affected by disease or other atypical stimulation leading to motion sickness, such as a boat bobbing in the waves or a spinning amusement park ride. Controlling for motion sickness is also an important issue for astronauts and jet pilots. Another example of an atypical stimulation of the vestibular organs occurs when too much alcohol has been consumed resulting in vertigo and nausea. In this situation, the alcohol alters the specific gravity of the endolymph in the semicircular canals, and this causes an abnormal vestibular response that is perceived as movement, even while standing or lying still.

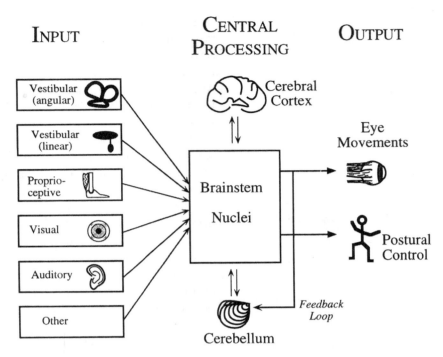

Figure 3–19. Overview of the components involved with balance and movement. Different sensory systems are processed by the brainstem, with connections to the cerebellum and cortex, to control eye movements, posture, and coordinated movements. From Goebel & Hanson, 1997, p. 44. Copyright 1997 by Thieme.

Semicircular Canals

The semicircular canals are responsive to rotational (angular) accelerations and decelerations of the head. Each of the three semicircular canals is most sensitive to rotation in a particular orthogonal plane of motion. Based on their orientation, the appropriate semicircular canal will respond when the head rotates left and right (x-axis), forward and backward (y-axis), or tilted toward each shoulder (z-axis); or more than one semicircular canal may respond to rotations in other spatial axes as typically occurs in everyday patterns of movement. As a simple example, the horizontal semicircular canals are most responsive to rotation of the head left and right, whereas the posterior and inferior semicircular canals are most responsive for forward and backward (pitch) and tilting left or right (yaw) rotations. In a normal system, the semicircular canals on both sides of the head work together

in functional pairs: The horizontal semicircular canal on the left side is paired with the horizontal semicircular canal on the right side; the superior semicircular canal on the left side is paired with the posterior semicircular canal on the right side; and the posterior semicircular canal on the left side is paired with the superior semicircular canal on the right side. These events are illustrated in Figure 3–20 for head rotations in the horizontal plane. During head rotation in one direction, the neural output of the semicircular canal on one side increases its neural discharge rate (relative to the spontaneous rate), while the paired semicircular canal on the other side decreases its neural discharge rate (Baloh, 1998). For example, horizontal head acceleration to the right produces an increase in the discharge rate from the right horizontal semicircular canal and a decrease in the discharge rate from the left horizontal semicircular canal. The vestibular nuclei in the brainstem

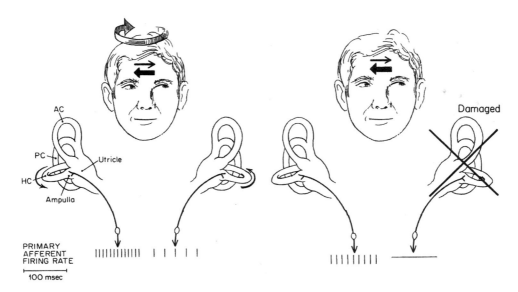

Figure 3–20. Schematic illustration of how activity (or lack of activity) from the two horizontal semicircular canals provides information to the brain. On the left side of the figure is a normal output that occurs with head rotation to the right. In this case, the right canal increases its discharge rate and the left canal decreases its discharge rate. On the right side of the figure, the output acts like a head turn to the right, but in this case the patient is not moving his head, and he may have resulting spontaneous eye movements and a sensation that the room is spinning. **AC**, anterior canal; **PC**, posterior canal; **HC**, horizontal canal. From Baloh, 1998, p. 36. Copyright 1998 by F. A. Davis.

integrate the neural information from the two sides in order to signal the direction of head rotation. Also shown in Figure 3–20 is the disruption in neural information from the side with a pathology, which sends inappropriate information to the central nervous system causing an imbalanced sensation.

As we learned in Chapter 1, the afferent nerves from the semicircular canals originate on the sensory hair cells in the cristae of the semicircular canals (within the ampullae). The hair cells have rows of stereocilia that are embedded into a gelatinous substance called the cupula. The rows of stereocilia are arranged from shortest to tallest; and next to the tallest row is a single large cilium called the kinocilium, which provides a functional orientation for excitation and inhibition. When the stereocilia are bent toward the kinocilium there is an increase in neural discharge rate (excitation), and when the stereocilia are bent away from the kinocilium there is a decrease in neural discharge rate (inhibition). When the head turns to the right,

the fluid in the semicircular canal applies force in the opposite direction because it lags behind the canal movement because of its viscous and inertial properties. This results in a deflection of the cupula that bends the stereocilia toward the kinocilium on the right side of the head and away from the kinocilium on the left side of the head. When the head rotation reaches a steady velocity, the relative differences in movement between the semicircular canals and the fluid no longer occur and the neural activity is once again in balance; however, additional accelerations or decelerations will result in renewed stimulation.

Utricle and Saccule

The utricle and saccule respond to linear accelerations and decelerations of the head, as well as maintain the body's orientation relative to gravity. The stereocilia of the maculae are covered by the otoconia, a gelatinous mass with calcium carbonate crystals. These calcium carbonate crystals have a higher specific gravity than the surrounding fluid, making them responsive to head position relative to gravity as well as changes that occur during linear head accelerations. The utricle is primarily responsive to linear motions in the horizontal plane (forward and backward or left to right), whereas the saccule is primarily responsive to linear motions in the vertical plane (up and down). Linear movements in other directions produce responses from combinations of these organs. The utricle and saccule on one side of the head work together with the utricle and saccule on the other side of the head to signal the direction of head movement by comparing which organ has increased its neural discharge rate and which has decreased its neural discharge rate. As with the semicircular canals, when the stereocilia are bent toward the kinocilium there is an increase in neural discharge rate above the spontaneous rate (excitation), and when they are bent away from the kinocilium there is a decrease in neural discharge rate (inhibition). The directional polarization of the kinocilia in the maculae is more complex than in the semicircular canals (see Figure 3–21). When the head movement reaches a steady velocity, the responses from the

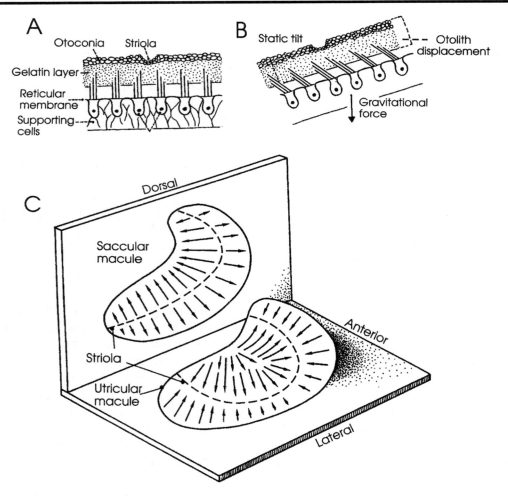

Figure 3–21. A–C. Functional polarization of the maculae in the utricle and the saccule. In the saccule, there are two groups of hair cells, functionally separated by the striola, and the kinocilia are directed away from the striola. In the utricle, there are also two groups of hair cells, also functionally separated by the striola; however, the kinocilia are directed toward the striola. From Barber & Stockwell, 1976. Copyright 1979 by Mosby Company.

maculae are back in balance, and ready for additional accelerations or decelerations.

Vestibulo-Ocular Reflex

The vestibular neural pathway has connections within the brainstem to neurons that control the extraocular muscles of the eyes, so that a clear visual image can be automatically maintained during head movement (Wright & Schwade, 2000). This pathway is called the *vestibulo-ocular reflex* (VOR). The VOR results in eye movements that are equal and opposite to the direction of head movements (Barber, 1984). As can be seen in Figure 3–22, the VOR for the horizontal semicircular canals involves afferent neurons from the vestibular nerve to the vestibular nucleus. From the vestibular nucleus, there are connections to the nucleus of the abducens nerve (6th cranial nerve), which controls the lateral rectus muscle of the eye on the opposite side of the head, and connections to the nucleus of the oculomotor nerve, which controls the medial rectus muscle of the eye on the same side of the head. The control of the eye muscles by the VOR is coordinated by the vestibular inputs from both sides of the head; one side is excitatory and the other side is inhibitory. For a head turn to the right (see Figure 3–22), the excitatory input from the right ear contracts the left lateral rectus and the right medial rectus, which makes the eyes move to the left. For a head turn to the left, the left vestibular pathway will be excitatory resulting in movement of the eyes toward the right. Because the eyes can only move a small distance in the orbit, there is an additional neural connection from the reticular formation that quickly brings the eyes back to the center (Wright & Schwade, 2000). These slow and fast eye responses, called *nystagmus*, continually repeat during the head rotation. Figure 3–23 shows a repeated pattern of nystagmus for head turn to the right. Nystagmus can be induced with clinical tests of vestibular function or may be abnormally present in certain vestibular disorders. Nystagmus can be measured with electrodes mounted next to the eyes that can record changes in the electrical potential, called the *corneoretinal potential*, as the eyes move. Recording

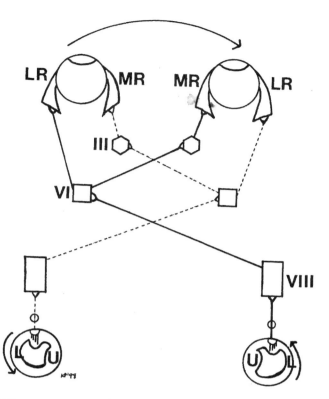

Figure 3–22. The vestibulo-ocular reflex pathway. In this example for a head turn to the right, the right ear horizontal canal is excitatory and moves the eyes to the left. **LR**, lateral rectus; **MR**, medial rectus. From Salvi et al., 2000, p. 81. Copyright 2000 by Thieme.

nystagmus is the basis of a clinical test of vestibular function called *electronystagmography* (ENG). Observing and/or recording eye movements under different conditions are very useful for assessment of many vestibular disorders.

Other Central Vestibular Connections

In addition to the VOR, the vestibular nuclei have connections to other sensory and motor systems. The vestibular system has important afferent and efferent connections with the cerebellum, where information from visual and proprioceptive systems are integrated for balance, coordination of

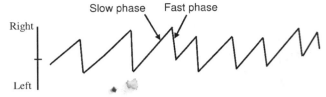

Figure 3–23. An example of nystagmus. Because the eyes can only move so far during a head turn, there is a central component that continually brings them back to center. Nystagmus has a slow phase due to the semicircular canal response and a fast phase due to the central (reticular formation) response. These responses can be observed by measuring (with electrodes around the eyes) how the corneoretinal potential changes with eye movements, or by video recording of eye movement.

movement, as well as control of eye movements. The vestibular system also has connections to the spinal motor system which result in a vestibulospinal reflex (VSR) that controls muscles in the neck, body, and limbs, especially important when the body makes unexpected changes in position relative to gravity. The vestibular system also has connections with the reticular formation of the autonomic nervous system, which influences respiration and gustatory or visceral reflexes. These vestibular pathways account for a person's nausea or vomiting from motion sickness, excessive alcohol, or vestibular disorders. Fortunately, the vestibular system is remarkably adaptive and many vestibular disorders involving the peripheral vestibular organs spontaneously recover or undergo

---

Synopsis 3–4

- Vertigo is an abnormal balance sensation mediated by the peripheral vestibular system in which there is a perception that things are spinning.

- The vestibular system relies on sensory information from the peripheral vestibular organs, as well as from the visual and proprioceptive systems, which is integrated in the brainstem, cerebellum, and cerebral cortex to control eye movements, posture, and limb movements in certain situations that change the position of the head.

- The semicircular canals are primarily responsive to rotational (angular) accelerations and decelerations of the head. Each of the three semicircular canals is most sensitive to rotation in a particular orthogonal plane of motion: The horizontal semicircular canal on one side is paired with the horizontal semicircular canal on the other side; the superior semicircular canal on one side is paired with the posterior semicircular canal on the other side. Input from one side of the head works with input from the other side to maintain balance and control during movement.

- The utricle and saccule maintain the body's orientation relative to gravity, and are also responsive to linear accelerations and decelerations of the head. The utricle is primarily responsive to linear motions in the horizontal plane (forward and backward or left to right), whereas the saccule is primarily responsive to linear motions in the vertical plane (up and down).

- Bending of the stereocilia within the peripheral vestibular organs is accomplished by head movement that displaces the gelatinous mass that covers the tops of the stereocilia. The utricle and saccule on one side of the head work together with the utricle and saccule on the other side of the head to signal the direction of head movement by comparing which organ has increased its neural discharge rate and which has decreased its neural discharge rate.

- The vestibular neural pathways within the brainstem have connections to the motor neurons of the cranial nerves that are involved with control of the extraocular muscles of the eyes, called the vestibulo-ocular reflex (VOR), so that a clear visual image can be automatically maintained during head movement.

- Observing and/or recording eye movements under different conditions are very useful for assessment of many vestibular disorders, and is part of the ENG battery of vestibular clinical tests. Nystagmus (repetitive slow and fast components of eye movements) can be measured with electrodes mounted next to the eyes that can record changes in the electrical potential, called the *corneoretinal potential*, as the eyes move.

- The vestibular system has central brainstem connections to the spinal motor system that result in vestibulo-spinal reflexes (VSR) to control muscles in the neck, body, and limbs when the body makes unexpected changes in position relative to gravity.

- The vestibular system also has connections with the reticular formation of the autonomic nervous system and can influence respiration and gustatory or visceral reflexes, as with motion sickness.

central nervous system reorganization, known as *vestibular compensation* (Vidal, De Waele, Vibert, & Muhlethaler, 1998).

References

Ballachanda, B. B. (1995). *The human ear canal.* San Diego, CA: Singular.

Baloh, R. W. (1998). *Dizziness, hearing loss, and tinnitus.* Philadelphia, PA: F. A. Davis.

Barber, H. O. (1984). Vestibular neurophysiology. *Otolaryngology-Head and Neck Surgery, 92,* 55–58.

Barber, H. O., & Stockwell, C. W. (1976). *Manual of nystagmography* (p. 27). St. Louis, MO: Mosby.

Békésy, G. (1960). *Experiments in hearing.* New York, NY: McGraw-Hill.

Borg, E., & Counter, S. A. (1989). The middle ear muscles. *Scientific American, 260,* 74–80.

Brownell, W. E. (1983). Observations on a motile response in isolated outer hair cells. In W. R. Webster, & L. Aitken (Eds.), *Mechanisms of hearing* (pp. 5–10). Clayton, Australia: Monash University Press.

Dallos, P. (1985). Role of cochlear outer hair cells. In M. J. Correia, & A. A. Perachio (Eds.), *Contemporary sensory neurobiology.* New York, NY: Alan R. Liss.

Dallos, P. (1986). Neurobiology of cochlear inner and outer hair cells: Intracellular recordings. *Hearing Research, 22,* 185–198.

Dallos, P. (1988). *Cochlear neurobiology: Revolutionary developments.* Rockville, MD: American Speech-Language-Hearing Association.

Davis, H. (1965). A model for transducer action in the cochlea. *Quantitative Biology, 30,* 181–190.

Durrant, J. D., & Lovrinic, J. H. (1995). *Basis of hearing science* (3rd ed.). Baltimore, MD: Williams & Wilkins.

Evans, F. (1975). The sharpening of cochlear frequency selectivity in the normal and abnormal cochlea. *Audiology, 14,* 436.

Geisler, C. D. (1998). *Sound to synapse.* New York, NY: Oxford University Press.

Gelfand, S. A. (2009). *Essentials of audiology* (3rd ed.). New York, NY: Thieme.

Goebel, J. A., & Hanson, J. M. (Eds.). (1997). *Clinical otology* (2nd ed.). New York, NY: Thieme.

Gold, T. (1948). Hearing II: the physical basis of the action of the cochlea. *Proceedings of the Royal Society of London, Series B: Biological Sciences, 135,* 492–498.

Gulick, W. L., Gescheider, G. A., & Frisina, R. D. (1989). *Hearing: Physiological acoustics, neural coding, and psychoacoustics.* New York, NY: Oxford University Press.

Kemp, D. T. (1978). Stimulated acoustic emissions from within the human auditory system. *Journal of the Acoustical Society of America, 64,* 1386–1391.

Khanna, S. M., & Leonard, D. G. B. (1982). Basilar membrane tuning in the cat cochlea. *Science, 215,* 305–306.

Kiang, N. Y. (1965). Discharge patterns of single fibers in the cat's auditory nerve. *Research Monographs, 35,* Cambridge, MA: MIT Press.

Kiang, N. Y. S., Liberman, M. C., Sewell, W. F., & Guinan, J. J. (1986). Single unit clues to cochlear mechanics. *Hearing Research, 22,* 171–182.

Liberman, M. C. (1978). Auditory nerve response from cats raised in a low-noise chamber. *Journal of the Acoustical Society of America, 63,* 442–455.

Liberman, M. C., Dodds, L. W., & Learson, D. A. (1985). *Structure-function correlation in noise-damaged ears: a light and electron microscopic study.* Paper presented at the NATO Advanced Studies Institute on Applied and Basic Aspects of Noise-Induced Hearing Loss, Lucca, Italy.

Liberman, M. C., Dodds, L. W., & Learson, D. A. (1986). Structure-function correlation in noise-damaged ears. In R. J. Salvi, D. Henderson, R. P. Hamernik, & V. Colletti (Eds.), *Basic and applied aspects of noise-induced hearing loss.* New York, NY: Plenum Press.

Møller, A. R. (1983). *Auditory physiology.* New York, NY: Academic Press.

Nedzelnitsky, V. (1980). Sound pressure in the basal turn of the cat cochlea. *Journal of the Acoustical Society of America, 68,* 1676–1689.

Rose, J. E., Hind, J. E., Anderson, D. J., & Brugge, J. F. (1967). Phase-locked responses to low frequency tones in single auditory nerve fibers in the squirrel monkey. *Journal of Neurophysiology, 30,* 772.

Sachs, M. B., & Abbas, P. J. (1974). Rate versus level functions for auditory-nerve fibers in cats: Tone burst stimuli. *Journal of the Acoustical Society of America, 56,* 1835–1847.

Salvi R. J., McFadden S. L., & Wang, J. (2000). Anatomy and physiology of the peripheral auditory system. In R. J. Roesner, M. Valente, & H. Hosford-Dunn (Eds.), *Audiology diagnosis.* New York, NY: Thieme.

Sellick, P. M., Patuzzi, R., & Johnstone, B. M. (1982). Measurement of basilar membrane motion in the guinea pig using Mossbauer technique. *Journal of the Acoustical Society of America, 72,* 131–141.

Shaw, E. A. (1974). Transformation of sound pressure level from the free field to the ear drum in the horizontal plane. *Journal of the Acoustical Society of America, 56,* 1848–1861.

Spoendlin, H. (Ed.). (1978). *The afferent innervation of the cochlea.* New York, NY: Academic Press.

Stuhlman, O. Jr. (1943). *An introduction to biophysics.* New York, NY: John Wiley and Sons/Chapman & Hall.

Vidal, P. P., De Waele, C., Vibert, N., & Muhlethaler, M. (1998). Vestibular compensation revisited. *Otolaryngology-Head and Neck Surgery, 119,* 34–42.

Wright, C. G., & Schwade, N. D. (2000). Anatomy and physiology of the vestibular system. In R. J. Roeser, M. Valente, & H. Hosford-Dunn (Eds.), *Audiology diagnosis* (pp. 73–84). New York, NY: Thieme.

Yost, W. (2000). *Fundamentals of hearing* (4th ed.). San Diego, CA: Academic Press.

PART II

CLINICAL AUDIOLOGY

We now switch our focus to the clinical assessment of hearing and the rewarding aspects of interacting with patients. In the following chapters you will learn about several tests used by audiologists to diagnose hearing loss, and you will be introduced to hearing aids as one of the treatments used by audiologists to help improve communication of patients with nonmedically treatable hearing loss. In this book, we prefer to use the terms patient, diagnosis, and treatment in the context of providing audiologic services; however, in some settings audiologists may prefer to use the terms client, evaluation, and management. While the audiologist does not use the audiologic results to diagnose auditory diseases, they often provide information to physicians about the hearing loss that is useful to the physician in making a medical diagnosis. In addition, the audiologic results directly bear on the audiologic treatment, including fitting hearing aids, aural rehabilitation, and/or tinnitus management.

Some of the tests covered in this book are behavioral measures, which require patients to make a judgment and perform a task like push a button when they hear a sound or repeat words that they are given. Some examples of behavioral tests include pure-tone audiometry and speech measures as described in Chapters 5 through 7. Other audiologic tests are physiologic measures, which do not require subjective judgments or responses by the patient; however, the patient must be cooperative and sit quietly or, in some cases, can even be asleep. Some examples of physiologic tests include tympanometry, acoustic reflexes, otoacoustic emissions, and auditory brainstem responses, which are described in Chapter 8. Behavioral measures are generally referred to as *subjective tests*, whereas physiologic measures are generally called *objective tests*. It is important to keep in mind, however, that many of the objective tests require the audiologist to make subjective decisions during the testing, and in most cases the audiologist is required to make subjective interpretations about the objective test data.

The audiologist needs to be keenly aware of when to refer the patient to a physician for medical management. Chapter 9 provides descriptions of some common hearing disorders and how they relate to the audiologic measures. One of the enjoyable aspects of audiology is the symbiotic relationships that can be established between the audiologist, physicians, and other health care providers. Working together with mutual respect provides the most complete care possible to those with hearing problems.

In many cases, there is no underlying medical condition related to the patient's hearing problems and the patient seeks services directly from the audiologist, who then takes primary responsibility for diagnosing and treating the patient regarding the hearing loss and its effects on communication. The audiologist is the most knowledgeable and appropriate professional to deal with the sensory and psychosocial aspects associated with hearing loss.

4

Pure-Tone Audiometry

After reading this chapter, you should be able to:

1. Discuss why pure tones are useful for assessing hearing and hearing loss.
2. Describe different types of audiometers and the functions of their basic components.
3. Describe the types of transducers used in audiometry and the advantages of each type.
4. Discuss the procedures for air conduction and bone conduction audiometry and how the thresholds obtained from these procedures are used to determine which parts of the auditory system are affected.
5. Describe the standard procedures for obtaining pure-tone thresholds.
6. Determine thresholds from hypothetical examples of threshold searches.
7. Discuss the variables that can affect thresholds and what can be done to accommodate and/or account for this variability.
8. Describe the methods for testing infants and toddlers using behavioral types of tests.

Now that you are equipped with the knowledge from previous chapters about basic acoustics and the anatomy/physiology of the normal ear, you can begin to learn how these principles are applied to the clinical assessment of a person's hearing ability. The measurement of a person's ability to hear different sounds is called *audiometry*. The term *audiometric* is used to describe different aspects pertaining to audiometry, such as audiometric results or audiometric testing. A basic hearing test, called *pure-tone audiometry*, involves finding the lowest sound pressure levels for different pure tones that a person is barely able to hear. The lowest sound pressure level of a pure tone to which a person reliably responds at least 50% of the time is called their *threshold* for that frequency. In pure-tone audiometry, pure-tone thresholds are obtained in a quiet environment for a range of frequencies, 250 to 8000 Hz, which is most relevant for speech sounds. Keep in mind, however, that most activities in the real world do not involve listening to barely audible pure tones in quiet test environments. Everyday sounds are much more complex, occur at moderate intensity levels, and are usually surrounded by background sounds. Although one's ability to hear depends on the processing of frequency, intensity, and temporal parameters of sounds, it can also be influenced by a variety of other non-acoustic factors, including maturation, cognition, motivation, and context.

Pure tones are used for basic testing for a variety of reasons. First of all, pure tones are relatively easy to produce and calibrate. In addition, since many types of hearing losses do not affect all the frequencies equally, the pattern of hearing loss as a function of frequency is often characteristic of certain types of hearing loss. For example, high frequencies are more affected than low frequencies for older persons with hearing loss due to aging. Pure-tone thresholds may also be useful when discussing how a patient's hearing loss might relate to his or her ability to hear different frequencies of speech sounds such as /f/, /s/, or /th/, which have relatively higher frequency components than other speech sounds.

It is important to keep in mind that while pure tones are relatively easy to generate, the actual testing of a patient requires considerable skill and experience in order to be able to recognize and adapt to different patient response abilities and patterns. The testing of an 18-month-old child, a mentally disabled young adult, an elderly person with dementia, or someone who is purposefully exaggerating a hearing loss are only some of the challenges that make audiometry interesting. An audiologist's ability to incorporate the pure-tone results and other test results (covered in later chapters) with information from the patient, and then make appropriate interpretations, impressions, and recommendations, are competencies that develop with time and experience.

Pure-tone audiometry is almost always part of the basic audiologic evaluation with cooperative patients and has been a key element in hearing testing since audiology's modern beginnings in the mid 1900s (Bunch, 1943, cited in Harrell, 2002). Pure-tone audiometric thresholds are used by audiologists in order to: (a) describe the amount of the patient's hearing loss, (b) determine which parts of the auditory system are involved, (c) determine if medical referral is needed, and (d) predict how the patient's hearing loss may relate to the ability to listen and communicate.

The Audiometer

The audiologist uses an instrument called an *audiometer* for many of the hearing tests. The first commercially available audiometer was developed in 1922 (Bunch, 1943, cited in Harrell, 2002). Today, there are different types of audiometers that are classified based on their capabilities and use. Although the appearance and operation of audiometers may differ depending on the manufacturer or model, they have similar functions and components.

Types of Audiometers

One class of audiometer is called a *diagnostic* or *clinical audiometer*. Some examples of diagnostic audiometers are shown in Figure 4–1. A diagnostic audiometer is an instrument capable of performing

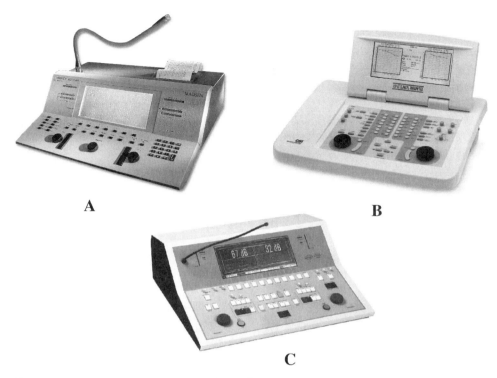

Figure 4–1. A–C. Some examples of two-channel diagnostic audiometers used for comprehensive clinical evaluations. **A.** Madsen Model Orbiter 922. **B.** Grason-Stadler Inc. Model 61. **C.** Interacoustics Model AC40. Photos courtesy of GN Otometrics (A), Viasys (B), and Interacoustics (C).

a variety of hearing tests, including pure-tone audiometry, and must conform to certain standards of operations, as specified by the American National Standards Institute (ANSI) for diagnostic audiometers. Diagnostic audiometers are available from a variety of manufacturers and come in a variety of shapes and sizes, including some which are designed for limited space and/or for portability. Many diagnostic audiometers (like those shown in Figure 4-1) have the option to save the patient response information through a RS-232 computer interface cable for storage and printing.

Computer-based audiometry is being more widely used for clinical testing. With the more sophisticated computer-based audiometers, the audiologist controls the testing with the computer keyboard and/or mouse. The audiometry software allows the computer to generate and control the delivery of the sounds (pure tones and speech materials), as well as the ability to store the patient's response, automatically analyze and print the results, and track patient databases. Some of the computer-based audiometry systems may also be interfaced with a more traditional audiometer instrument, thereby giving the audiologist the flexibility of testing with the audiometer instrument, the keyboard, and/or the mouse. Some examples of computer-based audiometry systems are shown in Figure 4-2.

Another type of audiometer is called an *automatic audiometer*. An automatic audiometer has the capability of automatically changing the signal level based on the response of the patient. Today, automatic audiometry usually refers to the use of computer-based systems that can automatically test one or more people at the same time, and is commonly used as an efficient way to assess workers in industrial settings. The original automatic audiometer, called a Békésy audiometer, allows the patient to control the level of the signal using a

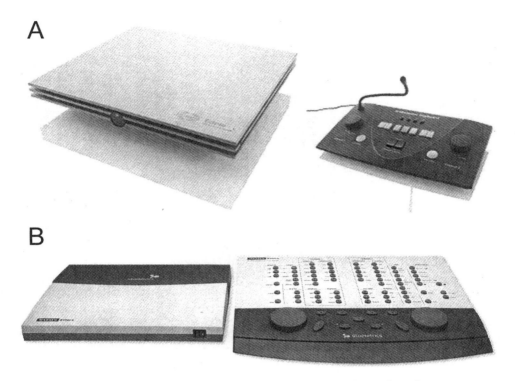

Figure 4–2. A and B. Some examples of computer-based audiometer systems. **A.** Interacoustics Equinox with instrument panel. **B.** Madsen Astera with instrument panel. Interfacing computers are not shown. Photos courtesy of Interacoustics (A) and GN Otometrics (B).

handheld response button while the tones are automatically changed from low to high frequencies. In Békésy audiometry, the patient holds down a button to increase the intensity of the tone until it is just barely audible, then releases the button to decrease the intensity until it is inaudible. The printout produces a tracing in one direction when the button is held down and then reverses direction when it is released. The patient's threshold is taken as the midpoint of the excursions. Békésy audiometry was popular through the 1970s but is not used much today in clinical testing, although it does have some useful diagnostic patterns when tracings are done for pulsed versus continuous tones and is sometimes used in laboratory settings. For more information on Békésy audiometry, see Jerger (1960) and Johnson (1977).

Another type of audiometer is called a *screening audiometer*. A screening audiometer is usually smaller, portable, and only uses limited pure

tones to assess hearing. A screening audiometer typically tests a limited range of frequencies, and the intensity levels are set at a selected level to determine if a patient passes or fails the screening (see Chapter 10 for more on hearing screening). A screening audiometer is typically used for doing hearing screenings in schools, in hospital rooms, or in other situations in which a patient cannot be tested in the audiology clinic. Speech-language pathologists, nurses, or those with an Audiometrist Certificate typically use screening audiometers.

Basic Components of Pure-Tone Audiometers

Table 4–1 lists the basic components of an audiometer (diagnostic and screening types). The basic functions of an audiometer are to produce pure

Table 4–1. Basic Functions and Components of a Pure-Tone Audiometer

Function	Component
Selects the frequency of the pure tone	Frequency selector
Changes sound pressure level of signal	Attenuator dial
Selects how the signal is delivered	Transducer selector
Directs signal to desired location	Router switch
Presents the signal to the patient	Interrupter switch
Indicates whether patient responded	Patient response indicator
Monitors/calibrates input level	VU meter

tones at selected frequencies (oscillator), change the intensity of the signal (attenuator), select how the signal is delivered to the ear (transducer), and direct the signal to a desired location (router). For example, a tester would set the oscillator frequency selector dial to 1000 Hz, set the attenuator dial to 40 dB,[1] select earphones as the transducer, and route the signal to the right ear. When ready, the tester pushes the interrupter switch to deliver the signal to the patient, and then the tester observes the patient to see if he or she responds. The patient can indicate that he or she heard the signal by either raising a hand or by pushing a response button that activates a patient response indicator on the audiometer. Diagnostic audiometers must always have two separate channels with all of the functions duplicated, since many of the hearing tests require that different signals be presented at the same time to the same or different ears. There are other functions and components of diagnostic audiometers that are specific for other diagnostic tests, some of which are discussed in later chapters. It is highly recommended that the tester get into a habit of reviewing the instrument manual that accompanies each audiometer in order to learn the specific details of the audiometer's op-

eration and to become familiar with all of its components and functions.

Transducers

The pure tones (or other test signals) are delivered to the patient through *transducers*, such as earphones. An audiometric transducer is a device that is capable of vibrating when activated by an electrical signal from the oscillator, thus converting (*transducing*) electrical signals into vibrations that can be heard. The transducers are connected to the audiometer, and the tester selects the desired transducer to which the signal is to be routed. Table 4–2 lists the different types of transducers used in audiometry. Earphones are color coded to indicate which ear is being tested; the red earphone should be used for the right ear (**R**ed = **R**ight) and the blue earphone should be used for the left ear. It is very important to be sure that the correct earphone is on the appropriate ear so that the audiometer routing switch corresponds to the ear to which you are actually sending the signal.

[1]You are probably thinking, "What is the reference value for this dB?" As you will learn later in this chapter, there is another type of decibel scale used in audiometry, called dB hearing level (dB HL). To simplify some of the concepts in this chapter, the dB reference may be omitted until dB HL is explained.

Table 4–2. Types of Transducers Used in Pure-Tone Audiometry

Transducer	Common Models	Corresponding Figure
Insert earphones	ER-3A, ER-5A, EARTone-3A	4–3
Supra-aural earphones	TDH-49, 50P	4–4
High frequency earphones	Sennheiser HDA200	4–5
Speakers	Various models	None
Bone conduction vibrator	B-71, B-72	4–6

Insert Earphone

An *insert earphone*, such as the Etymotic ER-3A or EARTone-3A, is the recommended transducer for most clinical testing today. The insert earphone was developed in the mid 1980s (Killion, Wilber, & Gugmundsen, 1985), to improve on the supra-aural earphones that have been aound much longer in clinical practice (see below for description of supra-aural earphones). Figure 4–3 shows a photograph of a patient wearing a set of insert earphones. The insert earphone has the electroacoustic diaphragm housed in a small case, which is attached by a clip to the patient's clothing. The signal is sent to the ear through a small tube held in place in the ear with a disposable foam cuff that is inserted into the ear canal. The foam cuff is compressed by hand prior to insertion into the ear canal and it expands, after insertion, to conform to the shape of the patient's ear canal. For sanitary purposes, the disposable foam cuffs are replaced for each patient. The proper placement of the insert earphone into the ear canal is important, and it should be inserted so that the outer edge of the foam cuff is just within the first bend of the ear canal.

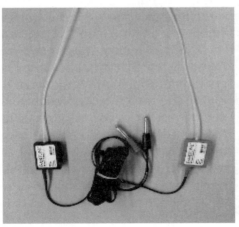
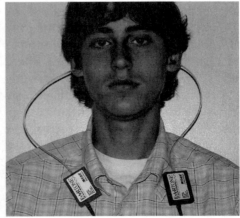

A   **B**

Figure 4–3. A. A set of insert earphones (ER-3A). **B.** Insert earphones properly placed for testing.

Supra-aural Earphones

A *supra-aural earphone*, such as the Telephonics TDH series (TDH-39, 49, 50P), was the standard earphone used in audiometry until the insert earphone was developed. Figure 4–4 shows a photograph of a patient wearing a set of supra-aural earphones. The supra-aural earphone has its electroacoustic diaphragm at ear level, which is covered with a rubber cushion that rests on the auricle. Supra-aural earphones are held in place with a headband designed to produce a specific tension. For sanitary purposes, the supra-aural earphone cushions are covered with disposable paper covers (or cleaned with an appropriate sanitary wipe). The proper position of the supra-aural earphone is to align the center of the earphone diaphragm with the opening of ear canal. An off-centered earphone can affect the delivery of higher frequencies, which have small wavelengths relative to the ear canal and thus may be partially blocked from entering the ear canal by improper supra-aural earphone placement. In some patients, a supra-aural earphone can close off (collapse) the ear canal, and the tester must be aware of this possibility when using this type of transducer. Inaccurate hearing thresholds due to temporarily collapsing the ear canal when using a supra-aural earphone are discussed in Chapter 5. In fact, the insert earphone was developed in order to avoid collapsing the ear canal, as well as to improve on some other limitations of the supra-aural earphone that are also discussed in Chapters 5 and 6.

Supra-aural earphones and insert earphones are designed to test frequencies from 250 to 8000 Hz; however, supra-aural earphones have about 5 dB higher maximum output than insert earphones. Supra-aural earphones are still used in situations where insert earphones are not available or when a patient is unwilling or unable to complete testing with the insert earphones. Supra-aural earphones must be used in patients who do not have ear canals (called atresia), patients who have profound hearing losses, or those with active drainage from the ears.

Ultra-High-Frequency Earphone

Another type of earphone is an *ultra-high-frequency (or circumaural) earphone*, such as the Sennheiser HDA200. Ultra-high-frequency earphones are used in special situations where the frequencies above 8000 Hz are to be evaluated.

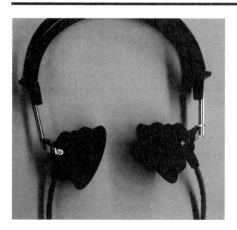
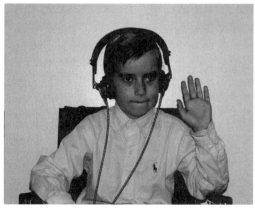

A　　　　　　　　　　　　B

Figure 4–4. A. A set of supra-aural earphones (TDH-50P). **B.** Supra-aural earphones properly placed for testing.

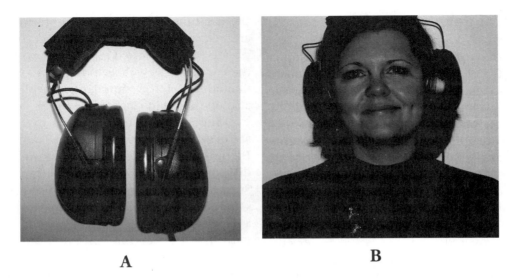

Figure 4–5. A. A set of ultra-high-frequency earphones (HDA200). **B.** Ultra-high-frequency earphones properly placed for testing.

The ultra-high-frequency earphone is housed in a larger cavity, which is designed to be positioned around the auricle so that it is less likely to move. Since the ultra-high frequencies have shorter wavelengths, proper position of the ultra-high frequency earphone is critical to avoid any effects related to the size of the ear canal. Figure 4–5 shows photographs of a set of ultra-high-frequency earphones and with the earphones placed on a patient.

Sound-Field Speakers

Speakers (or loudspeakers) are another type of transducer sometimes used in audiometry. Speakers are usually positioned in the corner of the test room a few feet away from the patient. When speakers are used for testing, it is referred to as *sound-field* or *free-field* testing. Speakers are used if testing a patient with hearing aids, since earphones are not able to be positioned over the ears while the patient is wearing hearing aids. Speakers may also be needed for testing the occasional patient who does not tolerate keeping the earphones

on his or her head, such as some young children. A limitation of testing in sound-field with speakers is that both ears will receive the sounds, so it is not possible to get ear-specific information. Whenever possible, it is recommended that hearing testing be done with earphones so that each ear can be tested separately. One should attempt to use earphones before resorting to sound-field testing. Even difficult patients and young children can often be convinced to wear the earphones with a little encouragement and demonstration.

Bone Conduction Vibrator

Another important type of transducer used in audiometry is called a *bone conduction vibrator*, such as the Radioear B-71. Figure 4–6 shows a patient wearing a bone conduction vibrator. The bone conduction vibrator has a plastic casing that is set into vibration by the pure tones. The bone conduction vibrator is placed against the skull behind the ear (on the mastoid bone) and held in place with a headband designed to produce a specific force on the skull. The bone conduction vibrator

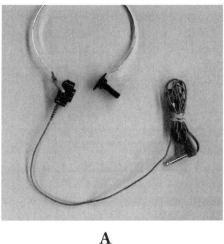
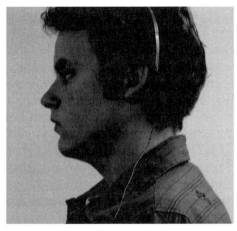

A   **B**

Figure 4–6. A. A bone conduction vibrator (B-71). **B.** Bone conduction vibrator properly placed for testing on the mastoid process. Notice that the bone conduction vibrator is placed on one side only and held in place with a headband.

should not touch the auricle and should be placed under the hair. The headband of the bone conduction vibrator is placed across the top of the head. Notice in Figure 4-6 that the bone conduction vibrator is a single transducer placed at one location on the skull rather than one for each ear. The bone conduction vibrator is not color coded and is switched from one side to the other. The bone conduction vibrator delivers the pure-tone vibrations to the skull, and these bone conducted vibrations stimulate the inner ears imbedded within the temporal bones of the skull. It is important to realize that when vibrations are delivered anywhere on the skull, both ears will receive these vibrations simultaneously because the bones of the skull act like a solid object. In order to obtain bone conduction thresholds from one ear at a time, a noise type sound, called a *masker*, may be needed in the other ear so it cannot hear the test tone being presented by the bone conduction vibrator. The specific clinical situations that require masking and the procedures for obtaining thresholds with masking are covered in Chapters 5 and 6. The bone conduction vibrator is useful for testing frequencies 250 to 4000 Hz and also has a more

limited intensity range than air conduction transducers because of the distortion that can occur with the bone conduction vibrator at higher frequencies and at higher intensities.

Air Conduction Versus Bone Conduction Testing

When earphones are used to deliver the sounds to the patient, it is referred to as *air conduction* (AC) testing. Air conduction testing stimulates the entire auditory system. The sounds begin as vibrations of air molecules at the outer ear and then proceed through the transduction process of the other parts of the auditory system. The overall amount of a patient's hearing loss is based on the results of AC testing, since this provides a measure of the entire auditory system and is the primary way in which hearing occurs. When the bone conduction vibrator is used to deliver sounds to the patient, it is called *bone conduction* (BC) testing. Bone conduction testing delivers the vibrations

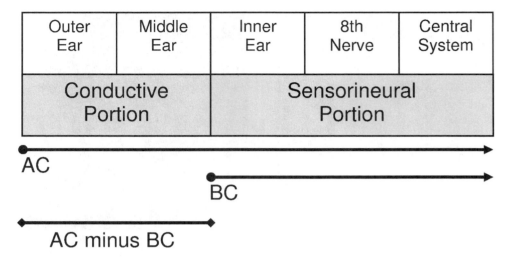

Figure 4–7. Illustration of the auditory pathways involved with air conduction (*AC*) and bone conduction (*BC*) testing. A hearing loss in the sensorineural portion of the ear affects AC and BC equally. A loss in the conductive portion of the ear is determined by the difference between testing by AC and BC, called the air–bone gap.

directly to the inner ear, which essentially bypasses the conductive (outer and middle ear) portions of the auditory pathway. The use of both AC and BC testing can help identify which part of the auditory system is involved in the patient's hearing loss.

Figure 4-7 illustrates how using both AC and BC testing can help determine which parts of the auditory system are involved in a patient's hearing loss. If a patient has a problem in the sensorineural part of the auditory system (inner ear, 8th nerve, and/or central) he/she would have the same amount of hearing loss when tested by AC and by BC since both types of testing include the sensorineural part of the ear. For example, a hearing loss in the inner ear would show up as an elevated threshold when tested by BC and the same amount of threshold elevation would show up when tested by AC. This is called a *sensorineural hearing loss*. As we will see in later chapters, there are additional diagnostic tests that allow us to determine if a sensorineural hearing loss is due to problems in the inner ear (sensory loss) or in the 8th nerve (neural loss). If a patient has a problem in the conductive portion of the auditory system, the BC conduction

threshold would be normal because BC testing bypasses the outer and middle ear. The patient with a problem in the conductive portion would have poorer AC thresholds than BC thresholds because AC testing includes the outer and middle ear (and all other parts of the auditory system). In order to determine the amount of the hearing loss that is related to the conductive portions of the ear, you must look at the difference in thresholds obtained by AC and BC testing, called an *air-bone gap*. If a patient has normal BC thresholds and an air-bone gap, it is called a *conductive hearing loss*. Of course, a patient could have more than one type of hearing problem at the same time, that is, there could be concomitant involvement of both the sensorineural and conductive portions of the auditory system. In that case, the patient would have a threshold elevation when tested by BC (reflecting a problem in the sensorineural portion) and a greater elevation in threshold when tested by AC, hence an air-bone gap (reflecting the additional involvement of the conductive portion). This type of hearing loss is called a *mixed hearing loss*. As you may already have surmised, BC thresholds should not be worse than AC thresholds because any changes in threshold due to the sensorineural portions of the ear, as reflected in the BC thresholds, would also be reflected in the AC thresholds. In clinical practice, however, testing variability may occasionally cause the BC thresholds to be slightly poorer than AC thresholds, but this does not generally have any clinical significance and is not called an air–bone gap.

The Test Environment

Diagnostic hearing testing must be done in a specially designed sound-attenuating test room (often called a "sound booth" or "test suite") that meets standards for permissible background noise levels suitable for audiometric testing (American National Standards Institute [ANSI], 1999). Figure 4–8 shows a picture of an audiometric test booth. The test booth walls are about 4 inches thick with sound absorption material inside and small holes in

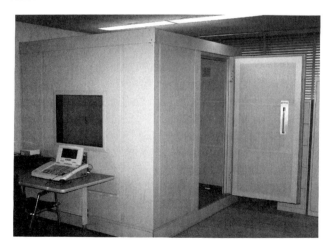

Figure 4–8. A single-room audiometric test suite. The patient is inside the room and the tester is outside the room. The tester's equipment is connected to the room through a connector panel, and there is a window to maintain visual contact. In many clinics, the tester is also in another similarly treated sound test booth that is connected to the patient's test booth.

the inside wall surface to absorb the sounds and reduce reflections. The test booth can be single walled or double walled (for more attenuation). The photo in Figure 4–8 is a single-room, single-walled test booth in which the equipment and tester are not inside the sound-attenuating environment. In this type of arrangement, the tester's environment must be kept relatively quiet while testing. A two-room test booth, which has a room for the patient and a separate room for the equipment and tester, is the preferred clinical arrangement. In either type of test booth, there is a window that allows the tester to be in visual contact with the patient and a control panel that allows the equipment to be connected from the audiometer to the patient's test booth.

The position of the patient in the test booth can be varied depending on the situation. The patient must be seated in such a way as to avoid any inadvertent visual cues by the tester, such as hand, head, or eye movements, facial expressions, or visible reflections. In order to reduce the possibility of inadvertent cues, the typical orientation would have the patient facing 45 to 90° away from the tester. However, for some patients the audiologist might prefer to have more direct eye contact to better read some of the patient's signs of confusion or to provide visual reinforcement. If performing sound-field testing with speakers, the orientation of the patient depends on the reason for using the speakers. For example, if pure-tone testing requires the patient to respond by turning toward the sound (e.g., when testing some toddlers), then the patient should be oriented 45 to 90° away from the loudspeaker so that a noticeable head-turn is observable. This can be done with one loudspeaker on one side of the room (the patient turns toward the loudspeaker when he/she hears a sound) or with a loudspeaker on each side of the room (the patient localizes the source of the sound by turning to the correct side). If interested in knowing whether or not the patient hears a sound without turning the head, the patient can be oriented toward the loudspeaker, which avoids direct visualization of the tester. Likewise, if testing a patient with hearing aids on, the patient should face the loudspeaker in order to have the sound directed into the microphone of the hearing aid.

Synopsis 4–1

- Pure-tone audiometry is a routine audiometric test whereby a patient's thresholds for pure tones are established over the frequency range 250 to 8000 Hz. Testing is performed with an audiometer in a sound-attenuating test booth. Special audiometers and earphones are needed for testing frequencies above 8000 Hz, called ultra-high-frequency audiometry. For clinical purposes, the test booth must meet ANSI (1999) standards for acceptable amounts of background noise in different frequency bands to allow testing with ears uncovered.

- Basic features of an audiometer include an oscillator to generate the pure tones, an attenuator to adjust the intensity, and switches to select the type of transducer and the ear to be tested. A variety of audiometers are available with different functions. The most common audiometer is a two-channel clinical audiometer capable of performing a comprehensive battery of audiometric tests. Clinical audiometers can be stand-alone instruments with or without computer storage capability, or can be entirely computer based.

- Audiometric transducers convert the electrically generated stimuli from the audiometer into acoustic stimuli, which are presented to the patient. Commonly used transducers include insert earphones (e.g., ER-3A), which are inserted part way into the ear canals, supra-aural earphones (e.g., TDH-50P), which rest on the auricles, and speakers, which present the pure tones in the sound field. Another transducer routinely used is a bone vibrator (e.g., Radioear B-71), which delivers the pure tones directly to the inner ear through vibrations in bones of the skull. Since both cochleae are embedded in the skull, both ears receive the vibrations from a single bone vibrator placed anywhere on the skull; therefore, to evaluate each ear separately with bone conduction testing, a masking noise must often be delivered to the non-test ear so that it cannot hear the test tone.

- Insert earphones have several advantages over supra-aural earphones, including situations in which masking of the non-test ear is required or when collapsed ear canals may be a problem. The audiometric consequence of temporarily collapsing the ear canals during testing will be discussed in Chapter 9.

- Thresholds obtained by AC are affected by damage anywhere along the auditory pathway, whereas thresholds obtained by BC reflect damage only in the sensorineural portions of the ear (and bypass the conductive pathways). The amount of hearing loss due to the conductive portion of the ear is determined by the air–bone gap.

- A hearing loss in the sensorineural portions of the auditory system (sensorineural hearing loss) is characterized by equal thresholds for AC and BC testing. A hearing loss in the conductive portions of the auditory system (conductive hearing loss) is characterized by normal BC thresholds and elevated AC thresholds (air–bone gap). A hearing loss in both the sensorineural portions and conductive portions (mixed hearing loss) is characterized by elevated BC thresholds and even greater loss in AC thresholds (air–bone gap).

- In order to reduce the possibility of inadvertent cues from the tester, such as hand, head, or eye movement, facial expressions, or visible reflections, the typical orientation would have the patient facing 45 to 90° away from the tester.

Procedures for Obtaining Pure-Tone Thresholds

In pure-tone audiometry, specific clinical procedures to determine thresholds have been standardized and are periodically updated (American National Standards Institute [ANSI], 1997, 2004; American Speech-Language-Hearing Association [ASHA], 1978, 2005). It is important for audiologists to use the same standardized procedures so that a patient's thresholds are reasonably consistent when obtained by different audiologists or from the same audiologist at different times. The standard clinical procedures for establishing pure-tone thresholds are based on what is called the modified Hughson-Westlake technique, first described by Carhart and Jerger (1959). Today, the modified Hughson-Westlake procedure for establishing clinical pure-tone thresholds is also commonly called the "up 5, down 10" (or "down 10, up 5") procedure, and is discussed in more detail below. While there are some variations among audiologists in how they apply the procedures, the following steps are typically followed:

1. Provide some clear instructions to the patient, such as: "We are interested in finding the faintest level at which you are able to hear sounds of different pitches. Listen carefully and be sure to press the response button (or raise your hand) as soon as you think you hear

a sound and release the button (or lower your hand) as soon as the sound goes away."

2. Place the appropriate transducer on the patient in the proper position (remember **R**ed = **R**ight). Do not allow the patient to put the transducer on or move it. Improper placement will result in inaccurate thresholds. Test AC before BC, and begin AC testing in the better ear if known or as reported by the patient.

3. Select the desired frequency. For AC testing, the recommended frequencies included in a basic hearing test are 250, 500, 1000, 2000, 3000, 4000, 6000, and 8000 Hz (ASHA, 2005). In addition, 750 and 1500 Hz should be tested if there is more than a 20 dB difference in thresholds between the adjacent octave frequencies. Testing usually begins with 1000 Hz because it is a mid-range tone, which is generally easier to perceive. The order for testing the other frequencies is not critical; however, the order suggested by ASHA (2005) is 1000, 2000, 3000, 4000, 6000, 8000, 500, 250 Hz. Retesting 1000 Hz is recommended in order to account for improvement due to practice effects with the other frequencies. For BC testing, the recommended test frequencies include 250, 500, 1000, 2000, 3000, and 4000 Hz (ASHA, 2005).

4. Present the pure tone by pressing and releasing the interrupter button. Most diagnostic audiometers have a pulse-tone option that presents pulsed tones when the interrupter switch

is activated. A series of pulsed tones is often used because they are easier to perceive and are more distinguishable from any ringing sounds the patient may have in the ears. The presentations of the tones or series of pulses should be 1 to 2 s in duration. There should be variable pauses (1 to 4 s) between presentations so that the patient is not able to predict the rhythm of the presentations.

5. Begin testing with a familiarization phase. This involves presenting the pure tone at a relatively easy level to hear (e.g., 30 to 40 dB above the estimated threshold of the patient), in order to allow the patient to become familiar with the task and to show the tester that the patient understands the task. If the patient does not hear the pure tone at the initial level, the level is increased in 20 dB steps until a response is obtained. The familiarization phase continues by decreasing the level of the pure tone in 10 dB steps until the patient no longer responds; this then marks the beginning of the threshold search phase. An alternate familiarization method is to present a tone at the lowest intensity level and gradually increase the level of the tone until the patient responds, and then decrease the level by 10 dB.

6. Begin the threshold search phase using the up 5, down 10 procedure. This means that the level is increased in 5 dB steps and decreased in 10 dB steps depending on the response of the patient. This threshold search procedure is an *ascending threshold procedure*, because the level is increased from below threshold. Since the beginning test level is below threshold from the familiarization phase, first increase the level of the pure tone in 5 dB steps until the patient responds. Then decrease the level of the pure tone in 10 dB steps until the patient does not respond. In other words, during the threshold search phase, the intensity level is increased by 5 dB whenever the patient does not respond and decreased by 10 dB whenever the patient does respond. The tester usually keeps mental track of "response" or "no response" in relation to the ascending trials. Keeping track of the patient's responses mentally may seem complicated; however, this ability becomes routine with practice.

7. Continue the tone presentations, using the up 5, down 10 procedure, until the threshold is established based on the following definition: A pure-tone threshold is defined as the lowest intensity level that the patient responds to in *at least 50%* of a series of ascending presentations, with at least two out of three required at a single level (ANSI, 2004; ASHA, 2005). Some audiologists in some situations may select threshold as the level in which they obtain two correct responses out of two presentations as long as there was zero out of two presentations at 5 dB lower. Generally, the interpretation of the procedure is that up to four presentations are required and that at least 50% be heard. Two out of three is about 67% which meets the definition of at least 50%. If the procedures are modified for other populations, such as young children or the disabled, or for any other reason, then be sure to indicate these along with the test results.

Examples of How to Establish Thresholds

Let's examine more closely the process of how to determine an accurate threshold. Let's say that after two ascending series (following the up 5, down 10 rules) the patient has responded 0% (0/2) at 35 dB and 100% (2/2) at 40 dB. At this point, you might be tempted to select 40 dB as the threshold, since 40 dB is the lowest level that the patient responded to at least 50% of the presentations (and 35 dB is less than 50%). However, this would not be an accurate threshold based on the recommended guidelines (ANSI, 2004; ASHA, 2005), which says that the patient must respond to at least two out of a minimum of three ascending trials. Suppose another ascending series was given in this example and the patient did not respond at 35 dB (0/3) and responded a third time at 40 dB (3/3); in this case, 40 dB would be the threshold. Actually, even if the patient did not respond at 40 dB in the third ascending series, 40 dB would be the threshold because there was no response at 35 dB (the purpose of the third trial was to see if 35 dB might be heard). Keep in mind the criterion that threshold is the lowest level in which the patient gives at least two correct responses out of three or four (if needed) presentations. In this example, the patient could have responded to the next two presentations at 35 dB, even though they did not respond to the first two presentations, and the threshold would have been 35 dB (2/4 responses). In either case, a third ascending series was necessary. If the patient did not respond to the third presentation at 35 dB you would not have to give the fourth presentation, since the best that they could do at 35 dB would be 1/4 responses. This is what is meant by four possible (or theoretical) presentations, and the threshold could be established with two out of three correct responses.

Let's look at some more examples of the steps used to establish threshold. Figure 4-9 shows three examples demonstrating how the presentation level was varied until an acceptable threshold was established following the rules described above. In Figure 4-9A, the testing started at 30 dB (trial 1) and the patient responded (+). Because the patient responded, the level was lowered to 20 dB (down 10) for trial 2 and the patient again responded (+). The level was lowered to 10 dB (down 10) for trial 3 and the patient did not respond (−). You should now be thinking that the threshold is somewhere between 10 dB and 20 dB. Now you begin the first ascending series from 10 dB by increasing the level in 5 dB steps; first to 15 dB (up 5) for trial 4 where the patient did not respond (−), and then to 20 dB (up 5) for trial 5 where the patient responded (+). At this point, there has been one ascending series with a response at 20 dB and no response at 10 dB or 15 dB. Trials 6 through 8 showed a similar response pattern following the rule of lowering the level by 10 dB following a response (+) and increasing the level by 5 dB when there was no response (−), and this second ascending series ended with a second response at 20 dB and no response at 10 or 15 dB. However, there is still the possibility that 15 dB could be the threshold if you were to give two more trials at that level (to satisfy the criterion that the patient had the opportunity to obtain at least *50% of the presentations out of a possible four presentations*). Trials 9 through 11 show the third ascending series in which the patient did not

respond at 15 dB (0/3) and did respond at 20 dB (3/3). Trial 11, technically, would not be required because you have already determined that the best score the patient could achieve at 15 dB would be 25% (1/4), and even if he/she did not respond at 20 dB in the third trial, he/she would have satisfied the criterion of two out of three. However, this last trial at 20 dB is usually included to complete the series, and in this example the patient again responded at 20 dB (3/3); thus, the patient's threshold would be 20 dB.

The example shown in Figure 4-9B started at the same level as in Figure 4-9A; however, this patient did not hear (−) the 30 dB presentation level, so the level was raised to 50 dB trying to find a level that is above the threshold for the familiarization phase of the procedure. At 50 dB (trial 2) the patient responded (+). You suspect that the threshold is somewhere between 30 and 50 dB. In trial 3, the level was lowered to 40 dB (down 10) and the patient did not respond (−). In trial 4, the level was raised to 45 dB (up 5) and the patient responded. In trial 5, the level was lowered to 35 dB and the patient did not respond. In trial 6 the level was raised to 40 dB and the patient responded. You now have one out of two responses at 40 dB, so additional trials are needed. The level was then lowered to 30 dB for trial 7 and the patient did not respond. The sequence continued until trial 12, where it was determined that there was more than 50% at 40 dB (3/4) and 50% would not be possible at lower levels even if a fourth presentation were given (already had 0/3 at 35 dB).

The example in Figure 4-9C follows the same rules of down 10 when the patient responded and up 5 when he did not respond; however, more trials were needed in this example because the patient was not as consistent as in the other two examples. In this case, the patient responded twice at 25 dB during ascending trials, but after a third ascending trial at 20 dB (trials 5, 8, 11) the patient had 1/3, so a fourth ascending series was needed. The patient did not respond to the fourth presentation at 20 dB (trial 14); therefore, the threshold was 25 dB. Notice how the threshold is not always 50%: In Figure 4-8A, the threshold is based on responses to 100% out of three ascending presentations at 20 dB and 0% at 15 dB; in Figure 4-9B, the threshold is based on responses to 75% out of four ascending

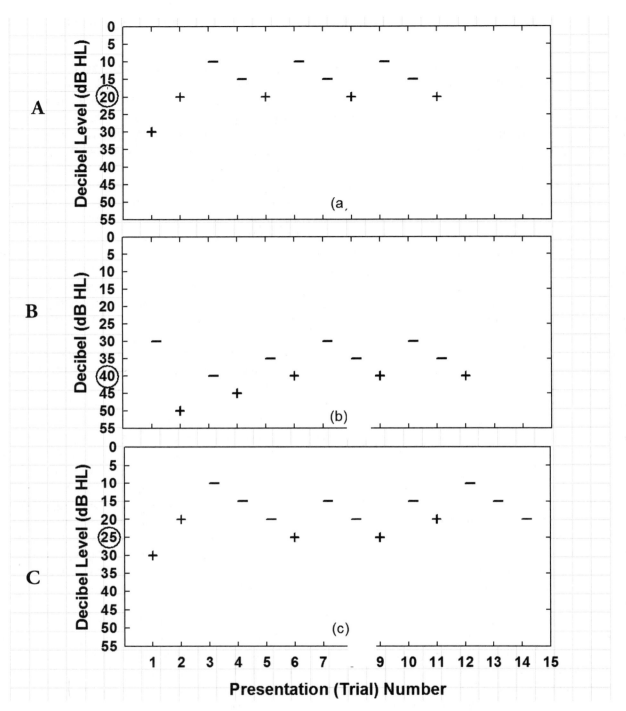

Figure 4–9. A–C. Hypothetical examples demonstrating the up 5, down 10 method to establish thresholds. The orientation of the dB levels is presented in this manner to be consistent with clinical hearing testing. In these three examples, threshold is based on the lowest level in which the patient responds to at least 50% of a possible or theoretical four presentations, and with a minimum of two out of three responses to ascending trials. A plus sign (+) indicates that the patient heard the tone and a minus sign (–) indicates that the patient did not hear the tone. After each trial in which the patient responds, the intensity of the signal is decreased by 10 dB, and after each trial in which the patient does not respond, the intensity is increased by 5 dB. For each of the three examples, the threshold is indicated by the *circled dB value*. See text for a detailed explanation for each of these examples.

presentations at 40 dB and 0% of three ascending presentations at 35 dB; in Figure 4–9C, the threshold is based on responses to 100% of three ascending presentations (3/3) at 25 dB and only 25% of four ascending presentations (1/4) at 20 dB.

Variables Influencing Thresholds

There is no absolute physiologic minimum response level that defines threshold, even for the same patient on different occasions (test-retest variability). There is some inherent variability when determining thresholds in a clinical setting, and this variability is related to a variety of factors. Remember, the thresholds you obtain in pure-tone audiometry are determined by monitoring the responses that the patient is willing to provide. All patients operate with some perceptual criterion that determines when to respond, and this criterion may be different across patients or even in the same patient on different days. Some patients may not want to make any mistakes and, therefore, choose to respond only when the auditory sensation is obvious. Other patients may not want to miss any of the sounds, so they tend to respond to questionably audible sounds. Thresholds can, in fact, be manipulated by the costs and rewards associated with a response. For example, if a person is told that he will earn one dollar for every signal detected, he will tend to respond more often and will end up with a lower threshold. On the other hand, if a person (or the same person) is told he will have to pay one dollar every time he responds when a signal was not presented, he will tend to respond less often and will have a higher threshold.

It would be nice if all patients were highly cooperative and consistent in their responses. The fact is, however, that most patients occasionally respond when a signal is not presented (false positives) and fail to respond to signals that they may have really heard or you expect them to hear (false negatives). Some of this lack of consistency is inherent in the concept of determining threshold. However, you should become cognizant of situations in which there are too many false responses or false negatives and learn to adjust your testing

strategy. The most important strategy is to be sure not to present the tones in a predictable pattern, so that the patient responds to an audible sensation instead of anticipating when you are going to present a tone. In addition, it is a good strategy to intersperse some longer (and variable) pauses between the presentations to get a sense of whether the patient has a tendency toward false positives. Most of the time, just giving patients some feedback and reinstructing them on what is expected of them may be sufficient. However, if there are too many false positives you might say, "Make sure you only push the button when you hear a tone," or for too many false negatives you might say, "Listen carefully and push the button even for the faintest sounds." In some cases, you might use a varying number (1, 2, or 3) of tone pulses instead of a continuous tone and ask the patient to push the button the same number of times that correspond to the number of pulses he heard. If there is a difference between the number of times the patient pushes the button and the number of pulses presented, that trial should be considered a false positive and treated the same as no response to that presentation trial.

You will, undoubtedly, observe other interesting response behaviors from your patients. For example, it is not uncommon to observe patients who give a "partial" response, for example, they cock their head and/or have an expression that conveys, "I think I hear something." This may be accompanied by holding their hand part-way up or "hovering" their thumb over the response button, not quite ready to push it. In most cases, the patient will produce the full response when the pure tone is raised 5 dB. It may be useful to reinstruct the patient with something like, "Go ahead and raise your hand all the way up (or push the button) even if you think you hear the sound." Of course, in some cases this may lead to increased false positives and one would need to revise the instructions again. You will also see some patients who keep their hand up or the button pushed while listening for the next sound. This behavior is usually extinguished with the next presentation or by giving them more instructions. A competent audiologist learns quickly to recognize and adjust for the nuances of the patient's behavior.

Pure-tone thresholds must represent a reliable and valid picture of the patient's hearing loss across frequencies and must be obtained in a reasonable amount of time. To be clinically useful, the goal of pure-tone audiometry is to obtain good estimates of the lowest levels the patient is willing to respond to consistently. To account for the inherent variations in thresholds, standardized procedures are used with a 5 dB step size, and test-retest variability of ±5 dB is acceptable and expected. The fact that pure-tone thresholds are repeatable within ±5 dB using the recommended procedures, even in different settings, makes them clinically robust. Pure-tone audiometry is highly effective at establishing reliable and valid thresholds in a relatively short period of time when performed by a competent audiologist using standardized procedures.

more responses from young children than pure tones. The use of narrowband noises or frequency-modulated tones (called *warble tones*) should be used when testing in the sound field in order to avoid effects from sound reflections off the walls of the test booth.

The following sections briefly describe some of the techniques used to behaviorally test pediatric patients from 6 months to 4 years of age. Behavioral hearing testing is not effective for infants less than 5 to 6 months age; for these younger infants, physiologic measures (see Chapter 8) are more appropriate to evaluate auditory function. For a more complete coverage of auditory development and testing of young children you should consult other more comprehensive books on pediatric audiology (Hayes & Northern, 1997; Madell, 1998; Northern & Downs, 2002).

Techniques for Testing Infants and Toddlers

For children under the age of 4 or 5 years, there are special considerations and procedures that are required when conducting pure-tone audiometry. While most of the auditory system is fully developed at birth, infants and toddlers undergo developmental changes in their ability to respond to sounds, and accounting for these changes is critical in order to be able to obtain valid measures of hearing thresholds. Equally important is the child's interest in the task and how well the audiologist can keep the child motivated through lots of verbal praise and/or other means of providing positive reinforcement. In many cases, having an assistant who interacts with the child in the test booth makes testing more efficient. It is also recommended that whenever possible, for all ages, testing should be attempted with earphones so that information can be obtained from each ear separately. When earphones are not tolerated, testing can be done with speakers in the sound field. Some audiologists prefer to use narrowband noises centered at different audiometric frequencies since they tend to elicit

Conditioned-Play Audiometry (Ages 2 to 4 Years)

Children between the ages of 2 and 4 years are very receptive to the task of listening and responding to sounds when they are incorporated into structured play-like activities. Testing children in this age range is usually very successful with an experienced audiologist who can engage the child in the task and can keep the child happy and motivated. It cannot be overemphasized how important it is for the audiologist to be enthusiastic and offer lots of positive reinforcement to the child, while at the same time being able to discern false positive or false negative responses, and quickly change activities as needed to keep the attention going. With an experienced audiologist, children in this age range can be tested by AC and BC, and they are capable of responding with thresholds similar to adults.

The technique for testing this age group is typically called *conditioned-play audiometry*. The child is asked to perform a fun activity whenever he hears the pure tone. Usually, the audiologist or assistant demonstrates what he/she wants the child to do. The play activities might be something like putting rings on a pole, putting blocks in a box, and/or flying toy airplanes to the hanger. This technique is a straightforward conditioning paradigm. The demonstration by the audiologist serves as the conditioning phase, familiarizing the child with what he/she will hear and teaching him/her what to do when the sound is heard. During the conditioning phase, the child should also demonstrate that he/she understands the task by correctly doing the activity when a suprathreshold tone is presented. If needed, the audiologist should help the child with the task when the tone is clearly audible and then have the child do it on his/her own when he/she hears the tone. Be sure not to allow the child to do the activity when the tone is not presented. The activity serves as a reinforcer to the child and is an indication of the child's response to the tone. Once the audiologist is confident that the child understands the activity, then the test phase begins. During the test phase, the sound intensity is varied using the standard procedure based on the child's response until a valid threshold is obtained. You have to work quickly with children of this age in order to obtain as much information as possible before they lose interest in the task. It is usually best to try to obtain a couple of thresholds in each ear, such as 2000 Hz then 500 Hz, and then add other frequencies back and forth between ears as time permits. In some cases, modification of the standard procedure to an "up 10, down 20" rule for intensity changes can be used to save time and get an estimate of their thresholds. Remember to document any modifications of procedures on the audiogram. For some children, usually those with other disorders, wearing the earphones and/or conditioning to the task are not successful in the clinic. In those cases, the parents might be taught to familiarize the child with the earphones and to the conditioning phase of the task while at home.

Visual Reinforcement Audiometry (Ages 6 Months to 2 Years)

For children as young as 6 months of age and toddlers who are not successfully conditioned to

perform conditioned-play audiometry, visual reinforcers have been found to be effective for obtaining thresholds to pure tones and/or narrowband noises (Moore, Wilson, & Thompson, 1977; Widen, 2011). When visual reinforcers are used in a conditioning paradigm, it is called *visual reinforcement audiometry* (VRA). The visual reinforcers are typically mechanical toys (e.g., animals) enclosed in tinted plastic enclosures and the tester activates a switch to light up and/or set the toy in motion. Presentation of the visual reinforces can also be done using flat screen monitors in the sound booth. The visual reinforcer is placed 45 to 90° away from the child's forward-facing position. The common method of VRA only requires a *unilateral head turn*: the child only has to look in one direction for the reinforcer regardless of the ear to which the sound is presented. Usually, clinics will have two toys stacked on top of each other and may switch the reinforcer to keep the child's interest longer. With flat screen monitors, different pictures are available to keep the child's attention if needed. For children older than 12 months, it is possible to test localization to sounds by placing the visual reinforcers on both sides of the child and teaching him to look to the side that corresponds to the sound he/she heard.

The conditioning procedure used for VRA is similar to that used in conditioned-play audiometry. It is best to try testing with earphones first in order to get ear-specific information, but testing can also be conducted in the sound field. Bone conduction testing can be performed if time permits. The VRA procedure begins by pairing an audible sound with the visual reinforcer and getting the child to look at the visual reinforcer. Often the visual stimulus itself will get the child to turn the head, but in some cases an assistant may be needed to direct (with enthusiasm) the child's attention to the visual reinforcer. The child's attention is then taken off the visual reinforcer by directing attention to other objects or another visual stimulus in front of him/her, often called "centering." When the child is not looking for the visual reinforcer, conditioning can continue by pairing the audible stimulus with the visual reinforcer until (usually after two or three times) the child is able to turn the head to look for the reinforcer when he/she hears the conditioning sound. The reinforcer must only be turned on after the child turns his or her head in response to a sound that was presented. Head turns without a sound presented should not be reinforced with the visual stimulus. Once the audiologist is confident that the child is performing the desired head turn in response to the sound, then the test phase begins. During the test phase, the sound intensity is varied using the standard procedure, based on the child's responses, until a valid threshold is obtained.

As with conditioned-play audiometry, it is usually best with VRA to try to obtain a couple of thresholds in each ear, such as 2000 Hz then 500 Hz,

and then add other frequencies back and forth between ears as time permits. In some cases, modification of the standard threshold search procedure to an "up 10, down 20" rule for intensity changes can be used to save time. For VRA and conditioned-play audiometry, the audiologist must learn to make decisions about whether the child might have a hearing loss or whether the child was unable to be conditioned to perform the task. In other words, was the child just not interested in the task or was it too difficult to perform? With a skilled tester and cooperative children, thresholds obtained using unilateral head-turn VRA are similar to those of adults (Diefendorf & Gravel, 1996; Widen, 2011; Wilson & Thompson, 1984).

Synopsis 4–2

- Thresholds are obtained using established guidelines called the up 5, down 10 procedure, where the level is increased in 5 dB steps when the patient does not respond and decreased in 10 dB steps when the patient does respond. In this procedure, thresholds are established in the ascending direction.

- Each threshold is defined as the lowest level in which the patient responds to at least 50% of a theoretical four presentations, with a minimum of two out of three responses to an ascending series of presentations.

- Thresholds can be affected by a patient's motivation or response criterion, which may be different across patients or even in the same patient on different days. A skilled audiologist must be aware of these patient variables and be able to adapt the testing strategy in ways that will produce valid and reliable thresholds.

- False positives (responding when tone is not presented) and false negatives (not responding to a tone that should be audible) are common response modes from many patients. Some variations in tone presentation rate and/or having them count pulses may be useful test modifications to help determine true response (responding when the tone is presented).

- Proper and clear instructions to patients are important. Be sure to let them know you are trying to find the faintest level of the tones that they can hear. Giving the patients feedback when they are doing the task correctly or reinstructing them when they are giving too many false positives or false negatives may reduce the false positives or false negatives.

- To be clinically useful, the goal of pure-tone audiometry is to obtain good estimates of the lowest levels the patient is willing to respond to consistently. When standardized test procedures are used, test-retest variability of ±5 dB for thresholds is expected and acceptable as valid measures of hearing sensitivity.

- Infants and toddlers who are 6 months to 4 years of age require special techniques to obtain behavioral thresholds. Conditioned-play audiometry, such as putting blocks into a bucket in response to hearing a sound, can be used for children 2 to 4 years of age. Visual reinforcement audiometry (VRA), using a unilateral head turn in response to hearing a sound, and then rewarding that behavior with an animated and/or lighted toy, can be used for children as young as 6 months of age. When successful, behavioral thresholds of children in these age ranges are similar to those of adults. However, careful decisions must be made by the audiologist in order to differentiate between whether the child actually has a hearing loss or whether he/she is only having difficulty performing the task.

- Children less than 6 months of age must be tested with physiologic measures. Several of these physiologic measures of auditory function are described in Chapter 8.

References

American National Standards Institute (ANSI). (1997). *Methods for manual pure-tone threshold audiometry.* ANSI S3.21-1978 (R1997). New York, NY: Author.

American National Standards Institute (ANSI). (1999). *Maximum permissible ambient noise levels for audiometric test rooms.* ANSI S3.1-1999. New York, NY: Author.

American National Standards Institute (ANSI). (2004). *Methods for manual pure-tone threshold audiometry.* ANSI S3.21-2004. New York, NY: Author.

American Speech-Language-Hearing Association (ASHA). (1978). Guidelines for manual pure-tone threshold audiometry. *American Speech-Language-Hearing Association, 20,* 297–301.

American Speech-Language-Hearing Association (ASHA). (2005). *Guidelines for manual pure-tone threshold audiometry.* Rockville, MD: American Speech-Language-Hearing Association. Retrieved January 10, 2008 from http://www.asha.org/policy/.

Carhart, R., & Jerger, J. (1959). Preferred method for clinical determination of pure-tone thresholds. *Journal of Speech and Hearing Disorders, 24,* 330–345.

Diefendorf, A. O., & Gravel, J. S. (1996). Visual reinforcement and behavioral observation audiometry. In S. E. Gerber (Ed.), *Handbook of pediatric audiology* (pp. 55–83). Washington, DC: Gallaudet University Press.

Gravel, J. S., & Hood, L. J. (1999). Pediatric audiologic assessment. In F. E. Musiek, & W. R. Rintleman (Eds.), *Contemporary perspectives in hearing assessment.* Boston, MA; Allyn and Bacon.

Harrell, R. W. (2002). Pure-tone evaluation. In J. Katz (Ed.), *Handbook of clinical audiology* (5th ed., pp. 71–87). Baltimore, MD: Lippincott Williams & Wilkins.

Hayes, D., & Northern, J. L. (1997). *Infants and hearing.* San Diego, CA: Singular.

Jerger, J. (1960). Békésy audiometry in analysis of auditory disorders. *Journal of Speech and Hearing Disabilities, 3,* 275–287.

Johnson, E. W. (1977). Auditory test results in 500 cases of acoustic neuroma. *Archives of Otolaryngology, 103,* 152–158.

Killion, M. C., Wilber, L. A., & Gugmundsen, G. I. (1985). Insert earphones for more interaural attenuation. *Hearing Institute, 36,* 34–36.

Madell, J. R. (1998). *Behavioral evaluation of hearing in infants and young children.* New York, NY: Thieme.

Moore, J. M., Wilson, W. R., & Thompson, G. (1977). Visual reinforcement of head-turn responses in infants under twelve months of age. *Journal of Speech and Hearing Disabilities, 42,* 328–334.

Northern, J. L., & Downs, M. P. (2002). *Hearing in children* (5th ed.). Baltimore, MD: Lippincott, Williams & Wilkins.

Widen, J. E. (2011). Behavioral audiometry with infants. In R. Seewald, & A. M. Tharpe (Eds.), *Comprehensive handbook of pediatric audiology*. San Diego, CA: Plural Publishing.

Wilson, W. R., & Thompson, G. (1984). Behavioral audiometry. In J. Jerger (Ed.), *Pediatric audiology* (pp. 1–44). San Diego, CA: College-Hill Press.

5

Audiogram Interpretation

After reading this chapter, you should be able to:

1. Explain three different ways to record pure-tone thresholds.
2. Describe the parameters of an audiogram and why dB hearing level (dB HL) is used for audiograms.
3. Describe how the occlusion effect and interaural attenuation are related to the use of insert earphones and supra-aural earphones.
4. Identify, from ANSI standards, the corresponding calibration reference values for different transducers.
5. Convert among dB HL, dB SPL, and dB SL (dB sensation level).
6. Identify air conduction (AC) and bone conduction (BC) thresholds for each ear from symbols on audiograms.
7. Recognize when masking of the non-test ear would be needed for AC and BC testing.
8. Describe a variety of audiograms using appropriate terms relative to type, degree, and shape of hearing loss.
9. Recognize audiograms that show thresholds at the limits of the equipment, tactile responses, or collapsed ear canals.
10. Calculate a pure-tone average (PTA) from the audiometric thresholds.

Proper documentation of information about a patient's hearing sensitivity is an integral part of the audiologist's evaluation. Understanding the results from a hearing evaluation is also important for other professionals so they can understand a patient's hearing ability in order to plan appropriate services. This chapter focuses your learning how to document pure-tone thresholds and how to describe and interpret the results of pure-tone audiometry. In addition, the concept of masking (putting noise into the non-test ear) is introduced in this chapter so that you can understand what the different unmasked and masked symbols used on an audiogram represent. A more complete discussion of masking, including how to perform masking, is covered in detail in Chapter 6.

To begin with, the patient's pure-tone thresholds are typically recorded on a graph called an *audiogram*. Figure 5–1 shows an example of an audiogram. While the actual size of an audiogram can vary, the aspect ratio (the ratio of the dimensions for the *y*-axis compared with the *x*-axis)

should be maintained so that a 20 dB change along the *y*-axis corresponds to a doubling of frequency (octave change) along the *x*-axis. For example, the distance from 20 to 40 dB along the *y*-axis should equal the distance from 2000 to 4000 Hz along the *x*-axis (American National Standards Institute [ANSI], 2004b; American Speech-Language-Hearing Association [ASHA], 2005).

Frequency is represented along the *x*-axis of the audiogram, beginning at 250 Hz and at equally spaced successive octave intervals (doubling of frequencies) up to 8000 Hz. Usually the inter-octave frequencies 3000 and 6000 Hz are also represented on the audiogram. Some audiograms include 125 Hz and/or 10,000 Hz; however, these frequencies are not usually tested during the basic hearing evaluation. If you need to test above 8000 Hz, an ultra-high frequency audiogram or numerical audiogram is used to document the thresholds for frequencies in specific increments, such as 10,000, 12,000, 14,000, and 16,000 Hz.

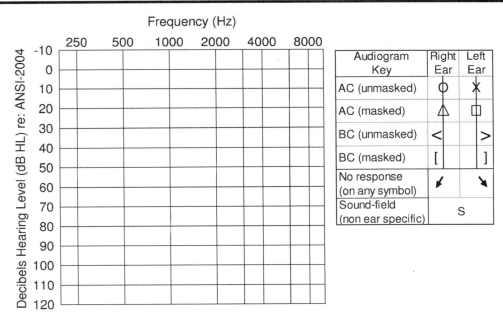

Figure 5–1. An example of an audiogram used to record pure-tone thresholds. An audiogram key, as shown on the right, is usually included with an audiogram to identify the symbols. **AC**, air conduction; **BC**, bone conduction.

Decibels of Hearing Level (dB HL)

The intensity levels of the test sounds are represented along the *y*-axis of the audiogram. You will notice that the intensity scale has the lowest intensity at the top of the graph and the highest intensity at the bottom of the graph. Also notice that the *y*-axis is labeled *decibels of hearing level* (dB HL), which is a different decibel scale from the dB SPL scale discussed in Chapter 2. The 0 dB HL line on the audiogram represents the lowest normal hearing level for each frequency averaged across normal hearing listeners. For each frequency, there is a corresponding dB SPL reference value for each 0 dB HL that is based on the known values associated with the threshold of audibility curve that you learned about in Chapter 2. As you recall, the different pure-tone thresholds require different amounts of dB SPL for normal hearing listeners (see Figure 2–15). The use of a dB SPL scale for

clinical testing would be somewhat cumbersome, since the same amount of hearing loss at different frequencies would be represented by different values in dB SPL, and the lines on the audiogram would not be linear. To simplify representation of hearing loss across frequencies, the threshold of audibility curve is normalized; in other words, the threshold of audibility curve is "straightened out" by creating a 0 dB HL at each frequency that is equal to the amount of dB SPL needed for normal hearing listeners for that frequency. The actual amount of dB SPL needed for 0 dB HL at each frequency is specified in standards developed by the American National Standards Institute (ANSI) or by the International Standards Organization (ISO) for pure-tone thresholds for normal hearing listeners. The ISO standards are used in countries other than the United States, but they are very similar to the ANSI standards.

Table 5–1 shows the 2004 American National Standards Institute (ANSI) *reference equivalent*

Table 5–1. Air Conduction and Bone Conduction Reference Values Corresponding to 0 dB HL, Also Called "Audiometric Zero," Based on ANSI S3.6 (2004). Air Conduction Reference Values Are in dB SPL re: 20 µPa. Bone Conduction Reference Values Are in dB Force re: 1 µN

Transducer	Model	Frequency (HZ)							
		250	**500**	**1000**	**2000**	**3000**	**4000**	**6000**	**8000**
Supra-aural phones[a]	TDH-50P	26.5	13.5	7.5	11.0	9.5	10.5	13.5	13.0
Insert phones[b]	ER-3A	17.5	9.5	5.5	11.5	13.0	15.0	16.0	15.5
Bone vibrator[c]	B-72	67.0	58.0	42.5	31.0	30.0	35.5	(40.0)	(40.0)
		6000	**8000**	**9000**	**10,000**	**11,200**	**12,500**	**14,000**	**16,000**
High frequency headphones[d]	HDA 200	17.0	17.5	18.5	22.0	23.0	28.0	36.0	56.0

[a]Calibrated with 6-cc coupler.
[b]Calibrated with an occluded ear simulator. Values are slightly different for HA-1 or HA-2 couplers (See ANSI standards).
[c]Calibrated with artificial mastoid for mastoid bone placement and with 40 dB effective masking to the non-test ear. Although bone conduction reference values are provided for 6000 and 8000 Hz, testing at these frequencies is not recommended (ASHA, 2005).
[d]Calibrated with a type 1 Adaptor. These values are considered interim standards.

threshold dB SPL (RETSPL) and reference equivalent threshold *dB force level* (RETFL) values as a function of frequency for different types of transducers (ANSI, 2004a). These values from the ANSI standards are the expected reference levels for 0 dB HL (a different one for each frequency and transducer). For pure-tone audiometry, the ANSI 2004 reference values are incorporated into the calibrations of the audiometer. For example, when the attenuator dial is set at 0 dB HL for 1000 Hz, using insert earphones, the audiometer is calibrated to produce an output that is equal to 5.5 dB SPL. When the attenuator dial is set at 0 dB HL for 500 Hz, using supra-aural earphones, the audiometer is calibrated to produce an output that is equal to 13.5 dB SPL. Each 0 dB HL becomes the average threshold value (based on normal hearing listeners) using the most current ANSI standards for pure-tone audiometry. By normalizing the threshold of audibility curve in this way, all of the numbers on the dB HL scale directly represent how many decibels a test signal is above the normal threshold of audibility at each frequency.

The ANSI and ISO periodically update their standards for pure-tone reference values. The audiograms in this textbook are based on the most recent ANSI standards reference levels (ANSI, 2004a,b). Notice in Figure 5–1 that the dB HL scale specifies that the audiometer was calibrated to the ANSI 2004 standards. Prior to the ANSI 2004 standards, calibration standards for audiometers were specified by ANSI in 1996 (ANSI, 1996). It is expected that an update of the ANSI standards will be coming in the next 2 to 3 years; however, the reference values do not change appreciably with the updates in ANSI standards for the existing transducers, but may include updates for newer transducers or updated models of existing transducers when necessary. For example, the ANSI 2004 standards provided RETSPLs for the ultra-high frequencies. Whenever new standards become available, any changes from previous standards should be incorporated into the calibration values of the audiometer and the new ANSI reference should be included on the audiogram.

The definition of 0 dB HL can also be illustrated with the basic formula used for decibel calculations: As you recall, whenever a sound is equal to its reference value, by definition this would equal 0 dB. The following calculation illustrates how the decibel formula would apply if you present the patient with 9.5 dB SPL, which is the ANSI reference value for 0 dB HL for 500 Hz using insert earphones:

$$\times dB\ HL = 10\ log\ (P1\ /\ P_{ref})$$

$$\times dB\ HL = 10\ log\ (9.5\ dB\ SPL\ /\ 9.5\ dB\ SPL)$$

$$\times dB\ HL = 10\ log\ (1)$$

$$\times dB\ HL = 10\ (0)$$

$$\times = 0\ dB\ HL.$$

Converting from dB HL to dB SPL, and vice versa, is a matter of adding or subtracting the ANSI reference values. For example, if a 500 Hz pure tone is presented at 40 dB HL using supra-aural earphones, how many dB SPL is that sound? The answer would be found in the following way:

$$\times dB\ SPL = dB\ HL\ (dial\ reading)\ plus\ the\ ANSI\ (2004)\ reference\ value$$

$$\times dB\ SPL = 40 + 13.5$$

$$\times = 53.5\ dB\ SPL.$$

Going the other way, if a 500 Hz pure tone is presented at 53.5 dB SPL, how many dB HL is that sound? The answer would be found in the following way:

$$\times dB\ HL = dB\ SPL\ minus\ the\ ANSI\ (2004)\ reference\ value$$

$$\times dB\ HL = 53.5 - 13.5$$

$$\times = 40\ dB\ HL.$$

Knowing how to do these conversions is useful for audiologists because sometimes audiologists work in dB SPL, such as when making measures during hearing aid fittings, and may need to relate these dB SPL values to a patient's audiogram in dB HL. Also, when making dB SPL measurements of different sounds, like speech or background noise, with a sound level meter, one may be interested in describing how those sounds relate to the patient's audiogram in dB HL.

Documentation of Thresholds

Let's now turn our attention to properly documenting the patient's thresholds on the audiogram. Figure 5-2 shows an audiogram with air conduction (AC) thresholds plotted for the right and left ears using symbols recommended by ASHA (1990, 2005). Audiograms are usually accompanied by a key (legend) that specifies what the symbols represent. In Figure 5-2, the right ear AC thresholds are denoted with a circle and the left ear AC thresholds are denoted with an X. While not required, these symbols may also be color coded to match the appropriate ear; red for the right ear and blue for the left ear. A useful way to learn to remember the AC symbols is "**R**ed = **R**ight = **R**ound." The AC

thresholds are centered on the vertical lines of the appropriate frequencies and the symbols are usually joined by solid lines. There are other symbols included in the key in Figure 5-2 that will be explained as we go along.

After obtaining AC thresholds, the bone conduction (BC) thresholds are usually obtained. Figure 5-3 shows the same AC thresholds as in Figure 5-2, but now the BC thresholds have also been plotted for the two ears. The BC symbols are usually not connected by lines. The BC symbols are placed to the side of the vertical line for each frequency. Notice that the right ear BC symbol (<) is placed on the left side of the line and the left ear BC symbol (>) is placed on the right side of the line. The reasoning for this BC symbol placement scheme comes from the idea that when one is looking at an audiogram while facing the patient, the right ear BC symbol lines up with the patient's right ear and the left ear BC symbol lines up with the patient's left ear. This strategy may require

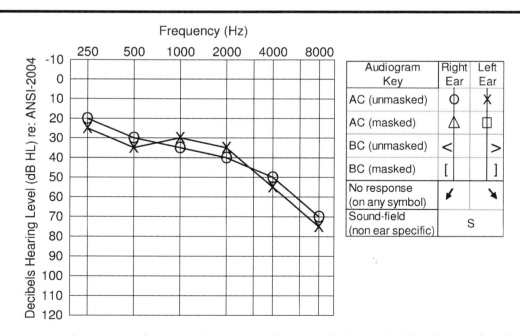

Figure 5–2. An audiogram with air conduction (*AC*) unmasked thresholds plotted for the right and left ears. AC thresholds are plotted on top of the frequency lines and are usually connected with a solid line. **BC**, bone conduction.

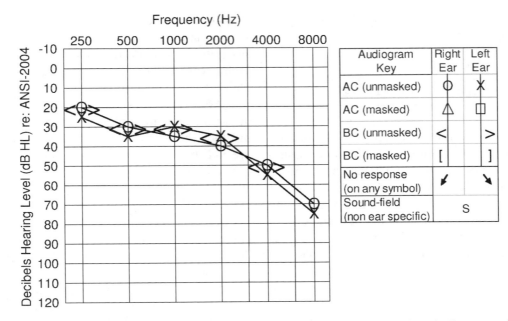

Figure 5–3. An audiogram with air conduction (*AC*) and bone conduction (*BC*) unmasked thresholds plotted for the right and left ears. The BC symbols are plotted to the right side of the frequency line when testing is done with the bone vibrator placed on the left ear and plotted on the left side of the frequency line when testing is done with the bone vibrator placed on the right ear. BC thresholds are not usually connected with a line.

some practice; however, it is very important to keep the concept straight when interpreting an audiogram so that you are sure you are describing the hearing loss for the appropriate ear.

The audiogram shown in Figure 5–3 has the thresholds for both ears plotted on a single audiogram. However, there are other ways to record audiometric thresholds. Figure 5–4 shows the same pure-tone thresholds recorded in three different formats. Instead of plotting the thresholds for both ears on the same audiogram (as in Figure 5–4A), the thresholds can be recorded on a two-panel audiogram, where the data for each ear are plotted on separate grids (Figure 5–4B). The data for the left ear are plotted on the right panel following the same logic described above for plotting BC symbols on different sides of the vertical lines. As a third alternative, the thresholds can be recorded as numbers in tabular form, sometimes referred to as a numerical audiogram (Figure 5–4C). Some audiologists prefer to record the thresholds in

tabular form while testing, and then transfer the data to an audiogram when finished. Computer-based programs usually allow the thresholds to be displayed and printed in any of the three formats. For the remainder of this book, the single-panel audiogram will be used for all of the illustrations and clinical cases.

Recognizing the Need for Masking

Look again at the audiogram key in Figure 5–4. Notice that each ear has two different symbols for AC and two different symbols for BC to indicate whether the pure-tone thresholds in the test ear were obtained *unmasked* (without noise presented in the non-test ear) or *masked* (with noise presented in the non-test ear). Many audiograms that you will encounter will have both unmasked and masked symbols; therefore, before you can

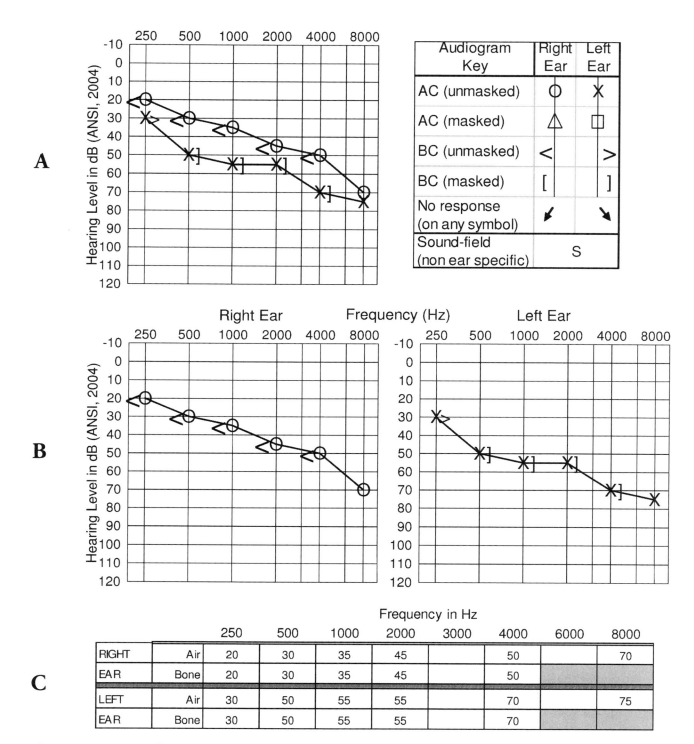

Figure 5–4. A–C. Illustrations of three different ways to record pure-tone thresholds. In **A**, both ears are plotted on a single panel audiogram. In **B**, a two-panel (or side by side) audiogram is shown, where each ear is plotted on a separate audiogram. The panels are arranged to correspond to the patient's ears as you look at them, that is, the panel on the left should correspond to the patient's right ear and the panel on the right should correspond to the patient's left ear. In **C**, the pure-tone thresholds are plotted in tabular or numeric format. **AC**, air conduction; **BC**, bone conduction.

learn to describe audiograms effectively, it is useful to have some knowledge about the need for masking in audiometry. In this section, a brief introduction to the need for masking is presented. More details about masking and an understanding of how to perform masking when needed are presented in Chapter 6.

To be clinically useful, it is expected that pure-tone testing will produce thresholds that are valid representations of the hearing sensitivity for the ear being tested. However, there are many conditions in pure-tone audiometry when the sound being presented to the test ear (TE) can be heard in the opposite non-test ear (NTE). One illustrative example of this problem is when testing is done with the bone conduction vibrator. Because both cochleae are embedded in the bones of the skull, they both receive the pure-tone vibrations fairly equally, even though the bone conduction vibrator is only placed on the mastoid behind one ear. This becomes especially problematic when the NTE has better hearing than the TE, since the patient will respond to the BC sound in the NTE, and this will produce invalid thresholds for the BC thresholds of the TE. When this situation arises, a noise stimulus must be put into the NTE to keep the NTE from hearing any of the pure tones that are presented to the TE. When masking noise is presented to the NTE, the patient is told not to respond to the masking noise stimulus and listen/respond only for the pure tones.

The process of putting noise into the NTE while measuring thresholds in the TE is called *clinical masking*. For clinical masking, the noise presented in the NTE is called the *masker* and the pure-tone thresholds obtained in the TE are called *masked thresholds*. Figure 5–5A shows an example of an audiogram with masked BC thresholds for the right ear. Notice the different symbols in the audiogram key for unmasked and masked BC thresholds for the right and left ears. Like the unmasked BC symbols, the masked BC symbols are placed to the appropriate side of the frequency line. When masked symbols are plotted on an audiogram they indicate that those thresholds for the TE were obtained with the appropriate amount of masking noise delivered to the NTE, so the NTE cannot be hearing the pure tone and one

is confident that the masked thresholds truly represent the hearing of the TE.

In Figure 5–5, the audiogram indicates that the patient has a sensorineural hearing loss in the right ear because the AC thresholds are the same as masked BC thresholds (as you learned in Chapter 4). However, if the right ear BC thresholds had not been obtained with masking in the left ear, the patient would have given unmasked BC thresholds for the right ear similar to those for the BC thresholds of the left ear. This occurs because the sound presented by BC on the right mastoid stimulates both ears, and the threshold one gets for the TE (right ear) is actually due to the patient hearing the tones by BC in the left ear. In this example, when pure-tone BC testing is done without masking in the left ear, the right ear shows an erroneous air–bone gap, since the patient actually has a sensorineural hearing loss. You can see, therefore, that it is important to use masking in some instances in order to obtain the true thresholds for the ear being tested.

You probably also noticed in the audiogram key that there are masked symbols for AC as well as BC. As it turns out, since the AC transducers are also in contact with the skull, at high enough intensities (around 50 to 60 dB HL or greater) the pure tones from these AC transducers can also vibrate the skull; and whenever vibrations are set up in the bones of the skull, the cochlea of the NTE will receive those vibrations (by BC). Figure 5–6 shows an example of AC pure-tone thresholds obtained without masking and then again with masking. Notice that the masked AC thresholds of the right ear (triangles) are poorer than the unmasked AC thresholds (circles). The unmasked AC thresholds (circles) in this case were actually due to the patient hearing the tones by BC in the left ear due to the vibrations of the skull.

It is fairly easy to visualize that when the bone vibrator is on the mastoid of one ear, the other cochlea can also be receiving the vibrations; and it should now be equally apparent that when pure tones are delivered by AC transducers at high enough levels they may be heard by BC from the better hearing NTE. The general guideline is that masking is needed for AC testing with supra-aural earphones when the presentation level of the tone in the TE is more than 40 dB above the BC

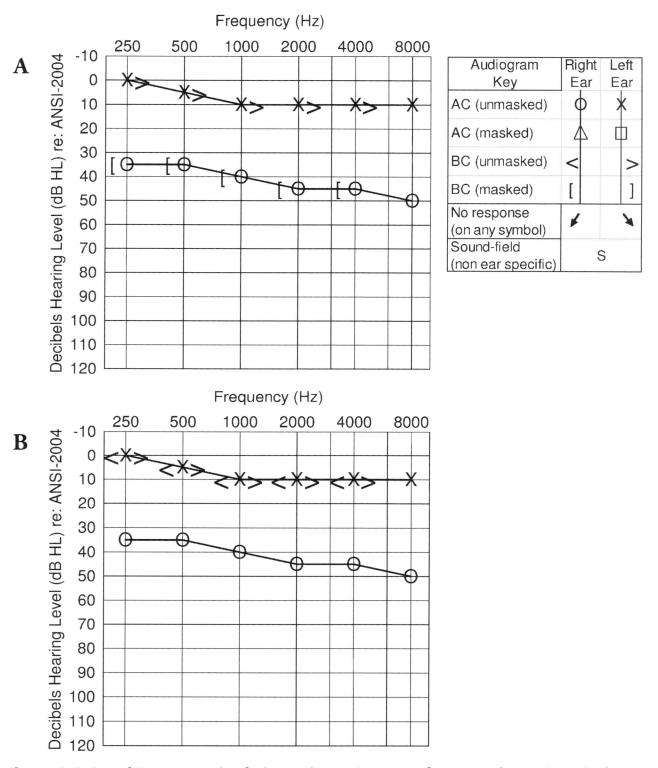

Figure 5–5. A and B. An example of why masking is important for proper diagnosis. In **A**, the patient's true masked bone conduction (BC) thresholds for the right ear indicate a sensorineural hearing loss (AC = BC). In **B**, the same patient's results are shown when obtained without masking, and indicate an invalid conductive loss (AC > BC). **AC,** air conduction.

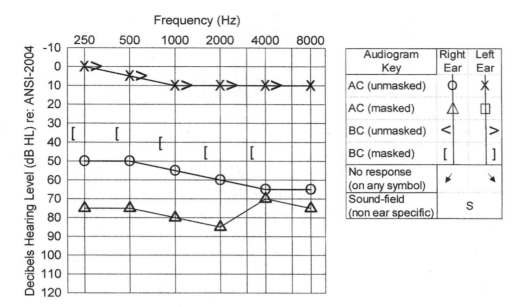

Figure 5–6. An example of why masking is important for proper diagnosis. The patient's true masked air conduction (*AC*) thresholds for the right ear are around 70–85 dB HL. The same patient's results are shown as they would be if obtained without masking, and incorrectly show thresholds to be at better hearing levels than the their true hearing thresholds.

threshold of the NTE. For insert earphones, due to less surface-area contact with the skull, masking is needed for insert earphone AC testing when the presentation level of the tone in the TE is more than 55 dB above the BC threshold of the NTE. For more on how to decide when to mask and how to perform masking, see Chapter 6. For now, these introductory concepts on masking are meant to give an understanding of why there may be masked symbols on an audiogram.

Synopsis 5–1

- An audiogram is used to graphically record a patient's audiometric information, especially pure-tone thresholds. Frequency is represented logarithmically along the x-axis in octave intervals from 250 to 8000 Hz. Intensity is represented along the y-axis in decibels of hearing level (dB HL). The proper aspect ratio for audiograms is 20 dB HL along the y-axis for each octave change in frequency along the x-axis.

- Decibels of hearing level (dB HL) are used on an audiogram to normalize the different dB SPL values that are associated with normal hearing for different frequencies. These normalized values for each frequency, called audiometric zero or 0 dB HL, are calibrated into the audiometer based on the most recent standards, currently ANSI 2004 reference values (ANSI, 2004a). The audiometer is calibrated for each transducer based on the standards so that 0 dB HL represents the average normal threshold levels (ANSI, 2004a).

- To convert from dB HL to dB SPL, add the value from the ANSI standard for the specific frequency and transducer to the dB HL. To convert from dB SPL to dB HL, subtract the value from the ANSI standard for the specific frequency and transducer from the dB SPL.

- The recommended symbols used on an audiogram are:

Audiogram Key	Right Ear	Left Ear
AC (unmasked)	Ọ	Ⅹ
AC (masked)	△	☐
BC (unmasked)	<	>
BC (masked)	[	]
No response (on any symbol)	↙	↘
Sound-field (non ear specific)	S	

- Pure-tone thresholds can be documented using a single-panel audiogram (data for both ears on same graph), a two-panel audiogram (data for each ear on a separate graph), or in tabular form.

- Testing by BC, and at high levels for AC, produces vibrations in the skull that can be heard through BC in both cochleae. Under these conditions, masking (and masked symbols) are required.

- Masking of the non-test ear (NTE) with narrowband noise is needed in those conditions where there is the possibility that the tone presented to the test ear (TE) may be heard through cross-hearing by BC in the NTE.

Describing Audiograms

We will now turn our attention to describing hearing losses based on patients' audiograms. In this section you will learn how to succinctly describe a person's hearing loss based on the pure-tone audiometric results. When describing the pure-tone audiogram, the following three types of information should be conveyed:

- Degree (amount) of hearing loss
- Type of hearing loss
- Shape of hearing loss

It is common practice to summarize, in brief sentences, the general characteristics of the pure-tone thresholds that are plotted on the audiogram. The sentences should be able to generate a mental picture of the audiogram, but not be so detailed as to be a repetition of all the audiometric thresholds. Information about each ear should be provided and significant differences across the frequency range should be noted. Although there are different ways to describe audiograms, the information presented in this chapter is generally accepted and commonly used in clinical practice. There is considerable leeway in the details and format that might be used to describe the same audiogram; there are many possible correct descriptions of a person's audiogram. In a sense this might be considered the "art of audiometry." However, there are also incorrect descriptions that you will want to avoid. You will learn to circumvent these mistakes as you go through the examples in this chapter.

Degrees of Hearing Loss

Describing the degree (or amount) of hearing loss from the audiogram means to apply some general descriptive term (e.g., mild) that corresponds to the decibel numbers associated with the patient's thresholds. The patient's AC thresholds are used to define the degree of hearing loss, since this would include hearing loss from all parts of the auditory system. The generally accepted classification scheme used to describe the degree of hearing loss is based on a continuum from normal to profound and, to a certain extent, reflects how those degrees of loss may affect communication (Clark, 1981; Goodman, 1965). The following terms are in common use to describe the degree of hearing loss (or hearing sensitivity):

−10 to 15 dB HL	normal
16 to 25 dB HL	normal for adults; slight or minimal in children
26 to 40 dB HL	mild
41 to 55 dB HL	moderate
56 to 70 dB HL	moderately severe
71 to 90 dB HL	severe
91+ dB HL	profound

Notice that the range 16 to 25 dB HL has different terms depending on whether the patient is an adult or a child. This is because children are still acquiring language and are in educational environments where a slight or minimal degree of hearing loss might have a greater impact than it would for an adult. It is also important to be cautious in assuming that these categories accurately apply to a patient's actual communication difficulty; they are merely a conventional and convenient way to describe the audiogram. This is particularly true of children where the above descriptive terms may not accurately reflect the extent of a child's problems or the parents' perceptions (Haggard & Primus, 1999). As you will see, each patient has a unique set of circumstances, perceptions, and underlying cause of his or her hearing loss. The pure-tone thresholds are only part of the puzzle that audiologists use in the overall evaluation of a patient.

It is quite common for the degree of hearing loss to change across the audiogram; therefore, the description should provide a general sense of how the degree of hearing loss changes across frequency. It is not required that each frequency be assigned a specific category. As you work through some of the examples, you will see that these categories are sometimes loosely applied over a range of frequencies and/or even cascaded. For example, a hearing loss may be described as being *moderately severe* to *severe* over a specified frequency range. Remember, the goal is to provide a summary description of the pure-tone thresholds, knowing that the details are available in the audiogram.

Types of Hearing Loss

To describe the *type of hearing loss* from the audiogram means to determine whether the hearing loss involves the conductive and/or sensorineural portions of the auditory pathways. Recall that the sensorineural portion of the auditory system refers to the cochlea, 8th nerve, and central pathways, whereas the conductive portion refers to the outer ear and middle ear. A hearing

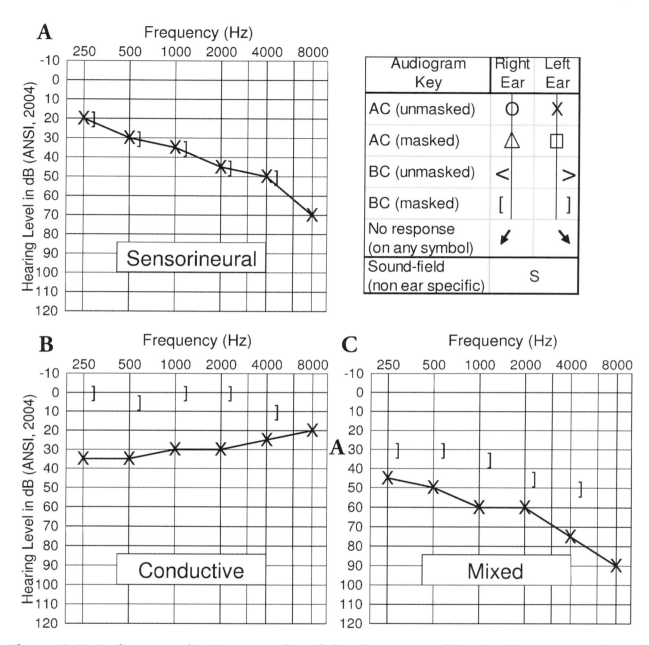

Figure 5–7. Audiograms showing examples of the three types of hearing losses: sensorineural (**A**), conductive (**B**), and mixed (**C**). See text for definitions of the different types. **AC**, air conduction; **BC**, bone conduction.

problem in the sensorineural portion of the auditory pathways would have the same hearing loss when tested by AC as when tested by BC. On the other hand, a hearing problem in the conductive part of the ear would have an air–bone gap, that is, normal hearing by BC and poorer hearing by AC. Of course, a hearing loss that occurs in both the sensorineural and conductive parts, called a mixed hearing loss, would have a loss by BC and an air–bone gap. Figure 5-7 shows examples of the three types of hearing losses (for one ear) that are commonly used when describing audiograms. The three types of hearing loss are defined as follows:

Sensorineural hearing loss:
Air-bone gap ≤10 dB

Conductive hearing loss:
Air-bone gap >10 dB; BC ≤25 dB HL

Mixed hearing loss:
Air-bone gap >10 dB; BC >25 dB HL

As you look at an audiogram, these definitions should be considered at each frequency. In many cases, there could be different types of hearing losses in different frequency ranges. For example, there may be a conductive hearing loss in the lower frequencies and a sensorineural hearing loss in the higher frequencies, and both types of hearing loss as a function of frequency should be included in the description of the audiogram.

As you can see, pure-tone audiometry can only grossly localize the problem to the conductive and/or sensorineural parts of the auditory system. Information from a battery of audiologic tests (covered in later chapters) can be used to better define the location and/or cause of the hearing loss.

Shapes of Hearing Loss

Describing the *shape of the hearing loss* from the audiogram means that you point out significant characteristics that convey a mental picture of how the thresholds look across the frequency range or across the two ears. For example, a hearing loss that is the same in both ears and the degree of hearing loss changes (at least 20 dB) across the frequency range might be described as "a bilateral sensorineural hearing loss, sloping from mild in the low frequencies to severe in the high frequencies." The term *bilateral* refers to both ears and "sloping" refers to the downward slope of the threshold curve on the audiogram. Figure 5–8 illustrates some general shapes of audiograms and the terms commonly used to describe those

shapes. Although not exhaustive, the following list of terms and descriptions of audiogram shapes are commonly used:

Bilateral	results similar in both ears
Relatively flat	within 20 dB across audiogram
Sloping	>20 dB per octave toward high frequencies
Precipitous	steeply sloping (e.g., >40 dB/octave)
Rising	improving from low to high frequencies
Notched	worse in a narrow region (typically 3 to 6 kHz)
Corner	residual hearing only in the lower frequencies

The term *unilateral* is sometimes used in reference to a hearing loss if it is only in one ear, and the term *asymmetric* is sometimes used when there is a significant difference in the hearing loss between the two ears. The use of unilateral in the description of an audiogram is not very useful since you would need to describe in which ear the hearing loss was; and the term asymmetric may not be useful since each ear would need its own description. There is considerable variability in how different audiologists convey the shape of the audiogram, and even greater variability in how words are combined to convey shape, degree, and type of hearing loss (the "art of audiology"). Undoubtedly, you will develop your own style for summarizing and describing audiograms. Conversely, when you are given a summary description of a person's hearing loss, you should have a good mental picture of the audiogram.

Sample Audiograms with Descriptions

In this section, there are four sample audiograms (Figure 5–9, Figure 5–10, Figure 5–11, and

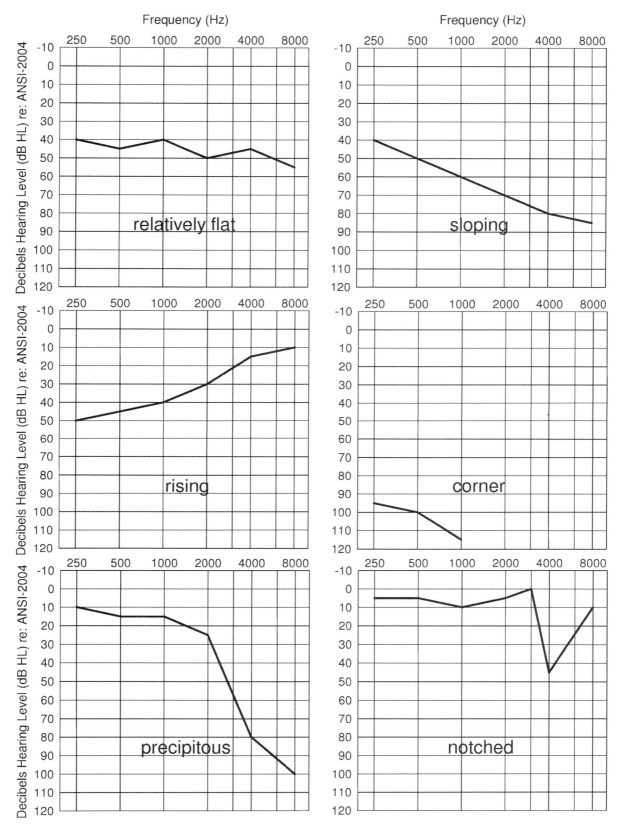

Figure 5–8. Audiogram configurations with common terms used to describe their shapes. See text for definitions of the terms.

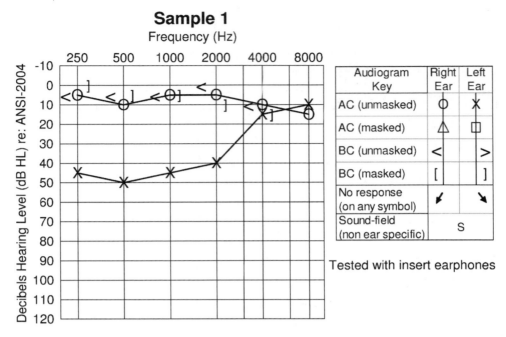

Figure 5–9. Audiogram sample 1. Two possible descriptions of the audiogram are: (a) Pure-tone threshold testing indicated a moderate conductive hearing loss through 2000 Hz rising to normal in the higher frequencies for the left ear. Hearing was within normal limits for the right ear. (b) Left ear showed a moderate conductive hearing loss through 2000 Hz. **AC**, air conduction; **BC**, bone conduction.

Figure 5–12). For each audiogram, there are examples provided on how the audiogram might be described. Remember, there are many correct ways to describe audiograms, some lengthier than others, and many different possibilities of word order. When describing an audiogram, the goal is to convey a summary of the audiogram for each ear and across the frequency range. Conversely, the description of the audiogram should conjure up a reasonably accurate mental picture of the audiogram. As you read the descriptions included with the sample audiograms you will notice that some descriptions include only the areas of the audiogram where there is a hearing loss (see Figure 5–9); this generally implies that the parts left out of the description are normal.

Additional Factors to Consider

No Response at Audiometer Limits

When the upper limits of the audiometer are reached and the patient does not respond, the appropriate symbols for AC and/or BC are plotted on the audiogram with arrows attached to the symbols. An example of this is shown on the audiogram in Figure 5–13. This patient has normal hearing in the right ear and masked AC and BC thresholds beyond the limits of the audiogram for most of the frequencies. It is common practice not to connect the AC symbols in regions where there are no responses (e.g., above 500 Hz in Figure 5–13).

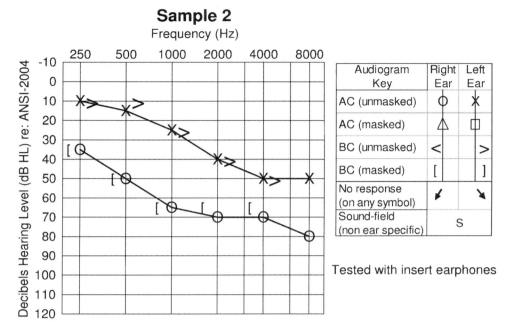

Figure 5–10. Audiogram sample 2. Two possible descriptions of the audiogram are: (a) Pure-tone threshold testing for the left ear indicated a sensorineural hearing loss that was mild at 1000 Hz sloping to moderate in the higher frequencies. The right ear showed a sloping sensorineural hearing loss that was mild at 250 Hz sloping to severe at 8000 Hz. (b) The left ear has mild to moderate high frequency sensorineural hearing loss with normal hearing in the lower frequencies. The right ear has a mild to moderate sensorineural hearing loss through 500 Hz sloping to severe at 8000 Hz. **AC**, air conduction; **BC**, bone conduction.

The purpose of the "no response" symbols on the audiogram is to show that testing was attempted at the limits of the audiometer, but that the patient actually has worse thresholds than indicated by the no response symbols and the audiometer was unable to test at high enough intensity levels to find the true threshold. In Figure 5–13, there is an appearance of an air–bone gap; however, it is important not to describe this as an air–bone gap because it is simply due to the difference in output limits for BC and AC. For the example in Figure 5–13, based on the audiogram alone, you cannot be sure if there is any involvement of the conductive portions of the ear (cannot determine if it is a mixed hearing loss) because you were not able to test masked BC any higher than 45 to 75 dB HL. Other information would be needed to help determine whether or not there was a conductive component. For Figure 5–13, can you predict where the unmasked BC and unmasked AC responses would have been?

Tactile Responses

Tactile (or *vibro-tactile*) *responses* are a result of the patient feeling the vibrations rather than hearing them (Nober, 1970). Clinically, tactile responses occur mostly by BC for 250 and 500 Hz. Tactile thresholds to BC have been shown to range from about 25 to 40 dB at 250 Hz and 55 to 70 dB at 500 Hz (Boothroyd & Cawkwell, 1970). As illustrated in Figure 5–14, tactile responses will result

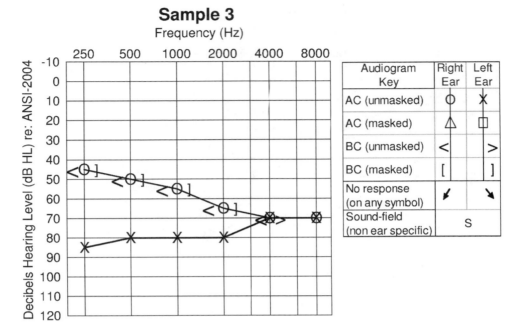

Figure 5–11. Audiogram sample 3. Two possible descriptions of the audiogram are: (a) Pure-tone threshold testing indicated a moderate to moderately severe sloping sensorineural hearing loss in the right ear. The left ear showed a severe, relatively flat, mixed hearing loss through 2000 Hz (with 40 dB air–bone gap at 250 to 15 dB air–bone gap at 2000 Hz), rising to a moderately severe sensorineural hearing loss in the higher frequencies. (b) The right ear has a sloping sensorineural hearing loss that ranges from moderate in the low frequencies to moderately severe in the mid to high frequencies. The left ear has a severe, flat hearing loss with a conductive (air–bone gap) component from 250 to 2000 Hz. **AC**, air conduction; **BC**, bone conduction.

in an air–bone gap that may falsely imply a conductive component to the hearing loss. You should always be suspect of tactile responses when testing BC in the low frequencies, especially when there is an apparent air–bone gap, and make note of it on the audiogram. Asking the patient if he or she felt the signal may also provide verification of tactile responses.

Collapsed Canals

Collapsed canals can occur in some individuals with reduced elasticity in the cartilaginous portion of the external ear canal when supra-aural earphones are used for testing. The collapsed canals

are only an artifact of the testing situation, whereby the force of the supra-aural earphone is enough to temporarily close off the ear canal. When the ear canal is collapsed by the earphone, it will reduce the intensity of the AC pure tones, but not the BC pure tones, and can result in an erroneous air–bone gap. Figure 5-15 shows an example of an audiogram that would suggest collapsed canals. The effects of a collapsed ear canal are usually seen in the mid to high frequencies, therefore showing up as a high frequency air–bone gap (true conductive hearing losses are usually in the low frequencies). Whenever there is a high frequency air–bone gap when using supra-aural earphones, the audiologist should be suspicious of a collapsed canal and use other means of testing, such

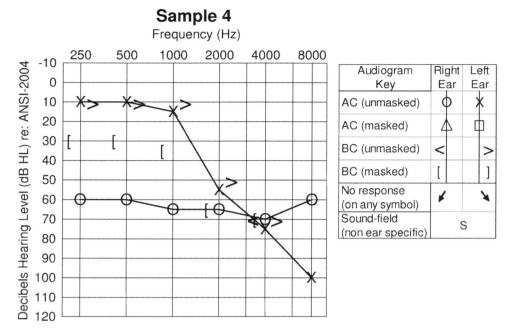

Sample 4

Figure 5–12. Audiogram sample 4. Two possible descriptions of the audiogram are: (a) Pure-tone threshold testing indicated a relatively flat, moderately severe hearing loss in the right ear which was mixed (30 dB air–bone gaps) through 1000 Hz and sensorineural from 2000 to 8000 Hz. The left ear has normal hearing through 1000 Hz with a sensorineural hearing loss that precipitously slopes to severe at 4000 Hz and profound at 8000 Hz. (b) The right ear has a moderately severe mixed hearing loss through 1000 Hz (30 dB air–bone gaps) and a moderately severe sensorineural hearing loss in the higher frequencies. The left ear has a moderate to profound sloping sensorineural hearing loss from 2000 to 8000 Hz. **AC**, air conduction; **BC**, bone conduction.

as insert earphones, hand-holding the supra-aural earphone loosely on the ear, or sound-field testing while masking the non-test ear.

Pure-Tone Average

Calculating a *pure-tone average* (PTA) for each ear is often done to provide a summary of the pure-tone thresholds over a particular frequency range most important for speech understanding. The PTA is calculated from the AC thresholds because the AC route includes all portions of the auditory system. The traditional PTA is the average of the thresholds at 500, 1000, and 2000 Hz. Other

calculations of PTA may be done in certain situations, including a four-frequency PTA (500, 1000, 2000, 3000 Hz) or a high frequency PTA (1000, 2000, 3000, 4000 Hz), especially when calculating percent of hearing handicap for compensation cases. A two-frequency PTA (e.g., 1000 and 2000 Hz) is sometimes used when there is a steep slope to the audiogram. Clark (1981) recommends using the three poorest thresholds between 500 and 4000 Hz. Whenever a PTA is calculated, the frequencies used should be noted.

The use of PTA is sometimes used for describing the degree of hearing loss; however, this author recommends describing degrees of hearing loss as they change across the entire audiogram. A single number (average) does not adequately

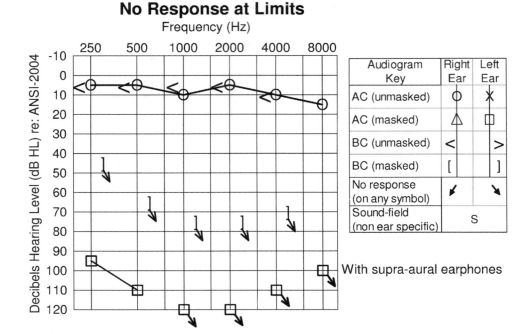

Figure 5–13. An example of an audiogram showing no responses at the limits of the equipment for the left ear bone conduction (*BC*) and air conduction (*AC*) thresholds. The appropriate symbols have an *arrow* attached to indicate that testing was performed up to the indicated maximum limit, but the patient did not respond at those levels. The differences between the AC and BC symbols do not imply any air–bone gaps since the actual thresholds for the left ear cannot be determined due to output limits of the transducers. The patient has a hearing loss in the left ear that is greater than that which could be tested. This audiogram might be described as having no useable hearing in the left ear.

reflect how the degree of hearing loss changes across the audiogram. For example, for a patient with normal hearing through 2000 Hz and a precipitous decline in thresholds in the higher frequencies, you would not want to leave the impression, based on the traditional PTA, that the patient has normal hearing.

Decibels of Sensation Level

"Oh my gosh," you are probably thinking, "another decibel!" Yes, there is another decibel used frequently in audiology, called *decibel of sensation level* (dB SL). For this decibel, the reference value is the actual threshold of the individual patient. In other words, 0 dB SL equals the patient's threshold (for any frequency or other threshold measure). As the dB SL increases above threshold (supra-threshold), the dB SL is an indication of how much the sound is above the patient's threshold. As you will see in later chapters, there are many audiologic tests that are done at a specific dB SL, which would require a different dB HL presentation level for different patients, depending on their thresholds. As an example, for Patient A, with a threshold of 20 dB HL at a given frequency, a tone at that frequency which is presented at 60 dB HL would be 40 dB SL (40 dB above the threshold). For Patient B, with a threshold of 40 dB HL, the same 60 dB HL tone would only be 20 dB SL (20 dB above the threshold). As another way of looking at this concept, suppose you want to evaluate how well a patient can hear comfortably loud speech.

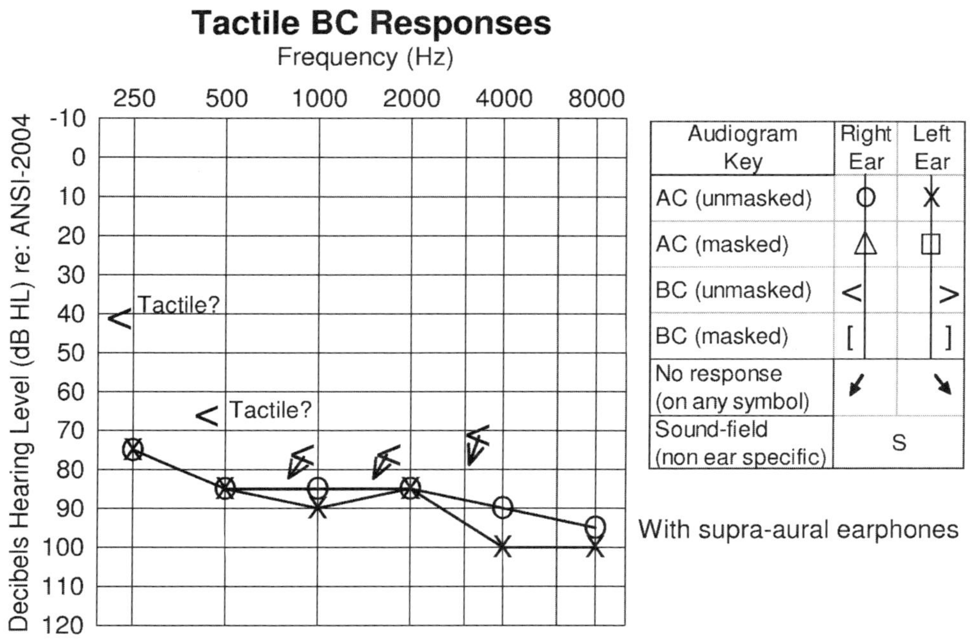

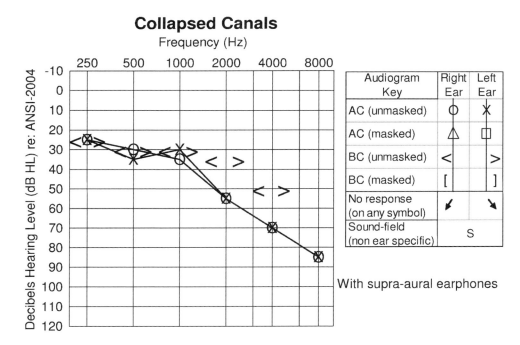

Tactile BC Responses

Figure 5–14. An example of an audiogram showing how to indicate the possibility that the low frequency bone conduction (BC) thresholds may be due to tactile sensations rather than auditory sensations. **AC**, air conduction.

Collapsed Canals

Figure 5–15. An example of an audiogram suggesting a false conductive hearing loss due to collapsed ear canals. The high-frequency air–bone gaps are characteristic of a temporary collapsed ear canal during the use of supra-aural earphones. Retesting with insert earphones should eliminate the air–bone gaps. **AC**, air conduction; **BC**, bone conduction.

Depending on the amount of hearing loss, each patient would need a different presentation level for the speech to be comfortably loud. Some audiologic tests are designed to be performed at a specific amount above a patient's threshold, for example 30 dB SL. For Patient A, that test would need to be presented at 50 dB HL (20 dB HL threshold + 30 dB SL); for Patient B, the test would need to presented at 70 dB HL (40 dB HL threshold + 30 dB SL). When referring to dB SL, you must always know the patient's threshold (reference). By definition, a signal presented at a patient's threshold is 0 dB SL.

Synopsis 5–2

- Descriptions of an audiogram should provide a concise summary of the type of loss, degree of loss, and shape of the loss as a function of frequency, without repeating all of the data that are on the audiogram.

- The following terms are in common use to describe the degree of hearing loss:
    - 10 to 15 dB HL   normal
    - 16 to 25 dB HL   normal for adults; slight or minimal in children
    - 26 to 40 dB HL   mild
    - 41 to 55 dB HL   moderate
    - 56 to 70 dB HL   moderately severe
    - 71 to 90 dB HL   severe
    - 91+ dB HL   profound

- The following terms are in common use to describe the types of hearing loss:
    - Sensorineural hearing loss: Air–bone gap ≤10 dB
    - Conductive hearing loss: Air–bone gap >10 dB; BC ≤25 dB HL; or ≤15 dB HL (child)
    - Mixed hearing loss: Air–bone gap ≥10 dB; BC ≥25 dB HL; or ≤15 dB HL (child)

- The following terms are in common use to describe the shape of hearing loss:
    - Bilateral   results similar in both ears
    - Flat   within 20 dB across audiogram
    - Sloping   >20 dB per octave toward high frequencies
    - Precipitous   steeply sloping (e.g., >40 dB/octave)
    - Rising   improving from low to high frequencies
    - Notched   worse in a narrow region (typically 3 to 6 kHz)
    - Corner   residual hearing only in the lower frequencies

- Some patients with severe to profound hearing loss may not respond at the limits of the audiometer. Because BC intensity limits are less than AC intensity limits, the difference does not indicate an air–bone gap, and the extent of any conductive involvement cannot be determined from the audiogram.

- Tactile responses, in which the patient feels the vibration rather than hears it, can occur for BC testing around 25 to 40 dB at 250 and 55 to 70 dB at 500 Hz. For patients with more than a moderate hearing loss, these tactile BC thresholds may appear as a false air–bone gap.

- Collapsed canals can occur in some patients with highly compliant ear canals when testing with supra-aural earphones. Collapsed canals are characterized by air–bone gaps that are present in the higher frequencies. Collapsed canals can be avoided by using insert earphones.

- A pure-tone average (PTA) is often calculated from the thresholds at 500, 1000, and 2000 Hz. In some cases with a steeply sloping hearing loss, when specified, the PTA can be calculated with two frequencies (500 and 1000 Hz).

- Decibel sensation level (dB SL) is another way of referencing the level of sounds that are presented to patients. The reference values for dB SL are the patient's own thresholds. By definition, 0 dB SL = patient's threshold.

References

American National Standards Institute (ANSI). (1996). *American National Standards specifications for audiometers.* ANSI S3.6-1996. New York, NY: Author.

American National Standards Institute (ANSI). (2004a). *American National Standards for audiometers.* ANSI S3.6 2004. New York, NY: Author.

American National Standards Institute (ANSI). (2004b). *Methods for manual pure-tone threshold audiometry.* ANSI S3.21-2004. New York, NY: Author.

American Speech-Language-Hearing Association (ASHA). (1990). Guidelines for audiometric symbols. *American Speech-Language-Hearing Association, 32*(Suppl.), 25–30.

American Speech-Language-Hearing Association (ASHA). (2005). *Guidelines for manual pure-tone threshold audiometry.* Rockville, MD: Author. Retrieved January 10, 2008 from http://www.asha.org/policy/.

Boothroyd, A., & Cawkwell, S. (1970). Vibrotactile thresholds in pure tone audiometry. *Acta Otolaryngologica, 69,* 381–387.

Clark, J. G. (1981). Uses and abuses of hearing loss classification. *ASHA, 23,* 493–500.

Goodman, A. (1965). Reference zero levels for pure-tone audiometer. *ASHA, 7,* 262–263.

Haggard, R. A., & Primus, M. A. (1999). Parental perceptions of hearing loss classification in children. *American Journal of Audiology, 8,* 83–92.

Nober, E. H. (1970). Cutile air and bone conduction thresholds in the deaf. *Exceptional Children, 36,* 571–579.

6

Clinical Masking for Pure-Tone Audiometry

After reading this chapter, you should be able to:

1. Understand why the non-test ear (NTE) needs to be masked to obtain true thresholds in the test ear (TE).
2. Know what is meant by interaural attenuation (IA) and the minimum IA values used for each transducer when making decisions about the need to obtain masked thresholds.
3. Recognize from the unmasked thresholds when masked thresholds must be obtained; apply the decision-making rules for masking when testing by bone conduction (BC) and air conduction (AC) using supra-aural earphones or insert earphones.
4. Describe the types of maskers used for pure-tone and speech testing.
5. Define effective masking (EM) and how maskers are calibrated in the audiometer.
6. Describe the occlusion effect (OE) and why this needs to be considered when masking.
7. Describe two advantages of insert earphones over supra-aural earphones as they relate to masking.
8. Define what is meant by a masking plateau and how much of a plateau is appropriate. Discuss why the width of the plateau is smaller when there is a potential bilateral moderate conductive loss.
9. Apply the specific steps for AC and BC masking using the plateau method for a variety of unmasked audiograms.
10. Define overmasking and masking dilemma, and recognize situations in which these may occur.

In Chapter 5, some basic principles of masking were presented so that you have an understanding of why unmasked or masked symbols are needed on an audiogram to represent a patient's pure-tone thresholds. To be clinically useful, it is expected that pure-tone testing will produce thresholds that are valid representations of the hearing sensitivity for the ear being tested; however, there are many testing situations in which the sound presented to the test ear (TE) can be heard in the opposite non-test ear (NTE). As you may recall, when testing by bone conduction at any intensity or when testing by air conduction at a moderate level and above, the sound vibrations occur in the skull and, therefore, can be received by both cochleae that are embedded in the bones of the skull. This becomes especially problematic when the NTE has better hearing than the TE, since the patient's response to the signal delivered to the TE could actually be a result of the patient hearing the signal by bone conduction in the NTE. To prevent the patient from responding to the pure tone that may be present in the NTE, a noise (called the masker) is delivered to the NTE by air conduction while presenting the pure tone to the TE. The patient is instructed not to respond to the noise that they will hear in one ear and to respond only when they hear the pure-tone. It is important to remember that the masker is always delivered by an AC transducer. If the masker is delivered by the BC transducer, then the masker would always be heard in both ears, making it impossible to get a true response from the test ear. By presenting the masking noise with an earphone, there is a range of masker levels (at least 40 dB HL with supra-aural earphones and at least 55 dB HL with insert earphones) that can be applied before the cochlea of the TE is stimulated by the noise. In other words, using insert earphones to present the masker to the NTE would allow at least 55 dB HL of noise to be used before there is any possibility of crossing over to the TE.

The process of putting noise into the NTE, while measuring thresholds in the TE, is called *clinical masking*. This chapter provides more details on when masking is needed and covers the step-by-step procedures to obtain masked thresholds. Several examples of how to obtain masked thresholds are given in this chapter; however, the reader is also referred to the companion workbook for more examples and practice with masking.

Maskers

The masking noises used in pure-tone audiometry are called *narrowband* (NB) *maskers*. For each audiometric test frequency, there is a corresponding band of noise (one-third-octave wide) centered on each of the audiometric frequencies. Depending on the frequency being tested, you would select the appropriate NB masker. For example, if the pure tone being presented to the TE is 1000 Hz, you would use a 1000 Hz NB masker in the NTE. In order to be able to deliver the NB masker into the NTE a two-channel audiometer is needed so that the pure tone can be routed through one channel to the TE and the NB masker routed through the other channel to the NTE. As mentioned earlier, the NB masker is always presented by AC to the NTE, preferably using an insert earphone, and the pure tone is presented to the TE by the other insert earphone (when testing AC) or by the bone vibrator (when testing BC). If the masker is presented using a supra-aural earphone during BC testing, the other earphone is placed on the temple next to the eye on the side of the TE.

As you will see in a later section, when doing speech testing you also must be cognizant of the possible need for masking to prevent the speech signals from being heard in the NTE. When masking is used for speech testing, a *speech masker* is used instead of a one-third-octave NB noise. The speech masker is a somewhat broader spectrum noise that encompasses the range of frequencies that are important for speech recognition. Masking procedures for speech testing are covered in Chapter 7.

The maskers are calibrated in terms of their *effective masking* (EM) *levels*. Effective masking is a calibrated amount of noise that will provide a threshold shift to a corresponding dB HL for the stimulus centered within the noise (Sanders, 1972; Yacullo, 1996). For example, 30 dB HL of effective masking will elevate the AC threshold of the corresponding pure tone to 30 dB HL. The required amounts of noise that correspond to 0 dB HL of effective masking for each frequency are set by the effective noise calibration levels for NB and speech maskers (ANSI, 1996). The ANSI (1996) masker levels are built into the audiometer (just as for 0 dB HL for the pure tones). In this way, the attenuator dial of the audiometer used to deliver the maskers directly correspond to the dB HL of effective masking. To illustrate, if the attenuator dial for the masker is set to 40 dB HL, it means that the masker can effectively elevate the AC threshold for the test signal (pure tone or speech) to 40 dB HL when presented in the same ear. The actual amount that the threshold changes, for a given dB HL of EM, will depend on the threshold. For example, if the patient's AC threshold is 30 dB HL, then putting in a 40 dB HL masker will elevate the patient's threshold *to* 40 dB HL, but the threshold change was only increased *by* 10 dB (40 dB HL effective masking minus 30 dB HL threshold). As you will come to see, it is very important to keep in mind that when you increase the AC threshold in the NTE with masking, you also increase the BC threshold by the same amount, but they both do not necessarily increase to the same dB HL. For instance, in cases where there is an air–bone gap in the NTE, this air–bone gap will remain. As an example, suppose the AC pure-tone threshold in the NTE is 50 dB HL and the BC threshold in the NTE is 30 dB HL (20 dB air–bone gap). When a NB masker is presented to the NTE by AC with an effective masking level of 60 dB HL, the AC threshold (in the presence of the noise) in the NTE will be elevated to 60 dB HL (a 10 dB increase in threshold) and, therefore, the BC threshold in the NTE will also increase by 10 dB to 40 dB HL (still a 20 dB air–bone gap).

When Is Masking Needed?

When testing by BC, it is fairly intuitive that vibrations are set up in the skull and, therefore, could be heard in both ears by BC. If the level of the BC signal occurring in the NTE is above the patient's BC threshold in the NTE, it would be audible to the patient and he/she would give a response that

does not represent the TE. Although not as intuitive as for BC testing, it is also the case that when presenting pure tones to the TE by AC at moderate to high levels, the sound vibrations are also created in the skull and could be heard in both ears by BC. If the level of the BC signal occurring in the NTE is above the patient's BC threshold in the NTE, it would be audible to the patient and she or he would give a response that does not represent the TE.

When testing by AC, the levels of the pure tone that can cause vibrations of the skull are different for supra-aural earphones and insert earphones. The differences are primarily dependent on the relative surface area of the skull that is exposed to the sound from each AC transducer; supra-aural earphones have a larger area of exposure than insert earphones. Supra-aural earphones can produce vibrations of the skull when presented at levels equal to or greater than 40 dB HL, whereas insert earphones can produce vibrations of the skull when presented at levels equal to or greater than 55 dB HL.

Interaural Attenuation and Cross-Hearing

It is easy to visualize that when the bone vibrator is on the mastoid process of one ear the other cochlea is also being stimulated. However, are both ears receiving the sound at the same intensity? In other words, is there some attenuation of the sound in the NTE as compared with the TE? Interaural attenuation (IA) is a term that is used to quantify the difference in the level of the signal level presented in the TE to the level of the signal level that occurs in the NTE (by BC). Another way of thinking about this is to ask how much greater does the level of the signal in the TE have to be before it is capable of being heard by BC in the NTE? Furthermore, of course, if the NTE is capable of hearing the sound presented to the TE, masking in the NTE would be needed in order to establish the true masked thresholds in the TE. Ranges of IA values have been determined for different transducers by several studies (e.g., Chaiklin, 1967; Coles & Priede, 1970; Sklare & Denneberg, 1987;

Studebaker, 1967). Figure 6–1 shows a comparison of IA values as a function of frequency for supra-aural earphones and insert earphones. The following are recommended minimum IA values for the different transducers adopted for this textbook:

BC IA (with bone conduction vibrator) = 0 dB

AC IA (with supra-aural earphone) = 40 dB

AC IA (with insert earphone) = 55 dB.[1]

Although studies have shown that there are slight variations in the IA as a function of frequency and across people, and because we cannot know each patient's actual IA, the minimum IA values are used in the clinic instead of the mean IA values so that we do not miss masking someone with IA below the average. Even though a patient's true IA might be higher than the minimum, it is better to mask in cases that might not need it than make a serious error by not masking the rare individual with the lowest (e.g., 40 dB) IA.

When the signal is delivered to the patient's TE and it is actually audible in the NTE, it is called *cross-hearing*. An important concept to keep in mind is that cross-hearing to the NTE always occurs by BC (Studebaker, 1962; Zwislocki, 1953). Whenever the NTE can hear the sounds through BC, masking is needed. For BC testing, cross-hearing to the NTE is a frequent problem and can occur whenever there is any difference in hearing between the two ears since IA = 0 dB. For AC testing, cross-hearing to the NTE can also be a problem when the difference between AC of the TE and BC of the NTE is greater than or equal to the IA for the specific transducer (IA ≥55 dB for insert earphones or IA ≥40 dB for supra-aural earphones).

Cross-hearing will occur when the IA is exceeded and if the pure-tone signal reaching the NTE is greater than the BC threshold of the NTE. In a clinical situation, to determine if cross-hearing might occur, you would compare the presentation

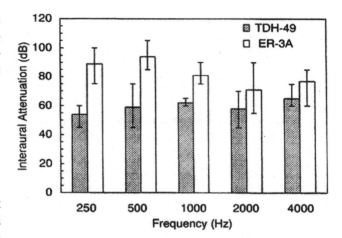

Figure 6–1. Comparison of interaural attenuation values for supra-aural earphones and insert earphones. From Sklare & Denneberg, 1987. From Sklare and Denneberg, 1987, p. 298. Copyright 1987 by Lippincott Williams & Wilkins.

level in the TE, either by AC or BC, to the BC threshold of the NTE. If the difference is greater than or equal to the minimum IA, then masking would be needed in the NTE in order to prevent possible cross-hearing. The reliance on minimum IA values allows one to decide if masking is necessary, but does not necessarily mean that the patient's actual IA is at that minimum level. In fact, most patients will have a higher IA, but we do not know, nor do we want to take the time to know, the IA value for each patient. In many cases, you can see from the unmasked thresholds on an audiogram that the patient's IA is higher than the minimum when you compare the unmasked AC threshold in the TE to the BC threshold in the NTE. For example, if a patient has an unmasked AC threshold in the TE of 65 dB HL and a BC threshold in the NTE of 5 dB HL, that patient's IA is at least 60 dB (and may even be more than 60 dB). However, masking would still be needed since 60 dB is greater than the recommended minimum IA.

---

[1]The IA values for insert earphones are not yet universally accepted or described in any standards. The IA values for inserts can vary depending on depth of insertion and also may be greater in the lower frequencies than in the higher frequencies. The minimum IA of 55 dB for all frequencies when using inserts is a recommendation by this author to provide a reasonable, yet conservative value, and to simplify the concept of masking with inserts by adopting one IA value for all frequencies.

Synopsis 6–1

insert = 55

- Testing the test ear (TE) anytime by BC and at moderate-to-high levels by AC produces vibrations in the skull that can stimulate, through BC, both cochleae.

- Interaural attenuation (IA) is the difference in the level of the test signal (by AC or BC) and the BC of the NTE.

- The recommended minimum IA values for the different transducers are:
  - BC IA (with bone conduction vibrator) = 0 dB
  - AC IA (with supra-aural earphone) = 40 dB
  - AC IA (with insert earphone) = 55 dB

- Cross-hearing can occur when the difference between the presentation level of the test sound in the TE (by AC or BC) and the BC threshold of the NTE exceeds the IA.

- Masking of the non-test ear (NTE) is needed in those conditions where there is the possibility that the tone presented to the TE may be heard through cross-hearing by BC in the NTE.

- For pure-tone threshold testing, one-third-octave narrowband (NB) maskers are used. For speech testing, wider spectrum speech maskers are used.

- Effective masking (EM) is the level of a noise masker that is sufficient to elevate a test sound centered within the specified masker to a specific dB HL (e.g., 50 dB EM will effectively mask out the test sound presented at 50 dB HL). The specific dB SPLs associated with the maskers for 0 dB HL are specified in the ANSI (2004) standards.

- Maskers are always delivered to the NTE by an AC transducer.

- When the threshold in the TE is obtained using masking, it is called the masked threshold. The masker is always presented to the NTE and masker levels are typically specified and recorded on an audiogram relative to the NTE.

Failure to properly use masking may lead to improper description of the type of hearing loss, the severity of the hearing loss, and/or which ear is responding. Audiologists are well trained to recognize the need for masking and the procedures to obtain masked thresholds. The following sections will describe the specific rules that determine when masking is needed for BC and AC.

Rules for When to Mask

If there is the potential for cross-hearing, then the NTE needs to be masked in order to obtain the masked threshold in the TE. To determine when masking is needed, you should compare the presentation level of the test tone in the TE, either by

AC or BC, to the BC threshold of the NTE (i.e., the unmasked BC threshold, which represents either ear). If that difference is greater than the minimum IA for the particular transducer, then masking would be needed in the NTE in order to prevent possible cross-hearing. The general guiding principle for deciding when to mask is:

Anytime the presentation level in the TE, whether by BC or AC, exceeds the minimum interaural attenuation value, the clinician must assume that the test signal can be heard by BC in the NTE and masking must be used.

When to Mask for Bone Conduction

Since there is no IA for BC (IA = 0 dB), you will never know which ear the unmasked BC threshold represents. In fact, the unmasked BC symbol is never ear specific and only represents the side on which the bone conduction vibrator was placed. This becomes problematic whenever there is a difference in hearing between the two ears. Masking is needed for BC whenever one ear has poorer AC thresholds than the other ear because the unmasked BC thresholds could be due to cross-hearing from the better ear (since the IA = 0 dB). Therefore, the rule to use to determine if masking is needed for BC is:

Whenever there is greater than 10 dB difference between the unmasked BC threshold and the AC threshold of the TE (an apparent air-bone gap), masking is needed to rule out the possibility that the BC threshold is coming from the NTE.

In Figure 6-2, some situations are shown that illustrate when BC masked thresholds would be needed as well as when they would not be needed. In Figure 6-2A, there is an air-bone gap in the right ear (poorer ear) when looking at the unmasked BC thresholds compared with the AC thresholds. In this case, you cannot be sure if the BC thresholds are from the right ear (TE) or from the left ear (NTE) and would need to use masking to determine the true BC thresholds for the right ear. The right ear masked BC thresholds could end up be-

ing anywhere from their unmasked levels up to the right ear AC thresholds. Figure 6-2B shows a situation where there are no air-bone gaps for either ear. In this case, masking is not necessary because the BC thresholds should not be any worse than the AC thresholds and the unmasked thresholds represent the lowest threshold possible for each frequency. In other words, when both ears have the same amount of sensorineural hearing loss, BC masking is not needed for either ear because masking will not significantly change the results.

There is another notable exception to the above rule for BC masking as illustrated in Figure 6-2C. In this case, if the masked BC thresholds are first obtained for the poorer ear, and they end up being poorer than the unmasked BC thresholds, the remaining (original) unmasked BC thresholds could only be from the better hearing ear and masking is usually not used even though there is more than a 10 dB air-bone gap. In other words, masking may not be used to obtain the left ear BC thresholds in the example shown in Figure 6-2C. Although this author typically would not mask in this type of situation, some audiologists would mask in order to be more precise, since there may be a small (5 dB) shift in the masked threshold simply due to the presence of noise in the NTE. This small shift is called central masking because it is thought to be due to some unexplained effect from the central nervous system.

When to Mask for Air Conduction

To determine whether you need to obtain masked AC thresholds, you compare the unmasked AC threshold of the TE to the BC threshold of the NTE (i.e., the unmasked BC threshold) for each frequency; if that difference exceeds the minimum IA (55 dB for inserts; 40 dB for supra-aurals), then cross-hearing could occur and masking must be used. Therefore, the rule to use to determine if masking is needed for AC is:

Whenever the difference between the unmasked AC threshold of the TE and the BC threshold of the NTE is greater than or equal to 55 dB (or 40 dB for supra-aural earphones), masking is

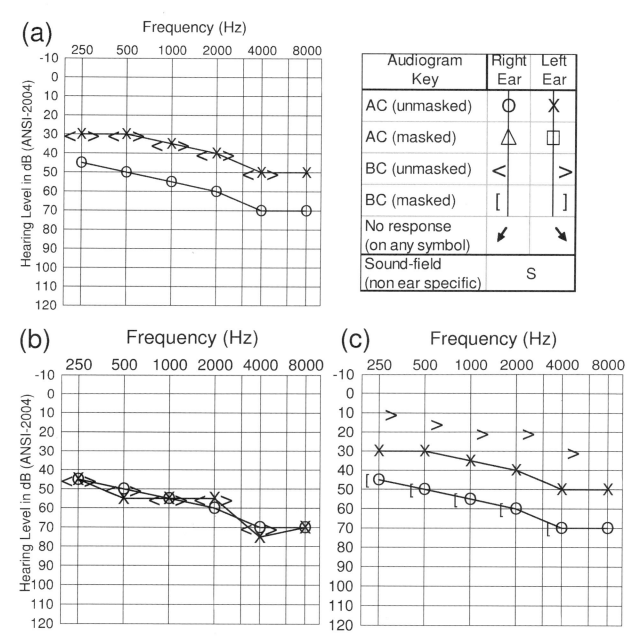

Figure 6–2. A–C. Examples of audiograms demonstrating situations where masking would be needed for bone conduction (*BC*) testing. In **A**, masked BC thresholds need to be obtained for the right ear because of the air–bone gaps. In **B**, masked BC thresholds are not needed because neither ear has an air–bone gap and BC thresholds are not usually any worse than air conduction (*AC*) thresholds. In **C**, the unmasked BC thresholds for the right ear (not shown) would be where the left ear BC thresholds are, and would incorrectly suggest an air–bone gap for one or both of the ears; however, in this case, when masked thresholds are obtained for the right ear they shift downward to the AC thresholds. In this case, even though there are air–bone gaps in the left ear, the unmasked BC thresholds must be from the left ear; therefore, the masked BC thresholds for the left ear need not be obtained.

needed to rule out the possibility that the AC threshold is coming from the NTE (by BC).

Examples Applying the Rules for Masking

Figure 6–3 shows three examples of audiograms with unmasked thresholds. In these examples, you should be able to apply the above rules to decide if any of the thresholds for AC or BC would have to be reestablished using masking. Each example has a table that indicates (+) where masked thresholds would be needed. In addition, each audiogram has an arrow that illustrates the possibilities for the masked thresholds at 1000 Hz. Similar arrows could be placed for all the other conditions that need masking.

In Figure 6–3A, all of the BC thresholds for the right ear need to be reestablished with masking because the unmasked thresholds could be from the left ear by BC (IA = 0 dB). Applying the rule for BC masking, there is more than a 10 dB difference between the right ear AC thresholds and the unmasked BC thresholds. The true BC thresholds for the right ear could be the same as the left ear BC thresholds if there is a conductive hearing loss, could be equal to the right ear AC thresholds if there is a sensorineural hearing loss, or could be anywhere in between the left ear BC thresholds and the right ear AC thresholds if both the conductive and sensorineural portions of the auditory system are involved. The only way to determine the true right ear BC thresholds is to mask the left ear with a noise presented to the left ear (through an earphone) so that the left ear cannot hear the pure tone.

In Figure 6–3B, all of the BC thresholds for the right ear would have to be reestablished with masking because the unmasked thresholds could be from the BC of the left ear BC (IA = 0 dB). In this case, however, there are also some AC thresholds (+) that exceed the 40 dB IA for supra-aural earphones when you compare the AC thresholds for the right ear to the BC thresholds for the left ear. Notice also that the arrows at 1000 Hz extend to the limits for BC (75 dB HL) and AC (120 dB HL) indicating that not much is known about the

hearing loss in the right ear based on the unmasked thresholds.

In Figure 6–3C, there is a potential air–bone gap for both ears. In this case, you would obtain the masked BC thresholds for one of the ears (usually the poorer of the two ears) and, depending on whether the masked thresholds stayed at the same level or not, the other ear may or may not need to be masked (recall the exception to the rule for BC masking). Notice in Figure 6–2C that the AC thresholds for the right ear do not need to be reestablished with masking because insert earphones were used and they have a higher minimum IA (IA = 55 dB). If supra-aural earphones had been used for the case in Figure 6–2C, masking would have been needed for the right ear AC thresholds because the minimum IA equals 40 dB. The higher IA values for an insert earphone are another important advantage over supra-aural earphone because masking for AC is not needed as often.

How to Mask for Air Conduction Thresholds

In this section you will learn how to perform a commonly used method of masking, called the *plateau method*, first described by Hood (1960). There are other masking strategies that can be used (e.g., Turner, 2004), as well as variations of the plateau method that work well if properly applied. There are many other resources on the plateau method that you may also want to consult (Gelfand, 2001; Martin & Clark, 2003; Silman & Silverman, 1991; Studebaker, 1964; Yacullo, 1996).

The objective of masking is to eliminate crosshearing of the NTE by presenting enough masking noise (by AC) to the NTE so that you are confident that the patient's response to the tone is a reflection of what he/she hears in the TE. The plateau method for obtaining AC masked thresholds begins by putting the masker into the NTE at 10 dB HL above the AC threshold of the NTE, commonly referred to as the *initial masking level* (IML). This initial masking level will raise the AC threshold in the NTE by 10 dB HL and will also raise the BC threshold in the NTE by 10 dB HL because

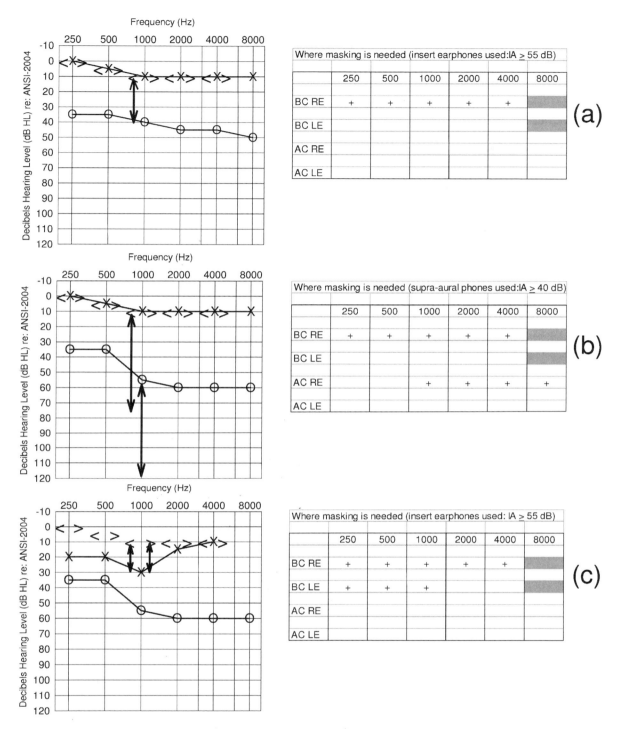

Figure 6–3. A–C. Three examples showing where masking would be needed based on the unmasked thresholds shown in the audiograms on the left. In the tables to the right, a plus (+) is used to indicate those frequencies where air conduction (*AC*) and/or bone conduction (*BC*) must be reestablished with masking. The *vertical arrows* on the audiograms represent the range of possible outcomes for the masked thresholds. In **A** and **C**, insert earphones were used to obtain the unmasked AC thresholds, assuming a minimum interaural attenuation value of 55 dB. In **B**, supra-aural earphones were used to obtain the unmasked AC thresholds, assuming a minimum interaural attenuation value of 40 dB. If insert earphones had been used for **B**, masking would not have been needed for AC testing due to the higher interaural attenuation. The left ear need not be obtained.

167

everything presented by AC affects all parts of the auditory system. With the plateau method, the tester keeps track of the patient's responses to the tone presented to the TE for different levels of masker presented in the NTE until becoming confident that cross-hearing is no longer a factor and the patient's threshold is a true threshold of the TE. The tester is confident that the response to the tone is from the TE when the threshold to the tone in the TE remains constant, called the *plateau*, for a range of increasing masker levels.

Let's look at the example in Figure 6–4, which shows an example of masking for the AC threshold at one frequency (500 Hz). The panel on the left (Figure 6–4A) shows the masking steps on an audiogram, and the panel on the right (Figure 6–4B) shows a masking profile similar to that used by Turner (2004) to track how the test ear threshold changes as a function of the masker level. The masking profile illustrates the relations between initial masking level, minimum masking level, and the plateau that are associated with the steps shown in Figure 6–4A. In clinical practice, audiologists usually keep mental track of where their progress is during the masking process. In Figure 6–4 (for 500 Hz), the difference between the right ear AC unmasked threshold compared with the left ear BC unmasked threshold is equal to the minimum 55 dB IA for insert earphones (60 dB unmasked AC threshold in TE minus 5 dB BC threshold in NTE) and, therefore, the NTE could be responsible for the patient's response to the tone. For this example, the right ear masked threshold needs to be obtained by putting the masker into the left ear. We start our masking process by putting an initial masking level (IML) of 20 dB HL into the left ear by AC. This will elevate the AC threshold in the NTE to 20 dB HL (an increase of 10 dB HL) and will also raise the BC threshold to 15 dB HL (also an increase of 10 dB HL). We then present the tone again to the TE at 60 dB HL (the unmasked AC threshold) to see if the patient still responds. If the original unmasked AC threshold response had been from the NTE, the patient will no longer be able to hear the tone at 60 dB HL with the 20 dB HL masker in the left ear because the difference between the tone presented to the TE and the elevated BC threshold (now 45 dB with masking) is

less than the minimum IA. However, at this point we do not know the patient's TE threshold because the patient no longer hears it at 60 dB HL. The next step is to raise the tone in the TE in 5 dB HL steps until the patient responds. In this example, you should be able to predict that the patient will respond at 70 dB HL because that is where the difference between the level being presented to the TE and the elevated BC threshold will again be 55 dB, thus reaching the minimum IA. But once again, you still do not know whether the response to the tone at 70 dB HL is from the TE or the NTE. The masking process continues by increasing the masker in the NTE by 5 dB HL steps and reestablishing threshold in the TE until sufficient masking has been applied. Masking is sufficient when the response in the TE compared with the elevated BC threshold in the NTE is less than the IA. You will know you have sufficient masking when the masker level is increased several 5 dB steps (e.g., 15 to 20 dB range) and there is no change in the threshold to the tone in the TE, which defines the plateau. For the example in Figure 6–4, after the patient responds at 70 dB HL, the masker is raised to 25 dB HL. The patient then responds to the tone at 75 dB HL (still from NTE?); the masker is raised to 30 dB HL and the patient responds at 80 dB HL (still from NTE?); the masker is raised to 35 dB HL and the patient responds again at 80 dB HL. Notice that, at this step, the threshold to the tone does not change even though the masker has been increased, so you know that you are 5 dB into the plateau. In clinical practice, it is recommended that a 15 to 20 dB plateau be established to be sure the NTE is sufficiently eliminated (some audiologists prefer establishing a 30 dB plateau if possible). In Figure 6–4, the masker is raised to 40 dB HL and the patient again responds at 80 dB HL; the masker is raised to 45 dB HL and the patient still responds at 80 dB HL. At this point, there is only a 40 dB difference between the level of the tone being presented in the TE (80 dB HL) and the elevated BC threshold in the NTE (40 dB HL), which is 15 dB less than the 55 dB minimum IA. We have established a 15 dB plateau and are now done masking for this frequency. It is good clinical practice to indicate on the audiogram the *final masking level* or range of masking levels used to

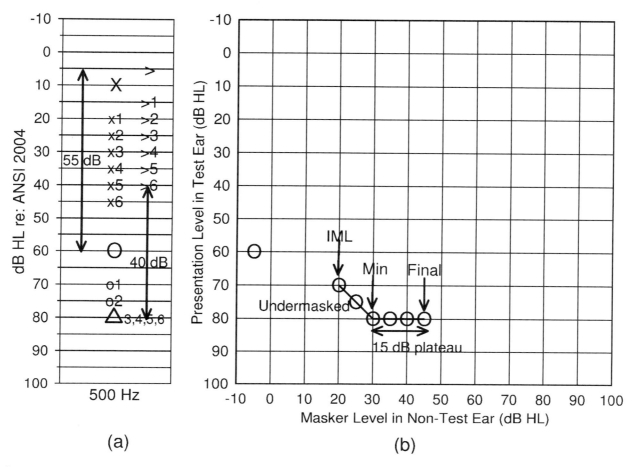

(a)   (b)

Figure 6–4. A and B. An illustration of the plateau method of masking. In this example, right ear unmasked air conduction threshold (*circles*) must be reestablished with masking to obtain the true right ear threshold (Δ). On the left is a representation of the audiogram at 500 Hz and on the right is a masking profile showing how the corresponding air conduction threshold in the test ear (*y*-axis) shifts as a function of masker level (*x*-axis). The *numbered symbols* on the audiogram represent the thresholds for successive masking steps. In this example, the masker is presented by air conduction to the left ear, so x1 represents the initial masking level; >1 is the elevation of the bone conduction threshold due to the x1 masker; and o1 is the air conduction response in the test ear in the presence of the x1 masker. The masking profile on the right shows the initial masking level (*IML*), the point where the plateau begins (*Min*), and the final masking level used (*Final*). The plateau is shown as a horizontal part of the masking profile where the test ear threshold does not change for increases in the masker presented to the non-test ear. On the audiogram portion, the corresponding plateau is indicated with the masked symbol with its corresponding series of masking steps where the threshold did not change (e.g., Δ3,4,5,6).

define the plateau. For this example, we would indicate on the audiogram the masked AC symbol (triangle) and a final masking level of 45 dB HL.

The range of masker levels from the initial masking level to where the plateau begins is called *undermasking* (also called "the chase"). The lowest level of masker on the plateau is called the *minimum masking level* or *change-over point*. A 15 dB plateau is adequate, although the plateau could be widened by adding more steps of masker.

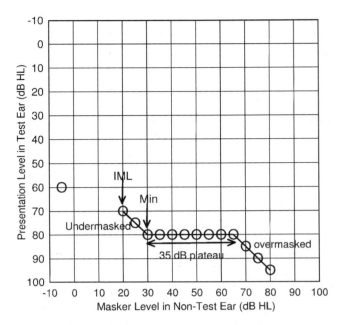

Figure 6–5. An expanded masking profile for the example from Figure 6–4 to illustrate that the plateau can be wider than the recommended 15 to 20 dB as the masker level is increased. When the masker level exceeds the interaural attenuation and is able to be heard in the test ear, overmasking occurs, as shown in the portion of the masking profile beyond the plateau where test ear thresholds again increase as masker level increases. See Figure 6–4 for an explanation on how to interpret the graph's symbols.

Some audiologists prefer to document a 20 to 30 dB plateau using 10 dB steps of the masker. This is shown in the masking profile in Figure 6–5, which is an extension of the example from Figure 6-4. Instead of stopping with a masker level of 45 dB HL, the masker is increased up to 65 dB HL, resulting in a 35 dB plateau. Although this wider plateau is not really necessary, it does illustrate the range of plateaus that you might see used by different audiologists. Of course, you do not want to put too much noise into the NTE, which might be uncomfortable for the patient. However, before we get too far and you think you can just put in as much noise as the patient can tolerate, you must realize that the noise masker itself can cross back

over to the TE if the IA is exceeded. When this occurs, it is called *overmasking,* and the masker will elevate (mask) the threshold to the tone in the TE and give a false threshold. This would always be the case if we were to present the masker by BC. Instead, we use AC transducers to present the masker so there is a range of masker levels (e.g., 55 dB HL for insert earphones; 40 dB HL for supra-aural earphones) that can be used before overmasking will occur. Again, the insert earphone has the advantage over supra-aural earphones because it has a wider range of masker levels possible before overmasking becomes a problem. In the examples given later in the chapter, you will see how overmasking can be a problem in some cases where there is an apparent air–bone gap in the unmasked thresholds for the NTE. Overmasking should never be a problem when there is a sensorineural loss in the NTE.

The main criticism of the plateau method is that in some cases you may go through a few unnecessary steps before arriving at the appropriate level of masking; however, it is better to be cautious with a few extra steps than to end up with the incorrect results, especially when learning how to mask. Once the masking concepts are mastered, you may choose to adopt other strategies to determine the proper amount of masking to put into the NTE. Regardless of which masking method is used, the following must serve as a guiding principle:

Sufficient masking noise must be presented to the NTE by AC in order to elevate the BC threshold in the NTE so that the tone presented to the TE can no longer be heard in the NTE.

To summarize, in order for you to know if the tone being presented to the TE by AC is actually being heard by the TE, you always need to compare the level of the tone being presented by AC in the TE to the BC threshold of the NTE (as elevated with the masker). If that difference is less than the IA, then the response to the tone must be coming from the TE because cross-hearing to the NTE can no longer be occurring. If the difference is equal to or greater than the IA, the response may still be coming from the NTE and more masking noise must be put into the NTE. At each step, the threshold to the tone is reestablished and a comparison is made between TE response level and the increased BC threshold in the NTE to determine if cross-hearing could be occurring. The process continues until cross-hearing is no longer possible. Again, your goal is to put enough masking (by AC) in the NTE so that the NTE cannot hear (by BC) the tone being presented in the TE.

How to Mask for Bone Conduction Thresholds

In general, the same masking procedures that are used for obtaining masked AC thresholds are used for obtaining masked BC thresholds, except the minimum IA value used is 0 dB. In clinical practice, masking for BC thresholds is performed much more frequently than masking for AC thresholds because of the 0 dB IA.

There is, however, an additional consideration that needs to be taken into account when masking for BC thresholds, and that is the *occlusion effect* (OE). When unmasked BC thresholds are obtained, the ear is said to be unoccluded (uncovered). The OE occurs during BC testing as a consequence of placing the AC transducer on/in the NTE, thus occluding the NTE.. The OE results in a noticeable increase in the intensity of low frequency tones presented by the bone vibrator, which translates into an improvement of the BC thresholds compared with the unoccluded condition (Studebaker, 1979; Tonndorf, 1972). You can easily experience the OE by alternately closing off (occluding) and opening (unoccluding) your ear by cupping your hands over your ear or pushing in the tragus while sustaining the vowel "eeee." With the ear occluded, the perceived sound is louder than when the ear is unoccluded. Figure 6–6 illustrates the concepts of the OE during BC testing. The source of the OE is the cartilaginous portion of the external ear canal, which can vibrate even during BC stimulation. When the ear is occluded with a supra-aural earphone (Figure 6–6A), the

sound created by the vibrations of the cartilaginous portion of the ear canal cannot escape the ear as they would in the unoccluded condition; therefore, the BC signal is actually heard louder because these vibrations within the ear canal send a small amount of energy into the ear by AC that combines with the energy created by BC. The OE is primarily of concern when using supra-aural earphones to present the masker to the NTE. An insert earphone, when properly inserted (Figure 6–6B), has a reduced or nonexistent OE because the foam cuff occupies much of the cartilaginous portion of the external ear canal so it does not have the capability of vibrating to the BC sounds (Yacullo, 1996). A reduced OE is yet another advantage of insert earphones over supra-aural earphones. However, the elimination/reduction of the OE with an insert earphone is dependent on its placement (Figure 6–6C). One can always determine the actual amount of any OE for each patient by obtaining BC thresholds unoccluded and occluded.

The OE only affects frequencies 250 to 1000 Hz, and the size of the OE increases as the frequency decreases. The mean OE for a supra-aural earphone varies slightly across studies and one can expect individual differences. Goldstein and Newman (1994) recommend OE values of 15 dB at 250 to 500 Hz and 10 dB at 1000 Hz. Roeser and Clark (2000) recommend 20 dB at 250 Hz, 15 dB at 500 Hz, and 5 dB at 1000 Hz. Yacullo (1996) recommends 30 at 250 Hz, 20 dB at 500 Hz, and 10 dB at 1000 Hz. For the examples in this textbook, the following OE values will be used for the supra-aural earphone:

250 Hz = 20 dB OE

500 Hz = 15 dB OE

1000 Hz = 5 dB OE.

As an audiometric example of the OE, suppose the unmasked (unoccluded) BC threshold at 500 Hz is found to be 20 dB HL. When the BC threshold is retested with the NTE occluded with a supra-aural earphone, but before any masking noise is added, the BC threshold might be improved to 5 dB HL,

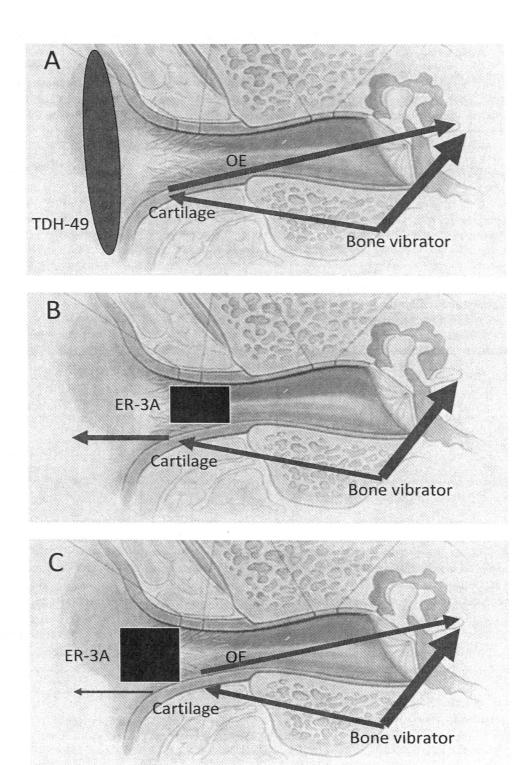

Figure 6–6. A–C. Illustration of the occlusion effect (*OE*). During bone conduction testing some vibrations occur in the cartilaginous portion of the external ear canal that produce some air-conducted energy which may or may not combine with the bone-conducted energy depending on the transducer occluding the ear. **A.** With supra-aural earphone on non-test ear (NTE). **B.** With proper depth of insert earphone in NTE. **C.** With shallow depth of insert earphone in NTE. See the text for explanation.

indicating an OE of 15 dB for that tone. The improvement in threshold is actually because the 20 dB HL BC tone is now equivalent to 35 dB HL due to the extra energy caused by the OE.

So how does one take into account the OE when obtaining masked BC thresholds? Since the occluded BC should have a lower threshold, this will create an artificial air–bone gap which must be taken into account when applying the masking noise. When using a supra-aural earphone to deliver the masker, the IML needs to be increased by the amount of the OE to elevate the BC threshold back to its original (unoccluded) starting point. Therefore, the IML would be presented at 10 dB above AC threshold in NTE, plus the amount of the OE. After correcting the IML for the OE, all of the rest of the masking steps are the same for BC as for AC.

Some audiologists prefer to adopt specific amounts to use for the OE based on average data from the literature; however, the actual size of the OE should be determined for each patient. This can be done by retesting the BC threshold in the occluded condition without masking and comparing it to the unoccluded threshold obtained during BC testing. Once you have the amount of OE, this amount is included in setting the IML. Alternately, you can track the occluded BC threshold in the NTE to decide when enough masking noise has been used to preclude the NTE from responding; both of these methods will require that the noise level be increased by the amount of OE, either at the beginning (IML) or at the end (FML), so that an adequate plateau is established. Also keep in mind that the OE, even with a supra-aural earphone, is offset with any conductive loss because air–bone gaps as little as 20 dB will preclude perceiving the increased intensity caused by the OE (Studebaker, 1979). So, in cases of a conductive loss in the NTE, the OE does not have to be added to the IM; however, enough noise needs to be included to establish an adequate plateau to insure that the NTE BC is sufficiently masked.

Step-by-Step Procedures for Masking with the Plateau Method

The plateau method of masking consists of a series of steps that will meet the above objectives. These steps can be adopted for AC or BC masking by appropriately adjusting for IML (adding in OE for BC masking) and for IA (55 dB[2] for inserts; 40 dB for supra-aural earphone; 0 dB for BC).

1. Present the appropriate NB masker to the NTE by AC at the initial masking level (IML):
   IML for AC testing = AC threshold of
   $\qquad$ NTE + 10 dB;
   IML for BC testing = AC threshold of
   $\qquad$ NTE + 10 dB +
   $\qquad$ occlusion effect (OE)

   Ask yourself: Is overmasking possible? Compare the initial masking level (by AC in NTE) to the BC threshold in the TE to see if it exceeds the minimum IA; if so, overmasking is a possibility. Overmasking is only going to be a possibility in cases where the unmasked thresholds show a moderate air–bone gap in both ears.

   1.1. If overmasking is not a possibility, go to step 2.

   1.2. If overmasking is a possibility, the patient's actual IA may be greater than the minimum IA, so see if you can establish a plateau. Go to step 7.

2. Present the test tone to the TE at the level of the unmasked threshold. Ask yourself: Does the patient respond?

   2.1. If the patient does not respond (and overmasking is not a possibility), you know that the original unmasked response had come from the NTE (by BC), so you are in the undermasking phase and still need to find the TE threshold; go to step 3.

   2.2. If the patient responds, you know that the masker is at the minimum masking

---

[2]This conservative minimum is based on the lowest IA, which occurs at 2000 to 4000 Hz. For lower frequencies, the minimum IA is at least 65 dB. Some audiologists may use IAs higher than 55 dB when considering masking for thresholds obtained with insert earphones.

level and the beginning of the plateau; go to step 4.

3. Raise the test tone in the TE in 5 to 10 dB steps until the patient responds.

   When the patient responds, compare the presentation level in the TE with the elevated (masked) BC threshold in the TE to see if it exceeds the IA or not:

   3.1. If the difference equals or exceeds the IA, the response could still be from the BC of the NTE, so you still need to find the true TE threshold (undermasking phase); go to step 4.

   3.2. If the difference does not equal or exceed the IA, you know that the masker is at the beginning of the plateau; go to step 4.

4. Raise the masker in the NTE by 10 dB HL (could use 5 dB HL, especially when suspecting a small plateau). Go to step 5.

5. Present the tone to the TE at the level where patient previously responded. Ask yourself: Does the patient respond?

   5.1. If the patient does not respond, you know that the previous response was from the NTE, so you still need to find the true TE threshold (still in undermasking phase); repeat steps 3 to 5.

   5.2. If the patient responds, you know that the response is from the TE because the masker has elevated the BC threshold of the NTE so that cross-hearing should not pose a problem. Go to step 6.

6. Repeat steps 4 and 5 until at least a 15 dB plateau has been established; record the TE masked threshold on the audiogram. It is also a good idea to record the maximum noise level (or range of noise levels) in the boxes at the bottom of the audiogram. It should be noted that some audiologists prefer to establish a wider plateau, for example, 20 to 30 dB HL, which is fine as long as overmasking does not occur. Clinically, there is no reason to increase the noise levels beyond what you consider needed to demonstrate an appropriate plateau. There is no need to find the patient's maximum masking levels (unless overmasking is a possibility in step 1).

7. (Use this step only if overmasking was a possibility in step 1): Present tone at the unmasked threshold in the TE. Ask yourself: Does the patient respond?

   7.1. If the patient does not respond, you do not know if the masker is crossing over and elevating the threshold in the TE; this is a masking dilemma. State on audiogram "Could not mask because minimum amount of masking may be overmasking (masking dilemma)."

   7.2. If the patient responds, he or she has an IA greater than the minimum IA and masking may be possible. Go to step 2.2, but keep in mind that the plateau may be narrow; for example, you may only be able to increase the masker by 5 or 10 dB before threshold starts increasing again (overmasking). Remember, there may be a narrower plateau with bilateral air-gone gaps.

Synopsis 6–2

- The rules for deciding if masking is needed are:
  - *BC masking:* Whenever there is more than a 10 dB difference between the unmasked BC threshold and the AC threshold of the TE (air–bone gap), masking is needed to rule out the possibility that the BC threshold is coming from the NTE.
  - *AC masking:* Whenever the difference between the AC threshold of the TE and the BC threshold of the NTE is greater than or equal to 55 dB (or 40 dB for supra-aural earphones), masking is needed to rule out the possibility that the AC threshold is coming from the NTE (by BC).

- Overmasking is the situation in which the level of the masker in the NTE can result in cross-hearing in the TE, thus precluding accurate threshold measures. The same IA values for the AC transducers apply to overmasking.

- Insert earphones have an advantage over supra-aural earphones in that masking is not needed as often because of the greater IA for the insert earphones. The greater IA is related to a smaller surface area of the insert earphone that is in contact.

- A popular method of masking is called the plateau method. This method effectively eliminates the NTE when the patient's response to the TE does not change for a series of increases in the level of the masker in the NTE. When overmasking is not a problem, a plateau of at least 15 dB is recommended; however, some audiologists prefer larger plateaus (e.g., 20 to 30 dB).

- In cases of bilateral conductive hearing loss, only a small (5 to 10 dB) plateau may be possible before overmasking occurs.

- When obtaining BC masked thresholds be cognizant of increasing the level of the lower frequency BC sounds due to the occlusion effect (OE). The OE occurs when placing the AC transducer on the NTE. The source of the OE is vibration of the cartilaginous portion of the external ear canal. The OE is higher with supra-aural earphones than with insert earphones placed at appropriate depth.

- The basic steps for the plateau method of masking include:
  - Present the masker to the NTE at an initial masking level (IML):

    IML for AC testing = AC threshold of NTE + 10 dB;

    IML for BC testing = AC threshold of NTE + 10 dB + occlusion effect (OE)
  - Find patient's threshold to the test sound in the TE for each masker level.
  - Continue process until patient's response to the test sound remains stable for a series of increases in the masker level (the plateau).

- A masking dilemma will occur when the initial masking level causes overmasking.

- Generally, it is better to obtain masked thresholds for the poorer ear first to reduce conditions that may be masking dilemmas.

Masking Examples

In this section, step-by-step instructions are presented to illustrate the plateau method of masking for four different situations. For each of the cases there is a single-frequency audiogram (with both the unmasked and masked thresholds) and a corresponding masking profile, like the one shown in Figure 6–4. Also introduced in these examples is a masking tracking table as part of each figure that the author has found useful to help students learn to apply the plateau method. A blank masking tracking table can be found in the companion workbook should you wish to make copies to practice masking. These examples are not exhaustive of the masking situations that may be encountered in clinical practice; however, they should illustrate concepts that will cover the majority of situations. For more examples and practice see the companion workbook.

The main goal when masking is to be confident that the NTE is not able to hear (by BC) the tone presented to the TE. If a masking plateau is established, this effectively means that the patient's response is no longer a result of the signal being heard in the NTE and represents the true TE threshold. In the following examples, the masker and tone are raised in 10 dB steps. Some audiologists may prefer to increase the masker and tone in 5 dB steps; however, keep in mind that 5 dB increases in masker would be needed when there is an air–bone gap in the NTE because there may only be a narrow plateau before overmasking occurs. It may take some effort to track all of the responses in these examples, but once the concepts are mastered, the steps flow faster when performing the masking on an actual patient. The first example has detailed steps; the subsequent examples are more cryptic (i.e., contain less explanation).

Example 1: Air Conduction Masking Resulting in a Worse Masked Threshold Than the Unmasked Threshold (from the NTE)

As Figure 6–7 shows, the unmasked right ear AC threshold, when compared with the unmasked BC, is greater than the minimum IA for supraaural earphones; therefore, the right ear masked threshold needs to be obtained. In this example, you can see that the final masked threshold (triangle) has worsened when compared with the unmasked right ear threshold (circle); therefore, you know that the unmasked right ear response was coming from the NTE (by BC) because the minimum IA was exceeded. The following steps would have been used to establish the masked right ear threshold. These steps correspond to

the information provided in the masking tracking table, and the undermasking and plateau can be seen in the masking profile. Note that the masker and tone are increased in 10 dB increments, and a 20 dB plateau is obtained.

1. IML = 10 dB HL (0 dB right ear AC threshold + 10 dB). This elevates the AC and BC threshold in the NTE to 10 dB HL.
2. Overmasking is not a possibility (10 dB of noise to 0 dB BC of TE <40 dB IA).
3. Present the tone to TE by AC at 50 dB HL (original unmasked threshold). Patient does not respond. This tells you that the RE AC unmasked response had been from the NTE (by BC).
4. Increase the tone in TE to 60 dB HL (noise still at 20 dB HL). Patient responds. Ask yourself: Could it be from NTE? In this case, the answer is "yes," because the difference between the presentation level of the tone in the TE when compared with the 10 dB BC masked threshold in NTE is 50 dB HL, which is not less than the patient's IA. You are in the undermasking phase.
5. Increase the masker to 20 dB HL; present the tone to TE at 60 dB HL. Patient does not respond. This tells you that the response the patient previously gave at 60 dB HL had been from the NTE (by BC).
6. Increase the tone in TE to 70 dB HL (noise still at 20 dB HL). Patient responds. Ask yourself: Could it be from NTE? In this case, the answer is again "yes," because the difference between the presentation level of the tone in the TE when compared with the 20 dB BC elevated threshold in NTE is 50 dB HL, which is not less than the patient's IA. You are still in the undermasking phase.
7. Increase the masker to 30 dB HL; present the tone to TE at 70 dB HL. Patient does not respond. This tells you that the previous response the patient gave at 70 dB HL had been from the NTE (by BC).
8. Increase the tone to 80 dB HL. Patient responds. Ask yourself: Could it be from NTE? In this case, the answer is again "yes," because

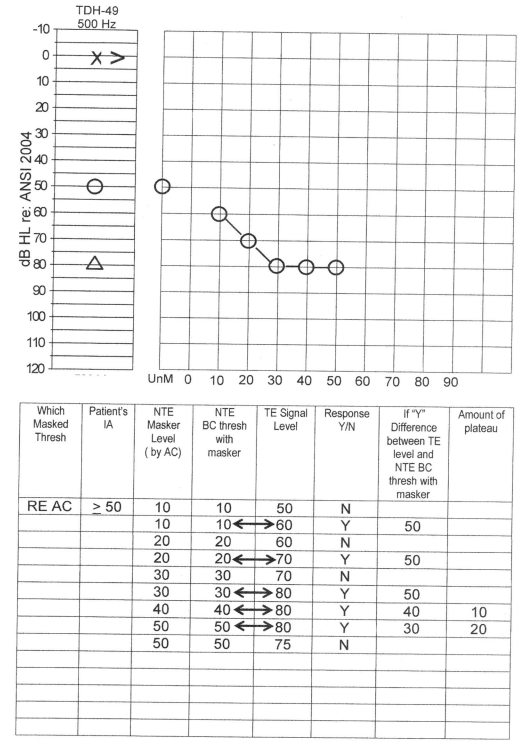

Which Masked Thresh	Patient's IA	NTE Masker Level (by AC)	NTE BC thresh with masker	TE Signal Level	Response Y/N	If "Y" Difference between TE level and NTE BC thresh with masker	Amount of plateau
RE AC	≥ 50	10	10	50	N		
		10	10 ⟷ 60		Y	50	
		20	20	60	N		
		20	20 ⟷ 70		Y	50	
		30	30	70	N		
		30	30 ⟷ 80		Y	50	
		40	40 ⟷ 80		Y	40	10
		50	50 ⟷ 80		Y	30	20
		50	50	75	N		

Figure 6–7. An illustration of the plateau method of masking used to establish the masked air conduction (*AC*) threshold for the right ear (*RE*). In the single-panel audiogram (*top left*), it can be seen that the true RE AC threshold (Δ) is worse than the unmasked threshold (*circle*). The masking profile (*top right*) along with the masking tracking table (*bottom*) illustrate the steps used to establish the masked threshold. See text for a description of the steps used in this example. **IA**, interaural attenuation; **NTE**, non-test ear; **TE**, test ear.

the difference between the presentation level of the tone in the TE when compared with the 30 dB BC elevated threshold in NTE is 50 dB HL, which is not less than the patient's IA. You are still in the undermasking phase.

9. Increase the masker to 40 dB HL; present the tone to TE again at 80 dB HL. Patient responds. Ask yourself: Could it be from NTE? In this case, the answer is "no," because the difference between the presentation level of the tone in the TE when compared with the 40 dB BC elevated threshold in NTE is now only 40 dB HL, which is less than the patient's IA. You now have a 10 dB plateau.

10. Increase the masker to 50 dB HL; present the tone to TE again at 80 dB HL. Patient responds. Ask yourself: Could it be from NTE? In this case, the answer is again "no," because the difference between the presentation level of the tone in the TE when compared with the 50 dB BC elevated threshold in NTE is now only 30 dB HL, which is less than the patient's IA. You now have a 20 dB plateau. If a wider plateau is desirable, then increase the noise again and retest the tone.

11. Because this example used 10 dB increases in the tone to the TE as each step, it is possible that the patient's threshold in 5 dB lower; therefore, present the tone to the TE at 75 dB HL to see if the patient responds or not. If so, 75 dB HL is their masked threshold; if not, 80 dB HL is their masked threshold.

12. Mark the masked right ear AC threshold at 80 dB HL and record a final masking level of 50 dB HL.

In summary, this is a case in which the unmasked RE AC threshold was not the true threshold, but instead was due to cross-hearing in the NTE. This became obvious when the original RE AC BC threshold of the TE had to be raised when masking was introduced to the NTE at the IML. After that point, the process was a repeated series of steps of increasing the masker, then increasing the tone, in 10 dB steps until the TE threshold remains stable for increases in the masker (plateau). Plateaus of 15 to 30 dB could have been established in this example.

Example 2: Bone Conduction Masking Resulting in a Sensorineural Loss

In Figure 6–8, the unmasked thresholds indicate a potential air-bone gap greater than 10 dB in the left ear, which means that the left ear BC threshold must be reestablished with masking. In this example, the patient actually has a moderate sensorineural hearing loss in the left ear. Because the left ear BC threshold will shift to the left ear AC threshold, there are several repeated steps (undermasking phase) until the plateau is established. The following steps are used to establish the masked BC threshold for the left ear. These steps can be observed in Figure 6–8.

1. IML = 60 dB HL (35 dB HL right ear AC threshold + 10 dB + 15 dB OE). This elevates the BC threshold in the NTE to 45 dB HL.

2. Overmasking is not a possibility (60 dB noise to 35 dB BC of TE <40 dB IA).

3. Present tone to TE at 35 dB HL (original unmasked threshold). Patient does not respond.

4. Increase tone in TE to 45 dB HL. Patient responds. Ask yourself: Could it be from NTE? In this case, the answer is "yes," because the elevated (masked) BC threshold in NTE is also at 45 dB HL.

5. Increase masker in 70 dB HL; present tone to TE at 45 dB HL. Patient does not respond.

6. Increase tone in TE to 55 dB HL. Patient responds. Ask yourself: Could it be from NTE? In this case, the answer is "yes," because the elevated BC threshold in NTE is also at 55 dB HL.

7. Increase masker to 80 dB HL; present tone to TE at 55 dB HL. Patient responds. Ask yourself: Could it be from NTE? In this case, the answer is "no," because the difference between the presentation level of the tone in the TE when compared with the 65 dB BC elevated threshold in NTE is now −10 dB (which is less than 0 dB minimum IA). You now have a 10 dB plateau. Notice here that the LE BC threshold is the same as the left ear AC threshold. Since BC is usually not poorer than AC, you know that you have probably reached the true BC

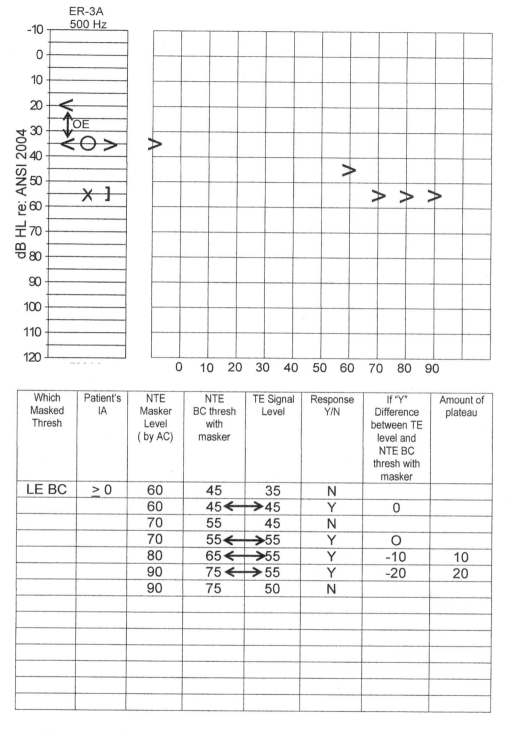

Which Masked Thresh	Patient's IA	NTE Masker Level (by AC)	NTE BC thresh with masker	TE Signal Level	Response Y/N	If "Y" Difference between TE level and NTE BC thresh with masker	Amount of plateau
LE BC	≥ 0	60	45	35	N		
		60	45 ⟷ 45		Y	0	
		70	55	45	N		
		70	55 ⟷ 55		Y	O	
		80	65 ⟷ 55		Y	-10	10
		90	75 ⟷ 55		Y	-20	20
		90	75	50	N		

Figure 6–8. An illustration of the plateau method of masking used to establish the masked bone conduction (*BC*) threshold for the left ear (*LE*). In the single-panel audiogram (*top left*), it can be seen that the true LE BC threshold (*]*) is worse than the unmasked threshold and shifts down to the left air conduction (*AC*) threshold (*X*) showing a sensorineural loss for the LE. The occlusion effect (*OE*) is also indicated on the audiogram. The masking profile (*top right*) along with the masking tracking table (*bottom*) illustrate the steps used to establish the masked threshold. See the text for a description of the steps used in this example. **IA**, interaural attenuation; **NTE**, non-test ear; **TE**, test ear.

threshold for the left ear; however, it is good practice to establish a plateau to account for any variability.

8. Increase masker to 90 dB HL; present tone to TE again at 55 dB HL. Patient responds. Ask yourself: Could it be from NTE? In this case, the answer is "no," because the difference between the presentation level of the tone in the TE when compared with the 75 dB BC elevated threshold in NTE is now −20 dB (which is less than 0 dB minimum IA). You now have a 20 dB plateau.

9. Present tone to TE at 50 dB HL since this level was skipped using the 10 dB increments. If they respond at 50 dB HL that is their threshold. If they do not respond at 50 dB HL, their threshold is 55 dB HL.

10. Mark the masked left ear BC threshold at 55 dB HL and record a final masking level of 90 dB HL.

In summary, this is a case in which the unmasked BC threshold was not the true left ear BC threshold. This became obvious when the original BC threshold of the TE had to be raised when masking was introduced to the NTE at the IML. From this point, the process is a repeated series of steps of increasing the masker, then tone, in 10 dB steps until the TE threshold remains stable for increases in the masker (plateau). A 30 dB plateau was obtained in this example, although a 20 dB plateau would have been sufficient.

Example 3: Bone Conduction Masking Resulting in a Conductive Loss

In Figure 6–9, the unmasked thresholds indicate a potential air–bone gap greater than 10 dB in the left ear, which means that the left ear BC threshold must be re-established with masking. In this example, the patient actually has a conductive hearing loss in the left ear. Because the left ear masked BC threshold is the same as the unmasked BC threshold (no undermasking/chase phase), there are fewer steps needed to establish the masked thresholds than in the previous example. The fol-

lowing steps are used to establish the masked BC threshold for the left ear. These steps can be observed in Figure 6–9.

1. IML = 35 dB HL (10 dB HL right ear AC threshold + 10 dB + 15 dB OE). This elevates the BC threshold in the NTE BC to 20 dB HL.

2. Overmasking is not a possibility (35 dB noise to 10 dB BC of TE <40 dB IA).

3. Present the tone to TE at 10 dB HL (original unmasked threshold). Patient responds. Ask yourself: Could this be from NTE? In this case, the answer is "no," because the elevated (masked) BC threshold in the NTE has been elevated to 20 dB HL, so the response at 10 dB HL is most likely from the TE. In this case, the IML already represents a 10 dB plateau since there was no shift in the original threshold with the masker 10 dB above the NTE threshold. The following additional steps are added to establish a wider plateau to account for any variability.

4. Increase the masker to 45 dB HL; present the tone to TE at 10 dB HL. Patient responds again. Ask yourself: Could it be from NTE? Again, the answer is "no," because the elevated (masked) BC threshold in the NTE is at 30 dB HL. You now have a 20 dB plateau.

5. Increase the masker to 55 dB HL; present the tone to TE at 10 dB HL. Patient responds again. Ask yourself: Could it be from NTE? Again, the answer is "no," because the elevated BC threshold in NTE is at 40 dB HL. You now have a 30 dB plateau.

6. Mark the masked left ear BC threshold at 10 dB HL and record a final masking level of 55 dB HL (if ending with a 30 dB plateau).

In summary, this is a case in which the original unmasked threshold was actually the true left ear BC threshold. This became obvious when the original BC threshold of the TE did not shift when masking was introduced to the NTE at the IML. At that point, you already had a 10 dB plateau. The process can continue by adding one or two additional steps of noise to widen the plateau. In this case, a 30 dB plateau was established, although a 20 dB plateau would have been sufficient.

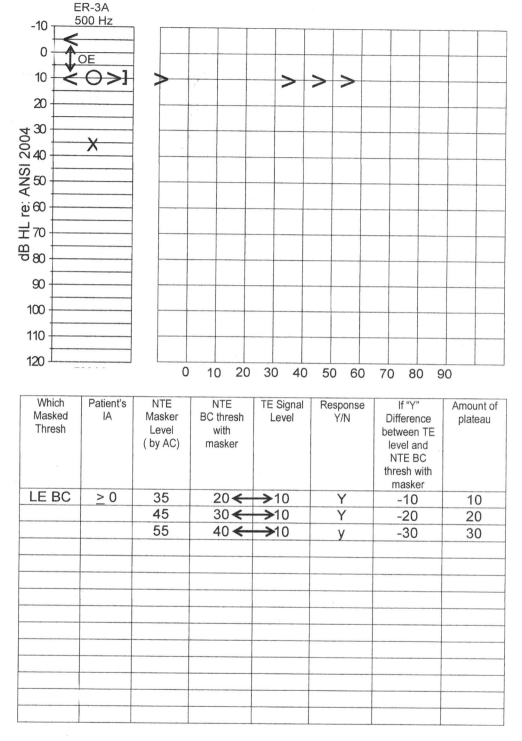

Which Masked Thresh	Patient's IA	NTE Masker Level (by AC)	NTE BC thresh with masker	TE Signal Level	Response Y/N	If "Y" Difference between TE level and NTE BC thresh with masker	Amount of plateau
LE BC	≥ 0	35	20 ←→10		Y	-10	10
		45	30 ←→10		Y	-20	20
		55	40 ←→10		y	-30	30

Figure 6–9. An illustration of the plateau method of masking used to establish the masked bone conduction (*BC*) threshold for the left ear (*LE*). In the single-panel audiogram (*top left*) it can be seen that the true LE BC (*]*) is the same as the unmasked threshold (>), which indicates a conductive hearing loss. The occlusion effect (*OE*) is also indicated on the audiogram. The masking profile (*top right*) along with the masking tracking table (*bottom*) illustrate the steps used to establish the masked threshold. See the text for a description of the steps used in this example. **IA**, interaural attenuation; **NTE**, non-test ear; **TE**, test ear.

Example 4: Masking Dilemma

In Figure 6–10, the unmasked thresholds indicate the possibility of a bilateral conductive hearing loss. In this example, one cannot be sure of which ear the AC or BC thresholds represent. One only knows that at least one of the ears has an AC threshold at the unmasked level and that the other ear could be the same or worse. The unmasked BC thresholds also indicate that at least one ear has BC threshold at the unmasked level and the other ear could be the same of worse, and one does not know the type of hearing loss in the poorer ear. In fact, this patient could have a profound sensorineural hearing loss in the poorer ear. To be able to answer these questions, masked thresholds must be obtained; however, as we will see, masked AC or BC thresholds cannot be obtained in this example due to a masking dilemma. In this type of situation, before concluding that it is a masking dilemma, masking is attempted using 5 dB increases in masker and tone in case a small plateau can be obtained. In this example, the steps would be the same for each ear. The first set of steps would be used to attempt to establish the masked AC thresholds for the left ear or right ear. The second set of steps would be used to attempt to establish the masked BC thresholds for the left or right ear. Both sets of steps (for either ear) can be observed in Figure 6–10.

For AC masked thresholds:

1. IML = 60 dB HL (55 dB HL right ear AC threshold + 5 dB). This elevates the BC threshold in NTE to 15 dB HL.
2. Overmasking is a possibility (65 dB HL to 0 dB BC of TE >45 dB IA) when using supra-aural earphones. The use of an insert earphone may allow a small plateau. When there is a possibility of overmasking you should always attempt masking because the patient may have a higher IA than appears from the unmasked thresholds, but be suspicious of a possible masking dilemma.
3. Present tone to TE at 55 dB HL (original unmasked threshold). Patient does not respond.

Note that if the patient had responded at this level, you may have the beginning of a small plateau.

4. Increase tone to 60 dB HL. Patient responds. Ask yourself: Could it be from NTE? In this case, the answer is "yes," because the difference between the presentation level of the tone in the TE when compared with the 15 dB BC masked threshold in NTE is 45 dB HL, which is not less than the patient's IA (45 dB). At this point, you are essentially in a masking dilemma; however, you should try a couple more steps to be sure a plateau cannot be established.
5. Increase masker to 65 dB HL; present tone to TE at 60 dB HL. Patient does not respond.
6. Increase tone to 65 dB HL. Patient responds. Ask yourself: Could it be from NTE? In this case, the answer is again "yes," because the difference between the presentation level of the tone in the TE when compared with the 20 dB BC masked threshold in NTE is still 45 dB HL, which is not less than the patient's IA.
7. Increase masker to 70 dB HL; present tone to TE at 20 dB HL. Patient does not respond.
8. Increase tone to 70 dB HL. Patient responds. Ask yourself: Could it be from NTE? In this case, the answer is again "yes," because the difference between the presentation level of the tone in the TE when compared with the 25 dB BC masked threshold in NTE is 45 dB HL, which is not less than the patient's IA. The same pattern would continue and never establish a plateau.
9. Indicate on the audiogram that "the initial masking may be overmasking (masking dilemma)." In this case, you cannot determine the true AC threshold for either ear. You can state that at least one ear has that degree of hearing loss, but you do not know which ear, and you do not know the degree of hearing loss in the other ear.

For BC masked thresholds:

1. IML = 60 dB HL (55 dB HL right ear AC threshold + 5 dB + 0 dB OE). This elevates the BC

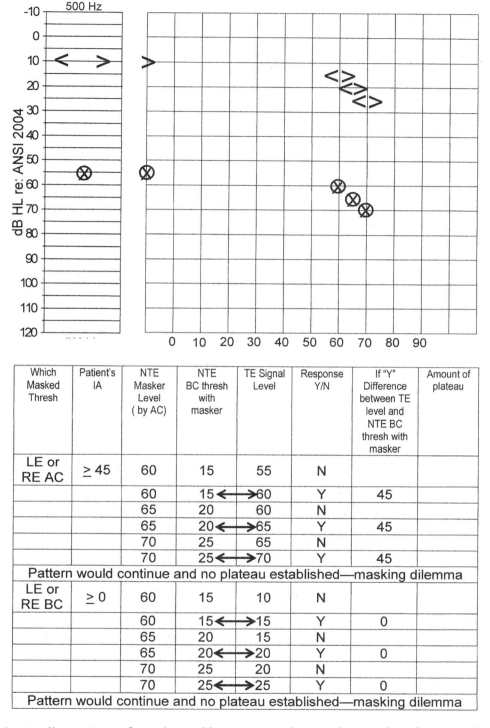

Which Masked Thresh	Patient's IA	NTE Masker Level (by AC)	NTE BC thresh with masker	TE Signal Level	Response Y/N	If "Y" Difference between TE level and NTE BC thresh with masker	Amount of plateau
LE or RE AC	≥ 45	60	15	55	N		
		60	15 ⟷ 60		Y	45	
		65	20	60	N		
		65	20 ⟷ 65		Y	45	
		70	25	65	N		
		70	25 ⟷ 70		Y	45	
Pattern would continue and no plateau established—masking dilemma							
LE or RE BC	≥ 0	60	15	10	N		
		60	15 ⟷ 15		Y	0	
		65	20	15	N		
		65	20 ⟷ 20		Y	0	
		70	25	20	N		
		70	25 ⟷ 25		Y	0	
Pattern would continue and no plateau established—masking dilemma							

Figure 6–10. An illustration of masking dilemmas. In the single-panel audiogram (*top left*) there is a bilateral moderate, air–bone gap based on the unmasked thresholds. The masking profile (*top right*) along with the masking tracking table (*bottom*) illustrate the steps attempted to establish the masked threshold for right ear (*RE*) or left ear (*LE*) and for air conduction (*AC*) and bone conduction (*BC*). In this example, for any of the thresholds, no plateau can be established, that is, the initial masking level was enough to cause overmasking. See the text for a description of the steps used for AC and BC for this example. **IA**, interaural attenuation; **NTE**, non-test ear; **TE**, test ear.

183

threshold in NTE to 15 dB HL. Notice there is no additional masker added for the OE because of the air–bone gap in the NTE.

2. Overmasking is a possibility (60 dB HL to 10 dB BC of TE >45 dB IA) when using supra-aural earphone. The use of an insert earphone may allow a small plateau.

3. Present tone to TE at 10 dB HL (original unmasked threshold). Patient does not respond. Note that if the patient had responded at this level, you may have the beginning of a small plateau.

4. Increase tone to 15 dB HL. Patient responds. Ask yourself: Could it still be from the NTE? In this case the answer is "yes," because the elevated (masked) BC threshold in NTE is also at 15 dB HL. At this point, you are essentially in a masking dilemma; however, one should try a couple more steps to be sure a plateau cannot be established.

5. Increase masker to 65 dB HL; present tone to TE at 15 dB HL. Patient does not respond.

6. Increase tone to 20 dB HL. Patient responds. Ask yourself: Could it still be from the NTE? In this case the answer is again "yes," because the elevated (masked) BC threshold in NTE is also at 20 dB HL.

7. Increase masker to 70 dB HL; present tone to TE at 20 dB HL. Patient does not respond.

8. Increase tone to 25 dB HL. Patient responds. Ask yourself: Could it still be from the NTE? In this case the answer is again "yes," because the elevated (masked) BC threshold in NTE is also at 25 dB HL. The same pattern would continue and never establish a plateau.

9. Indicate on the audiogram that "the initial masking may be overmasking (masking dilemma)." In this case, you cannot determine the true BC thresholds for either ear. You can state that at least one ear has a conductive loss, but you do not know which ear.

In summary, for situations in which there is a potential bilateral air–bone gap, you should suspect a possible masking dilemma. As you can surmise from Figure 6–10, each time a "yes" was obtained, the difference between the presentation level in the TE when compared with the elevated (masked) BC threshold in the NTE still equaled the patient's IA (45 dB) and you could not conclude that it was for the TE. With additional increases of masker and subsequent increases in TE (AC or BC) threshold, not even a small plateau could be established in this particular case. However, when faced with the potential for a masking dilemma, masking should always be attempted, because the actual patient's IA may be higher than the minimum seen based on the unmasked thresholds. In some cases, a small (e.g., 10 dB) plateau may be established and provide some evidence of the true thresholds. See the companion workbook for more examples with small pateaus. As indicated earlier, in cases where there is a difference in the AC thresholds between the two ears, it is best to try to obtain masked responses from the poorer ear first because the IML would be lower in the better ear, and if the masked BC thresholds of the poorer ear reveal a shift (e.g., sensorineural loss), then the original unmasked BC would represent the other ear and masking would not be needed, thus avoiding any masking dilemma. If you had attempted to obtain masked thresholds first for the better hearing ear, the IML would be more likely to show a masking dilemma. Ultimately, however, you may need to attempt masking in both ears.

References

American National Standards Institute (ANSI). (1996). *American National Standards specifications for audiometers.* ANSI S3.6-1996. New York, NY: Author.

American National Standards Institute (ANSI). (2004a). *American National Standards for audiometers.* ANSI S3.6 2004. New York, NY: Author.

Chaiklin, J. B. (1967). Interaural attenuation and cross-hearing in air-conduction audiometry. *Journal of Auditory Research, 7,* 413-424.

Coles, R. R. A., & Priede, V. M. (1970). On the misdiagnosis resulting from incorrect use of masking. *Journal of Laryngology and Otolaryngology, 84,* 41-63.

Gelfand, S. A. (2001). *Essentials of audiology*. New York, NY: Thieme.

Goldstein, B. A., & Newman, C. W. (1994). Clinical masking: a decision-making process. In J. Katz (Ed.), *Handbook of clinical audiology* (4th ed., pp. 109–131). Baltimore, MD: Williams & Wilkins.

Hood, J. D. (1960). The principles and practice of bone-conduction audiometry. *Laryngoscope, 70*, 1211–1228.

Martin, F. N., & Clark, J. G. (2003). *Introduction to audiology*. Boston, MA: Allyn & Bacon.

Roeser, R. J., & Clark, J. G. (2000). Clinical masking. In R. J. Roeser, M. Valente, & H. Hossford-Dunn (Eds.), *Audiology diagnosis* (pp. 253–279). New York, NY: Thieme.

Sanders, J. W. (1972). Masking. In J. Katz (Ed.), *Handbook of clinical audiology* (1st ed., pp. 111–142). Baltimore, MD: Williams & Wilkins.

Silman, S., & Silverman, C. A. (1991). *Auditory diagnosis: Principles and applications*. San Diego, CA: Academic Press.

Sklare, D. A., & Denneberg, L. J. (1987). Technical note: Interaural attenuation for tubephone insert earphones. *Ear and Hearing, 8*, 298–300.

Studebaker, G. A. (1962). On masking in bone-conduction testing. *Journal of Speech and Hearing Research, 5*, 215–227.

Studebaker, G. A. (1964). Clinical masking of air- and bone-conducted stimuli. *Journal of Speech and Hearing Disorders, 29*, 23–35.

Studebaker, G. A. (1967). Clinical masking of the non-test ear. *Journal of Speech and Hearing Disorders, 32*, 360–367.

Studebaker, G. A. (1979). Clinical masking. In W. F. Rintelmann (Ed.), *Hearing assessment* (pp. 51–100). Baltimore, MD: University Park Press.

Tonndorf, J. (1972). Bone conduction. In J. V. Tobias (Ed.), *Foundations of modern auditory theory* (Vol. II, pp. 197–237). New York, NY: Academic Press.

Turner, R. G. (2004). Masking redux ii: a recommended masking protocol. *Journal of the American Academy of Audiology, 15*, 29–46.

Yacullo, W. S. (1996). *Clinical masking procedures*. Baltimore, MD: Allyn & Bacon.

Zwislocki, J. (1953). Acoustic attenuation between the ears. *Journal of the Acoustical Society of America, 25*, 752–759.

7

Speech Audiometry

After reading this chapter, you should be able to:

1. Describe how to calibrate the speech materials using the VU meter and discuss why this must be done each time testing is performed.
2. Describe how to perform and interpret the speech recognition threshold (SRT) test using two procedures (Downs & Minard, and ASHA).
3. Define what is meant by the speech banana and explain how the different speech sounds are affected by different degrees of hearing loss.
4. Describe how to use a count-the-dots audiogram to help the patient understand his hearing loss and how it might be applicable to differential diagnosis.
5. Describe how to perform a supra-threshold test for word recognition score (WRS) and discuss issues related to selecting the presentation level(s) for WRS testing.
6. Graph performance intensity functions (PI–PB) for cochlear versus 8th nerve disorders and calculate the rollover ratios.
7. Calculate WRS using whole word and phoneme scoring, and determine whether two WRS values are significantly different from each other, or whether a WRS is suggestive of a cochlear or 8th nerve disorder.
8. Describe the Hearing in Noise Test (HINT) and Quick Sentence in Noise Test (QuickSin).
9. Discuss variations that are used for speech testing of children.
10. Perform masking for speech testing when needed.

Speech audiometry is the method used by audiologists to evaluate how well a patient can hear and understand specific types of speech stimuli. As mentioned in the previous chapters, the lowest levels at which we can hear pure tones are not very representative of what we listen to in our real-world environments. Most patients do not begin to notice their hearing loss until they are having trouble understanding speech, or when a family member notices that the person is having trouble communicating. Speech tests provide a formal way to determine the patient's ability to recognize speech, albeit in a controlled environment. Speech audiometry can also contribute to the diagnosis of different hearing disorders. For example, a problem in the cochlea can have a fairly predictable relation between shape of the audiogram and understanding of speech, whereas a problem in the 8th nerve often results in significantly poorer speech recognition than would be suggested by the audiogram. It is not unusual for two persons with identical audiograms to have different degrees of difficulty recognizing or processing speech. Results of speech tests are used to compare and validate pure-tone thresholds, compare recognition ability between the two ears, and/or monitor changes across time. Speech audiometry can also help determine whether a patient is an appropriate candidate for hearing aid use or to compare how a patient performs with different hearing aids or hearing aid settings. Speech audiometry includes two basic types of speech tests: (a) the establishment of a speech threshold and (b) a measure of speech recognition ability performed at a level above the threshold (*suprathreshold*). This chapter describes some of the basic speech tests routinely performed during an audiometric evaluation, and discusses ways to interpret these measures.

Speech Testing Equipment and Calibration

Speech audiometry can be performed using the same comprehensive diagnostic audiometer that is used for pure-tone testing. The speech materials are presented to the patient through the speech channel of the audiometer. Figure 7–1 shows the main components of an audiometer used for speech testing. The speech channel has options for the tester to present the speech materials by talking into a microphone, called *monitored live voice* testing, or by using *recorded speech materials* presented through an externally connected device such as a compact disk (CD) player or computer. Recorded speech materials are generally recommended because of their consistency and ability to be standardized, which improves comparisons across testing sessions or different patients. However, monitored live voice testing is acceptable in situations where flexibility is needed in presenting the speech materials to patients who may need some modifications in the speed of presentation, may have limited vocabularies, or are being assessed for auditory-visual speech perception abilities. The specific procedures and speech materials used for the different speech measures are described within the different types of speech measures presented in the following sections.

The audiometer's speech channel is calibrated to meet the American National Standards Institute (ANSI) standards for normal speech threshold based on the average value from a group of normal hearing listeners, which establishes the reference value for 0 dB HL. Because words and sentences vary in intensity, the ANSI reference

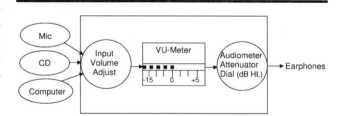

Figure 7–1. Block diagram showing the major components of a clinical audiometer that are used for speech testing. Speech materials can be delivered by microphone (*Mic*), compact disk (*CD*), or computer. The input volume must be adjusted until the volume unit (*VU*) meter peaks at zero so that the audiometer attenuator dial reading (dB HL) is in calibration.

Table 7–1. Air conduction reference values for speech channel corresponding to 0 dB HL (audiometric zero) based on ANSI S3.6 (2004). Air conduction reference values are in dB SPL re: 20 µPa. Expected calibration levels are 12.5 dB above the reference value for a 1000 Hz calibration tone for the respective transducer.

Transducer	Model	1000 Hz	Speech Correction	Calibration dB SPL
Supra-aural phones[a]	TDH-50P	7.5	12.5	20.0
Insert phones[b]	ER-3A	5.5	12.5	18.0

[a]Calibrated with 6-cc coupler.
[b]Calibrated with occluded ear simulator. Values are different for HA-1 or HA-2 couplers (ANSI, 2004).

level for speech testing is calibrated by presenting a 1000 Hz pure tone through the speech channel so that the measured output is 12.5 dB higher than the calibration dB SPL value at 1000 Hz for the appropriate transducer (Table 7–1). The additional 12.5 dB SPL value for speech calibration (above the RETSPL for 1000 Hz) is to compensate for the fluctuations of energy levels inherent in speech material. For recorded speech materials, there is always a calibration tone (1000 Hz) that is played at the beginning of the compact disk that is used to set the calibration.

Whether presenting the speech materials by monitored live voice or by external devices, it is very important to adjust the presentation level of the materials before testing so that they are appropriately calibrated in dB HL. In other words, variations in the level of the tester's voice or the distance from the microphone can alter the level of the signal being delivered to the patient. For recorded materials, the externally connected devices also have their own variable output levels that need to be compensated for so that the audiometer's attenuator dial is an accurate representation of the dB HL being presented to the patient. Adjusting the calibration of the speech channel is a required step each time speech testing is performed, including each time different recorded materials are used. Adjustment of the speech channel is done by monitoring a *volume unit* (VU) *meter*, a meter that is readily visible on the audiometer

(see Figure 7–1). As the materials are being presented, the VU meter has an indicator that fluctuates with the level of the incoming signal. The VU meter has a midpoint labeled 0 dB, which represents the point where the speech channel is in calibration and, therefore, the presentation level of the speech material is equal to the value on the audiometer attenuator dial. The tester can adjust the input volume knob to control the level of the speech material being delivered to the audiometer. The typical VU meter has a range that goes from −20 dB to +5 dB relative to the calibration point at 0 dB. For example, when speech materials are being presented and the VU meter is at −5 dB, it means that the level of the speech materials is 5 dB lower than it should be, and the tester must then adjust the input volume knob by increasing the level by 5 dB in order to peak the VU meter at 0 dB to be at the calibrated output level. When the VU meter peaks at 0 dB, the audiometer attenuator dial is properly calibrated so that 0 dB HL is equal to the dB SPL needed for normal listeners' threshold for speech (ANSI, 2004).

For recorded materials, once the calibration level of the VU meter is set using the 1000 Hz calibration tone, no further adjustments are needed while testing that patient with those specific speech materials; however, the VU meter must be reset to the appropriate calibration tone each time a new patient is tested or a different set of recorded speech materials is used. For monitored live voice testing, the tester must pre-adjust the VU meter by presenting some words and getting the VU meter to peak at 0 dB when a word is presented. The tester must continuously monitor the VU meter throughout the test to ensure that fluctuations in the output level are not occurring.

Speech Threshold Measures

One of the goals of speech audiometry is to find the lowest level at which a patient is able to produce a response to speech stimuli, which is called the *speech threshold*. Speech stimuli are generally more familiar to a patient than pure tones, and in cases where pure tones are not successful or contaminated by false positives or false negatives, speech thresholds may provide the only information about the patient's degree of hearing loss. Some audiologists prefer to start the hearing evaluation with speech measures to get an idea of where to expect the pure-tone thresholds.

The speech threshold is measured on the same dB HL scale as the pure-tone thresholds, and the degree of hearing loss for speech can be described by the same categories used for degree of hearing loss for pure-tone audiometry (see Chapter 5). The frequencies of speech stimuli generally fall within the 300 to 6000 Hz region of the audiogram, and measures of speech thresholds can provide an estimate of the thresholds in those frequencies most important for speech. Keep in mind, however, that the speech threshold is primarily representative of those frequencies where the patient has the best hearing; thus, the speech threshold is not able to predict the shape of the audiogram.

Another important use of the speech threshold is as a cross-check with the pure-tone thresholds. The speech threshold is usually equal to or slightly better than the pure-tone average (PTA), but should be within 10 dB HL of the PTA. If there is more than a 10 dB difference between the speech threshold and the PTA, then a determination of why there is a difference should be explored. When the speech threshold and the PTA do not agree, you should explore the following possibilities:

Could the discrepancy be due to the shape of the audiogram? For steeply sloping audiograms, are there one or two frequencies that could be providing the cues for the speech threshold?

Could the discrepancy be related to limited proficiency in the language or a foreign dialect?

Were the speech materials properly calibrated with the VU meter?

Were the pure-tone thresholds purposely exaggerated or contaminated in some way by response bias? See Chapter 9 for more information on the use of speech threshold for evaluation of exaggerated (functional) hearing loss.

Speech Recognition Threshold

The speech procedure most often used to determine the speech threshold is called the *speech recognition threshold* (SRT).[1] The SRT procedure uses two-syllable compound words, called *spondee words*, that can be presented with nearly equal intensity and/or stress on each syllable, such as railroad, baseball, doormat. The words are presented so that the VU meter peaks at 0 dB for each syllable and there should not be any excessive voice inflection on either syllable. For monitored live voice testing, it takes some practice to be able to properly present the spondee words. The spondee word list most commonly used today for SRT measurement is based on materials developed at the Central Institute of the Deaf (CID). The CID W-1 word list consists of 36 spondee words. The following are some examples of the spondee words from the CID W-1 word list:

---

[1]The term *speech recognition threshold* is preferred over older terms such as *speech reception threshold* or *spondee recognition threshold* (ASHA, 1988).

airplane	iceberg	sidewalk
birthday	mousetrap	stairway
cowboy	oatmeal	sunset
farewell	playground	toothbrush
hardware	railroad	woodwork

Although basic SRT measures are almost always performed with spondee words, sentence materials are also available for speech threshold testing, especially in noise (see Hearing in Noise Test later in this chapter).

The SRT requires the patient to correctly recognize the presented words. The tester varies the presentation level of the words to find the lowest level at which the patient can recognize at least 50% of a series of spondees. Recorded materials or monitored live voice are acceptable for SRT testing and there are no appreciable differences in threshold between the two methods (American Speech-Language-Hearing Association [ASHA], 1988). For SRT testing, the spondee words are usually presented without any preceding *carrier phrase*, such as, "Say the word." Most audiologists use monitored live voice for SRT testing (Martin, Champlin, & Chambers, 1998). There are several different procedures in use for establishing the SRT. Most procedures have the following features in common: (a) spondee words are used, (b) the patient is first familiarized with the list of words at a comfortable listening level and the words not correctly identified are omitted from the test list, (c) a block of words is presented at each level, (d) the increase or decrease in presentation level follows specific rules (and may be different depending on the procedure), and (e) the threshold is the lowest level that estimates the point where at least 50% of the presented words are correctly recognized. Some SRT procedures are *descending methods* in which the words are first presented above a patient's estimated threshold and blocks of words are presented at descending levels. Other SRT procedures are *ascending methods* in which the words are presented below the estimated threshold and the blocks of words are presented at ascending levels. Most SRT methods have an initial phase that quickly searches for an approximation of the patient's threshold and establishes a starting level for the threshold determination. The reason for the initial phase is to save time presenting too many words at levels that are too far below or too far above the patient's actual threshold. The "up 5, down 10" method used for pure-tone threshold testing is used by some audiologists and has been described by Martin and Dowdy (1986); however, this bracketing procedure is not part of any standard or guideline for obtaining an SRT. In the following paragraphs, two different SRT procedures will be described in more detail; an ascending threshold procedure by Downs and Minard (1996) and a descending threshold procedure by ASHA (1988). The interested reader is referred to Chaiklin and Ventry (1964) for an additional descending SRT procedure.

The Downs and Minard Method for Obtaining the SRT

The Downs and Minard (1996) method for obtaining an SRT is a relatively fast and easy procedure to perform, and in their study, the authors demonstrated that their procedure produced results similar to those of other SRT procedures. The following steps are performed for the Downs and Minard SRT procedure (refer also to Figure 7–2A):

1. Familiarize the patient with the spondee words at a comfortable listening level.
2. Instruct the patient that the words may sound very faint and they are to repeat the words back to you.
3. Begin by presenting one spondee at the lowest audiometer setting or at least 30 dB below previously known speech threshold or PTA (or at 0 dB HL if estimate is unknown); continue presenting one spondee at ascending 10 dB steps until the patient repeats a spondee correctly.
4. Decrease the level by 15 dB (to get below threshold again): This is the start level for the ascending threshold search.
5. At the start level and at ascending 5 dB HL steps, present blocks of two, three, or four spondees as needed until patient repeats two spondees correctly: This level is the SRT.

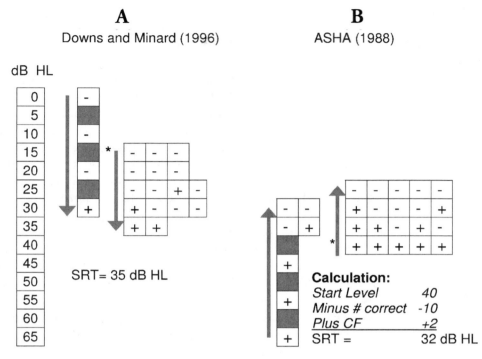

Figure 7–2. Illustration of how speech recognition threshold (SRT) is obtained using **(A)** the Downs and Minard (1996) procedure and **(B)** the ASHA (1988) procedure. The Downs and Minard procedure is an ascending method and the ASHA procedure is a descending method. Both methods have an initial phase to determine the start level for the test phase. The *boxes on the left* of each procedure illustrate the steps to find the start level, and the resulting start level is indicated by the *asterisk*. The *boxes on the right* of each procedure illustrate the threshold search phase. The boxes represent the number of words presented at each level. The *minus signs* represent words not correctly identified and the *plus signs* represent words correctly identified. In this example, the SRT is equal to 35 dB HL using the Downs and Minard procedure and 32 dB HL using the ASHA procedure. See text for explanation of both procedures. **CF**, correction factor.

Notice that this procedure does not require all four words to be presented at any level. The level is increased by 5 dB HL whenever there is no longer the possibility that the patient could get two out of the possible four correct. For example, if he or she misses the first three words, there is no longer the possibility that he or she could get two out of four correct, so the level would be raised by 5 dB HL and a new block of words presented. On the other hand, if he or she gets one of the first three words correct, then the fourth word must be presented to see if he or she could get two out of four correct (50%). On the rare occasion when the patient gets two correct at the original start level, the start level is reduced by 10 dB HL and the procedure begins at the new start level.

The ASHA Method for Obtaining the SRT

The ASHA (1988) method for obtaining SRT presents blocks of five words at each level, descending from the lowest level at which the patient responds to 100% of the words down to the level where she or he responds to 0% of the words. The SRT representing the 50% correct level is interpolated using statistical principles and requires a quick calculation after completion of the test to determine the SRT. The following steps are performed for the ASHA SRT procedure (refer also to Figure 7–2B):

1. Familiarize the patient with the spondee words at a comfortable listening level.
2. Instruct the patient that the words may sound very faint, and he is to repeat the words back to you.
3. Begin by presenting one spondee at 30 to 40 dB above the patient's previously known speech threshold or PTA (or 50 dB HL if estimate is unknown); continue presenting one spondee at descending 10 dB HL steps until the patient misses the spondee . At that level present a second spondee and, if necessary, continue to decrease in 10 dB steps until two spondees are missed at a single level.
4. Increase the level by 10 dB (to get above threshold again): This is the start level for the descending threshold search.
5. Present blocks of five spondees at the start level and then at descending 5 dB steps, keeping track of how many spondees are correctly identified and how many are not correctly identified for each block of five spondees at each level. If the patient does not get five out of the first six spondees, the start level should be increased by 10 dB and the process repeated.
6. Continue descending in 5 dB steps until the patient misses all five spondees.
7. The SRT is equal to the start level, minus the number correct across all blocks, plus a 2 dB correction factor (start level–number correct + 2). The ASHA procedure can also be done using 2 dB descending steps with two spondees

presented at each level and applying a 1 dB correction factor.

Speech Detection Threshold

A *speech detection threshold* (SDT), sometimes referred to as a *speech awareness threshold* (SAT), is a speech threshold measure that determines the lowest level at which a patient can simply detect speech rather than correctly recognizing the speech. The SDT is usually 5 to 10 lower than the SRT because the SDT only depends on the patient reacting to the most audible frequency of the presented word. The SDT is only used when an SRT cannot be obtained, such as with adults with severe to profound hearing loss, young children, patients with speech or language impairments, or physically/mentally challenged patients. The choice of speech materials for obtaining a SDT is not that critical; they can be familiar two-syllable words, such as "hello," familiar phrases such as "Can you hear me?," nonsense syllables such as "ba ba ba," continuous discourse such as reading a passage, and/or spondee words. Familiarizing the patient to the speech is also not required when obtaining a SDT. Generally, the intensity of the speech is adjusted in an ascending direction from below threshold until the patient responds in some instructed manner (raises hand) or by using a head-turn visual reinforcement audiometry VRA procedure. The SDT can also be established with some bracketing procedure, such as the up 5, down 10 method used for pure-tone thresholds (ASHA, 1988). When considering the SDT as a cross-check with PTA, one must take into account whether there is good agreement with the best frequency threshold between 250 and 4000 Hz. If the SDT is more than 20 dB lower than the average of the best two-frequency average, then either measure should be suspect and the discrepancy should be resolved (Brandy, 2002). When the SDT is obtained instead of the SRT, it should be clearly indicated and reported on the audiogram report, and the type of speech stimuli used should also be specified. The SDT is a poor indication of the shape of a person's hearing loss, as it only reflects the best hearing frequency.

Synopsis 7–1

- Speech audiometry is part of the basic audiologic evaluation. Speech tests are used to validate pure-tone results, compare speech abilities between the two ears, monitor changes over time, and as a measure of hearing aid suitability and/or performance.

- Speech testing is performed by selecting appropriate options from the clinical audiometer. Speech materials can be presented by monitored live voice (MLV) through a microphone circuit, recorded materials through a compact disk (CD), or digitally generated by computer, all of which can be interfaced with the audiometer. Recorded or computer-generated materials should be used whenever possible.

- To compensate for variations in voice level at the microphone or output settings on the CD player, the tester must preset the level being delivered to the patient by making volume adjustments through peaking a VU meter at zero, the point at which the speech channel is in calibration. This must be done for each patient and for each test to ensure that the dB HL reading displayed on the intensity dial represents the correct output level. In addition, annual electroacoustic calibrations of the speech channel must be performed in order to conform to the ANSI standard for speech, which is 12.5 dB SPL higher than the ANSI standard for a 1000 Hz pure tone for each transducer.

- One of the basic speech measures is the determination of a speech recognition threshold (SRT). This test uses common two-syllable words called spondees. The patient is first familiarized with the words at a comfortable listening level and then the spondee threshold is established. While there are several methods in use for determining the SRT, the Downs and Minard (1996) procedure or the ASHA (1988) procedure is recommended by this author. In the Downs and Minard procedure, begin 30 dB below the estimated threshold or at the lowest level on the audiometer and give one spondee at each 10 dB increment until the patient gets one spondee correct: Decrease 15 dB and then give two, three, or four spondees at each 5 dB increment until the patient gets two spondees correct; this level is the SRT.

- For those patients for whom the SRT test is too difficult, a speech detection threshold (SDT) can be obtained. The SDT is only a test of the lowest level at which the patient detects speech and does not require recognition. The SDT is usually obtained using and ascending procedure and/or applying the up 5, down 10 threshold search procedure similar to pure-tone threshold testing. The SDT reflects the patient's best pure-tone threshold and does not provide much information about the shape of the audiogram or the ability to recognize speech.

- The primary purpose of the SRT or SDT is to cross-check with the pure-tone thresholds when they are available or to provide some limited information about hearing thresholds when the pure-tone thresholds are not obtainable.

- The SRT should be within 10 dB of the patient's PTA. If the difference between SRT and PTA is more than 10 dB, it could indicate that the patient is exaggerating his pure-tone hearing loss; however, be sure to rule out the possibility of it being related to the steep slope of the audiogram (compare with a two-frequency PTA), language or dialect issues, or improper peaking of the VU meter.

Suprathreshold Speech Recognition

Although the SRT is useful for describing hearing loss and for cross-checking with the PTA, a threshold for speech is not representative of the levels that people listen to speech in their real environments. People generally listen to speech at a comfortable conversational level or at other suprathreshold levels depending on the situation, and they are often listening to speech in a variety of noisy situations.

Different speech sounds have different intensity and frequency ranges. For example, most vowels are lower in frequency and higher in intensity. Normal conversational level for speech is considered to be about 50 dB HL and is based primarily on the intensity level of the vowels; however, normal variations in the levels of the other speech sounds result in an approximate range of 20 to 50 dB HL for normal conversational level of speech. For a normal hearing listener, 50 dB HL would be about 25 to 50 dB above his threshold (dB SL). Figure 7–3 shows a simplified illustration of how the acoustic features of speech are distributed on the audiogram when spoken at a normal conversational level.

The shaded region in Figure 7–3 represents the range of the speech sounds associated with conversational-level speech. This shaded region is often referred to as the *speech banana* due to its general shape. As a first approximation, the vowels have the highest intensities, and the consonants, especially the fricatives (e.g., /f/, /s/), have the lowest intensities. Keep in mind, however, that the acoustic properties of speech show considerable variations in the frequency content for many of the different speech sounds. Additionally, recognition of speech depends on more than just detecting a specific frequency, such as: (a) recognition of vowels depends on the first and second formants, (b) recognition of some consonants (e.g., /b/ vs. /g/ vs. /d/) depends on the first and second formants of their associated vowels, (c) many voiced consonants and nasals have two or three energy bands, (d) consonant frequencies can vary depending on the preceding and following sounds (coarticulation), and (e) differences occur across talkers, especially across gender.

Figure 7–4 shows an audiogram with the speech banana at a normal conversational level (50 dB HL) for a patient with a mild high frequency hearing loss. In this example, many of the higher frequency components of consonant sounds (e.g., f, s, th, t, z, v), which have relatively low intensity levels, fall below the patient's thresholds. This patient may confuse words, such as *fight* or *sight*. Different degrees of hearing loss will result in different acoustic features being more or less audible to the patient. As shown in Figure 7–5, a patient with a moderately-severe hearing loss would not be able to hear most of the speech sounds when spoken at a normal conversational level. Figure 7–6 shows another example for a patient with a low frequency hearing loss.

Making general comparisons of the patient's thresholds to the speech acoustic information can

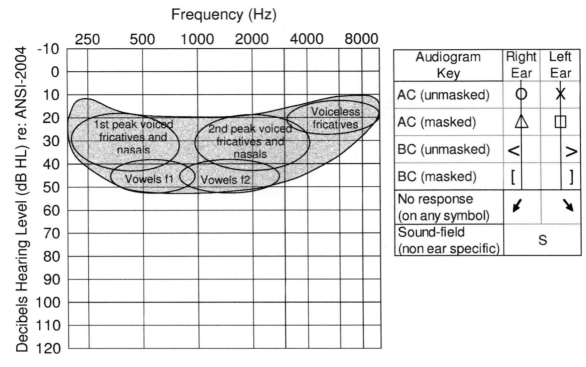

Figure 7–3. A simplified representation of how different types of speech sounds are distributed across the audiogram during average conversational level (50 dB HL). The overall outline is typically referred to as the speech banana.

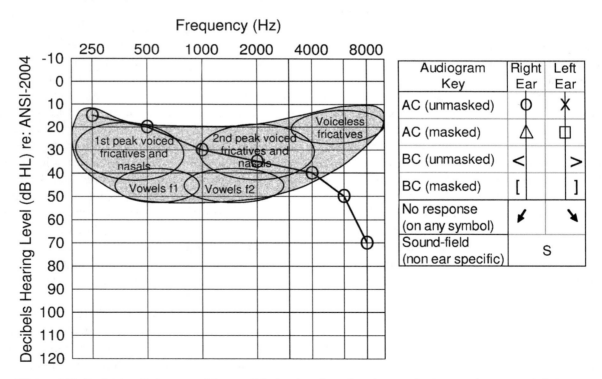

Figure 7–4. An audiogram with a mild sloping hearing loss relative to the speech banana at a normal conversational level (50 dB HL). This patient may hear people talking, but may have some difficulty understanding some words because the high-frequency speech sounds (e.g., fricatives) are inaudible.

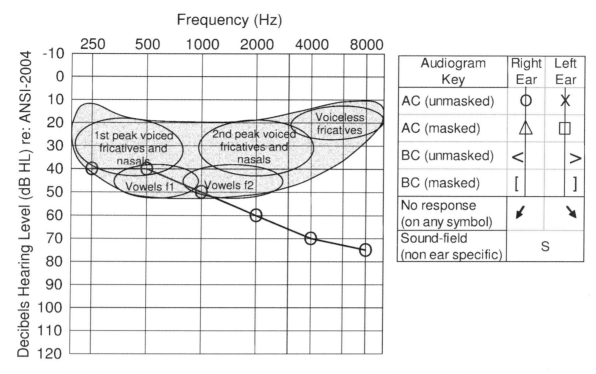

Figure 7–5. An audiogram with a moderate to severe sloping hearing loss relative to the speech banana at a normal conversational level (50 dB HL). Because most of the speech sounds are inaudible, this patient may have a very difficult time understanding conversations at normal levels.

be useful when discussing the hearing loss with the patient so that she or he can get an idea about why he might be having some difficulties understanding what is being said. Figure 7–7 shows a simplified, although less correct, representation of the speech sounds on an audiogram. This type of representation of the speech banana is often included on an audiogram as a simple and easily understood way to explain to a patient what parts of the speech she or he can or cannot hear.

Count-the-Dots Audiogram

As discussed above, it is often helpful to describe to a patient how a hearing loss might be expected to affect his hearing of speech in the real world by using the speech banana on the audiogram. Obviously, this is a very general approach and does not give any quantifiable information. Finding a

systematic way to predict speech understanding based only on the speech spectrum has been the subject of research for quite some time. The earliest attempts to predict overall speech intelligibility was done by Fletcher (1950) and French and Steinberg (1947), and this was known as the *articulation or audibility index* (AI); this was later revised and renamed the *speech intelligibility index* (SII) (ANSI, 1997). The basic principle of the SII lies in the fact that as less of the speech spectrum becomes audible (by external filtering or by the presence of a hearing loss), speech intelligibility gets poorer. In addition, some frequency regions contribute more to intelligibility than others. The different frequencies within the speech stimuli are divided into a number of bands that are given weightings based on their importance to the overall recognition of the speech stimuli. The SII results in a number that ranges from 0.0 (none of the speech acoustic information is available) to 1.0 (all

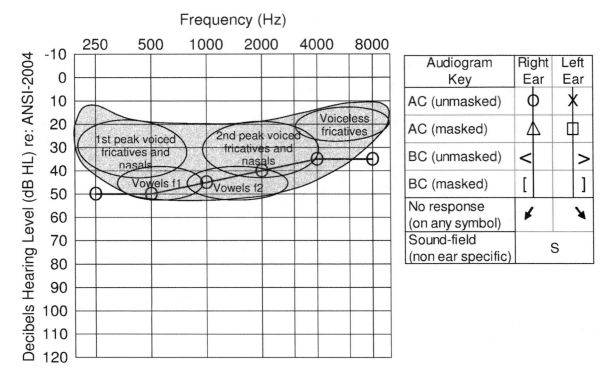

Figure 7–6. An audiogram with a moderate low frequency and mild high frequency hearing loss relative to the speech banana at a normal conversational level (50 dB HL). The patient may barely hear people talking because he is unable to hear the louder vowel sounds, and he may also have difficulty understanding conversation because of the loss of high frequency consonant information.

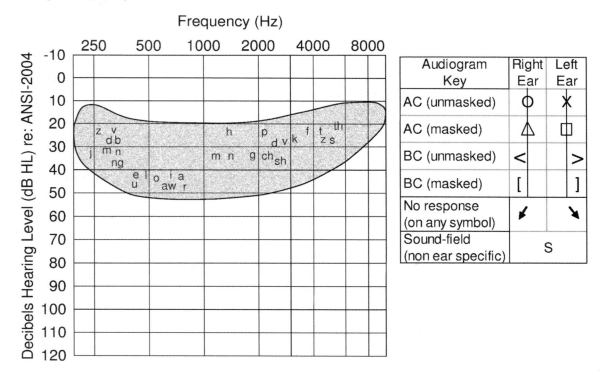

Figure 7–7. A simplified representation of the speech banana on the audiogram for common speech sounds. This format, although not very accurate, is often used by audiologists to convey results to patients.

of the speech acoustic information is available). Actual calculations of the SII take into account a variety of listening conditions and speech parameters, which are put into a complicated mathematical formula to derive a number that represents the amount of speech information that is usable to the listener. Figure 7–8 shows a hypothetical plot of the percent of correct word recognition as a function of the SII value. This illustrates how a normal hearing listener might respond to single-syllable words as the amount of acoustic information is increased or decreased. As you would expect, as the amount of the available acoustic speech information increases, the better the speech recognition. The exact shape of the curve will depend on the type of speech stimuli used and the parameters included in the calculation of the SII.

For clinical purposes, the calculations of the AI or SII in their original forms are much too burdensome. However, clinical versions of the SII

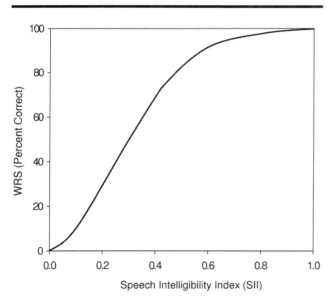

Figure 7–8. An illustration of how the speech intelligibility index is plotted for word recognition score (*WRS*). The curve represents a hypothetical example for normal hearing listeners. As the SII decreases (due to a reduction in usable acoustic information), there is a corresponding decrease in the WRS.

concept have evolved that are much simpler and easier to use to determine how different degrees of hearing loss affect the useable speech acoustic information and how this might predict speech recognition. Essentially, the clinical versions to predict a patient's useable acoustic information assign a weighting to the audiometric frequencies that reflect their contribution to the overall importance to speech recognition. These weightings are represented on an audiogram as dots, known as a *count-the-dots audiogram*. Those frequencies that have a greater contribution to speech recognition have more dots. Figure 7–9A shows an example of a count-the-dots audiogram developed by Humes (1991). In this illustration, there are 33 dots distributed across the frequencies 250, 500, 1000, 2000, and 4000 Hz, with a higher number of dots representing a higher weighting for speech recognition. For example, there are more dots at 2000 and 4000 Hz than at lower frequencies. For the hearing loss shown in Figure 7–9A, the SII would be estimated by counting the dots that occur higher than the patient's thresholds and multiplying by 0.03 (21 dots × 0.03 = 0.63). Other versions of the count-the-dots audiograms differ primarily in how they assign the weightings and/or how many dots are included (e.g., Mueller & Killion, 1990).

A slightly different approach for clinically estimating the patient's useable acoustic information was described by Pavlovic (1988), as shown in Figure 7–9B. In this approach, instead of using dots to represent the speech spectrum, the speech area is defined by a range of intensity levels in normal speech as it relates to the speech spectrum at 500, 1000, 2000, and 4000 Hz. This method assumes that normal speech has 30 dB of intensity range available at each of the four frequencies, resulting in a total of 120 dB of speech intensity information available across these four speech frequencies. The SII is calculated by dividing the audible portion of the speech spectrum by 120 dB. For the same hearing loss as in Figure 7–9A, using the Pavlovic method, you would estimate the SII by adding up how many decibels are above the patient's threshold and divide by 120 dB (80 divided by 120 = 0.66). The count-the-dots audiogram and the speech spectrum audiogram are convenient ways to provide feedback to the patient

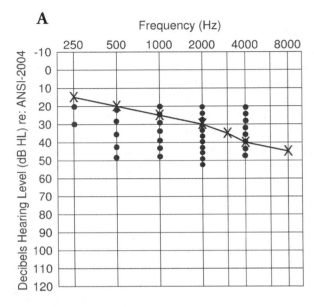

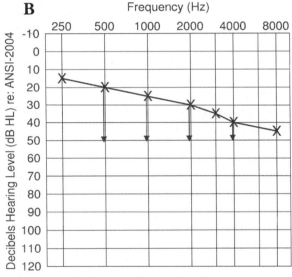

Figure 7–9. A. A count-the-dots simplification of the speech intelligibility concept as developed by Humes (1991). The speech information is divided, in a weighted fashion, across the audiogram by 33 dots. Each dot contributes 3% to the intelligibility (33 dots × 3% = 99%). For the hearing loss shown, there are 21 dots above the patient's threshold, which would result in 63% of the acoustic information being audible (and 36% inaudible). **B.** Another adaptation of the speech intelligibility concept as developed by Pavlovic (1988). The speech information is divided into 120 dB of speech information based on the 30 dB range available at each of the four frequencies (500, 1000, 2000, 4000 Hz). For the hearing loss shown, there are 80 dB of acoustic information available above the patient's thresholds, which would result in 66% (80 dB/120 dB) of the acoustic information being audible (and 34% inaudible). As illustrated in these examples, both methods are comparable for the same hearing loss.

about the amount of speech signal that he or she is able to use or not use. For the above example, you might tell the patient that he is having some difficulty communicating because he or she is not receiving about a third of the speech frequency information.

The count-the-dots audiogram (or SII) has been used more with hearing aid comparisons, but can be quite useful in diagnostic applications.

Keep in mind, however, that using the count-the-dots audiogram is only an assessment of how much of the speech stimulus the patient is able to hear (or not hear) and that it is based on the parameters at conversational levels of speech. Relying only on the pure-tone audiogram to predict a patient's speech recognition has not been adopted as a routine procedure in the clinical setting; however, this approach may become more widely used in the future as more validation studies are done. For the present, there are other clinical procedures to measure speech recognition ability that are typically included as part of the basic audiometric evaluation and are discussed later in this chapter.

Most Comfortable and Uncomfortable Loudness Levels

Most of us prefer to listen to sounds at comfortable levels and we tend to avoid listening to sounds at uncomfortable levels. Audiometrically, we often establish the level (dB HL) at which a patient prefers to listen to speech, called the *most comfortable loudness level* (MCL), as well as the level at which a patient finds speech to be too loud, called the *uncomfortable loudness level* (UCL) or *loudness discomfort level* (LDL). Information about a patient's MCL and UCL may be helpful in selecting the appropriate level at which to do speech testing. The most common way to determine a patient's MCL and UCL is to use categorical ratings where the patient is asked to judge the loudness for increasing presentation levels of words or sentences according to the following eight categories (a list of these categories is given to the patient):

8. Uncomfortably loud
7. Loud, but OK
6. Comfortable, but slightly loud
5. Comfortable
4. Comfortable, but slightly soft
3. Soft
2. Very soft
1. Cannot hear

As you will see later in this chapter, and in the chapter on hearing aids, information about patients' MCL and UCL are useful in order to assess their ability to understand supra-threshold speech and to evaluate how much range they have before speech becomes uncomfortably loud. The UCL represents the upper end of the range for a person's hearing. Measures of UCL are important for hearing aid fittings in that the hearing aids must be programmed to limit their output to just below the patient's UCL. The normal hearing person's MCL for speech is generally between 40 and 50 dB HL and the UCL for speech is usually somewhere between 75 and 95 dB HL. For patients with hearing loss, the MCL for speech is usually somewhere between the SRT and UCL. It is difficult to establish a single level to represent a patient's MCL because most people have a range of values that sound comfortable to them. The amount of useable hearing for a patient, called his *dynamic range*, is the difference between the SRT and the UCL. In cochlear hearing losses, it is typical for the patient to have a UCL for speech at the same level as for those with normal hearing; however, since the patient has an elevated SRT, the resulting dynamic range is greatly reduced (Kamm, Dirks, & Mickey, 1978). Figure 7–10 illustrates how the dynamic range is affected by type of hearing loss.

Suprathreshold Speech Recognition Procedures

Supra-threshold speech testing is an audiometric procedure used to evaluate how well a patient can recognize speech at one or more levels above his SRT. Speech recognition tests are usually done with single-syllable words or single-syllable nonsense words, although sentence materials have been developed and can be used in addition to word tests or instead of word tests when necessary. Supra-threshold speech recognition tests are an important part of the audiometric evaluation.

Word recognition testing uses single-syllable words, which are phonetically or phonemically balanced lists of single-syllable words (consonant-vowel-consonant), called PB words. The goal of the word recognition test is to obtain a *word recognition score* (WRS). The two most popular PB word lists in use today are the CID W-22 set of word lists (phonetically balanced) developed by Central Institute for the Deaf, and the NU-6 set of word lists (phonemically balanced) developed at Northwestern University. The PB word lists were

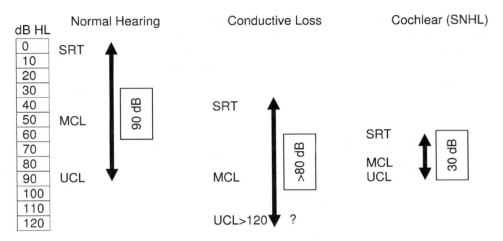

Figure 7–10. Illustration of the dynamic range for speech for a normal hearing ear, a conductive hearing loss, and a cochlear hearing loss. The dynamic range for speech is the difference between the speech recognition threshold (*SRT*) and the uncomfortable loudness level (*UCL*). Most notable is the greatly reduced dynamic range (e.g., 30 dB) seen with cochlear hearing losses. **MCL**, most comfortable loudness level; **SNHL**, sensorineural hearing loss.

constructed to approximate the frequency of occurrence for different speech sounds as they normally occur in the English language. The PB words are usually presented in an *open-set* format, meaning that the patient is not aware of what words are to be presented. In some situations, the PB words can be presented with and without patient looking at the tester in order to assess their ability to recognize words with visual cues compared with auditory cues only. Other single-syllable materials available for speech recognition testing include the California Consonant Test, the CUNY Nonsense Syllable Test, the High Frequency Word List, and the Computer-Assisted Speech Perception Assessment Test (CASPA). Because of the sensitivity of the WRS to the variations in the different speech sounds, and in order to insure consistency across tests and patients, it is highly recommended that WRS testing be done with recorded materials (remember to calibrate the VU meter). A carrier phrase, "Say the word . . . ," is normally included as part of the word recognition testing. Also, because the WRS is one of recognition, familiarizing the patient with the words is not done.

The WRS is reported as a percentage of correctly identified items. There are two ways to score the results for word recognition tests. One way is to count the number of words that are correctly identified and convert this to a percentage of the number of words presented, called *whole word score*. Another way is to count the number of phonemes, called *phoneme score*, where each phoneme (initial consonant, vowel, final consonant) in each word is scored, and convert this to a percentage of the number of phonemes presented. The number of items used to obtain the WRS is not standardized. In clinical practice, lists of 50 words (full lists) or lists of 25 words (half lists) are usually used. However, it is important to keep in mind that as the number of test items decreases, the variability increases; and as the variability increases, larger differences between scores must occur to be statistically significant (see Critical Differences in WRS Based on Binomial Distribution later in this chapter). Although many audiologists use lists of 25 words to save time, the larger associated variability, as well as the loss of phonemic balance associated with a half-list, makes the use of whole word scoring with 25 words less meaningful. On the other hand, a list with 50 words decreases the associated variability, but takes longer to administer. However, by using phoneme scoring there may be a better tradeoff between variability and the time to administer the test. With phoneme scoring for WRS, a half-list (25 words) has 75 items that are scored, and this larger number of items reduces the variability and saves time compared to presenting a list of 50 words. Phoneme scoring may also give a better representation of the patient's overall ability to understand speech because you can see the type of phoneme errors being made. Regardless of the chosen method, it is important to indicate on the audiometric worksheet the number of words used and whether the WRS is based on whole word or phoneme scoring so that any changes in the patient's ability over time are calculated using the same scoring format.

Selection of the Presentation Level for WRS Testing

The selection of the presentation level is an important consideration for WRS testing. There is no agreed-upon approach for selection of WRS test level, and this is still an area of debate. Often times, only one WRS is obtained for each ear (at one supra-threshold intensity level); however, a more complete assessment of speech recognition ability can be done by testing WRS at more than one intensity level and/or in the presence of background noise. One thing to keep in mind is the question you are trying to answer. For example, obtaining WRS at 50 dB HL (normal conversational level) might be done in order to demonstrate to the patient how his or her hearing loss affects his or her ability to understand normal levels of conversational speech or show him or her how amplification may be expected to provide an improvement or to plan some rehabilitation. On the other hand, one might be interested in knowing the patient's best WRS by testing at one or more supra-threshold levels. Historically, WRS testing was performed at 40 dB above the patient's SRT (40 dB SL). This level was based on data showing normal-hearing listeners

achieve maximum word recognition when words are presented at or above 30 dB SL, and those with cochlear hearing losses reach maximum word recognition at or above 40 dB SL (Maroonroge & Diefendorf, 1984). Although 40 dB SL is still often used by audiologists, this approach must be interpreted with caution because it may not be the optimal level for patients to achieve their best performance. As Figure 7–11 shows, for sloping hearing losses, more of the speech banana would be audible if WRS testing were to be performed at a higher intensity level, in this case at 50 dB SL (90 dB HL), than if testing were to be performed at 40 dB SL (75 dB HL). If the WRS is only obtained at 40 dB SL, one may underestimate the patient's ability to understand speech when wearing a hearing aid. Brandy (2002) suggested that for sloping hearing losses the WRS could be presented 40 dB above the patient's PTA of 500, 1000, 2000, 3000, and 4000 Hz, rather than 40 dB above the SRT.

Additionally, in many cases with moderate to severe hearing losses, one may not even be able to present words at 40 dB SL because this level would be above the patient's UCL (Kamm et al., 1978). It follows then that to obtain an estimate of the patient's best speech recognition, WRS testing should be done at the highest level possible without being uncomfortable. Guthrie and Mackersie (2006) found maximum word recognition scores were obtained when the testing level was at UCL minus 5 dB (UCL-5 dB) or at 20 dB above the pure-tone threshold at 2000 Hz.

Testing for WRS at a single high intensity level may create its own problem, especially when evaluating patients with a possible 8th nerve problem. For example, patients with an 8th nerve disorder characteristically show poorer speech recognition performance at high intensities than they do for somewhat lower levels. For these type of patients, if WRS is only tested at one presentation level, such as UCL-5 dB, the WRS may give a misleading account of the patient's word recognition ability, since the score may be better if the patient were to be tested at a lower level. One solution to this issue is to perform WRS tests at more than one level in order to get a complete picture of how the patient performs and to estimate their maximum WRS, as discussed in the following sections.

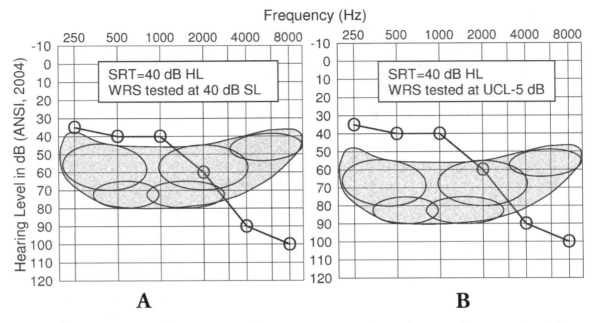

Figure 7–11. A. and B. Illustration of how an increase in word recognition test level from 80 dB HL (40 dB SL) to 90 dB HL (UCL-5 dB) can provide more acoustic information at a more audible level, and this may result in a higher word recognition score (*WRS*) for the same person. **SRT**, speech recognition threshold.

Performance-Intensity Function for WRS

The optimal way to determine the patient's best word recognition ability is to perform the WRS test at multiple presentation levels. This is usually done with PB words at three to five presentation levels, called a *performance-intensity function for PB words* (PI–PB function). By graphing how the patient's WRS changes with presentation level, you can better estimate the patient's maximum speech recognition ability, called PB_{max}. Figure 7-12 shows examples of PI–PB functions for a normal hearing listener and a patient with a mild degree of cochlear hearing loss. For both PI–PB functions, you can see that as the presentation level is increased there is a rise in the WRS. At some point, the WRS reaches a maximum whereby further increases do not improve the word recognition scores. The point where the curve first levels off is the PB_{max}. Notice that the cochlear hearing

loss in this case would not have demonstrated a true PB_{max} if testing was only done at 40 dB SL (70 dB HL). Unfortunately, a PI–PB function is often not performed clinically because of the additional time required. However, a more contemporary speech recognition test, called Computer-Assisted Speech Perception Assessment Test (CASPA), developed by Boothroyd (1999), offers promise for obtaining a PI–PB function in a reasonably short time period. The CASPA uses phoneme scoring as a way to increase the number of test items without increasing the test time. The CASPA uses only ten words at each presentation level, resulting in 30 scored phonemes at each level. The presentation of the word lists and the calculations of the phoneme and/or word scores are done by the computer software. Because the test is more efficient, multiple levels can be tested in a shorter time period than possible with traditional PI–PB testing. The CASPA has 16 different word lists balanced for phonemes and inter-list equivalency (Mackersie,

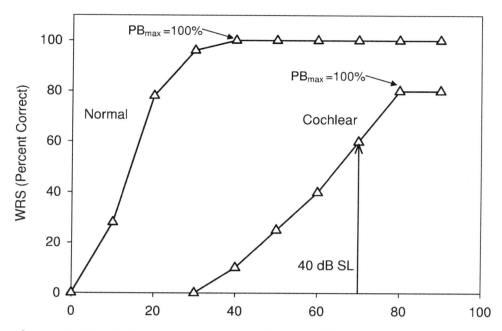

Figure 7–12. Performance intensity function (PI–PB function) for a normal hearing listener and a patient with a mild cochlear hearing loss. WRS testing was done at multiple intensity levels to determine the maximum performance (*PB$_{max}$*). The PB$_{max}$ is the point where the function begins its plateau. Notice that in this example if testing had only been done at 40 dB SL, the PB$_{max}$ would have been underestimated.

Boothroyd, & Minniear, 2001). Although designed for hearing aid assessment using multiple levels with and without noise, the CASPA is also useful for diagnostic applications to quickly determine the patient's PB$_{max}$ using multiple level testing.

In summary, the selection of the presentation level or levels for WRS testing must consider the points discussed above. There are many options for selecting the presentation level for WRS testing, including: (a) 40 dB above the SRT, (b) 40 dB above the three- or four-frequency PTA, (c) 20 dB above 2000 Hz threshold, (d) at the patient's MCL, (e) at 85 dB HL, (f) at UCL-5 dB, (g) at 50 dB HL (normal conversational level), or (h) at multiple levels. Certainly, more research is needed to determine the optimal presentation level or levels to test for WRS. The ultimate decisions the audiologist makes will depend on the individual patient, as well as the information the audiologist wants to obtain with the speech measures.

Procedure for Obtaining WRS

Testing for WRS includes the following recommended procedures:

1. Select the presentation level
   a. Multiple-level testing with the CASPA is recommended. This will rapidly provide a PI–PB function and establish PB$_{max}$.
   b. If only one level is to be performed, consider the question being asked. For maximizing acoustic information available to the patient, use UCL-5 dB.
   c. For each level of testing, determine if masking is needed in the non-test ear (see later section on how to mask for speech).
2. Present one or more recorded list of PB words (e.g., NU-6 list).
3. Keep track of patient's correct and/or incorrect responses.

4. Calculate the WRS as a percentage of correct responses:
   a. For whole word scoring, the percentage would be equal to the number of words correct / 25 × 100 for a list with 25 words, or the number of words correct / 50 × 100 for a list with 50 words.
   b. For phoneme scoring, the percentage would be equal to the number of phonemes correct / 75 × 100 for a list of 25 words, or the number of phonemes correct / 150 × 100 for a list of 50 words. Note: the NU-6 is recommended, especially if using phoneme scoring.
5. Repeat the test at a 20 dB lower presentation level (especially if suspicious of 8th nerve involvement). If the WRS is the same or worse at the lower level, then use the score obtained at the higher level as the WRS (PB_{max}). If the WRS is better by more than 8% at the lower level, additional testing at lower levels is required to define the PB_{max} and determine if there may be significant rollover (see section below on PI–PB Rollover). Testing should continue with additional 10 dB decrements in presentation level until PB_{max} is obtained. Calculate the PI–PB rollover ratio (see later section in this chapter).

Obtaining the WRS is a routine part of the audiologic evaluation and can be used to: (a) estimate how a patient's hearing loss affects speech understanding at comfortable listening levels, (b) compare performance between the two ears, (c) compare performance across time, and (d) provide a more relevant stimulus to assess how a patient performs with a hearing aid.

Synopsis 7–2

- The distribution of speech sounds at a normal conversational level ranges from 20 to 50 dB HL, with consonants being softer and vowels being louder. The distribution of frequencies in speech sounds is more complex and variable; however, the voiceless fricatives (s, f, th, sh, ch) are generally the highest in frequency and lowest in intensity, and can be a significant factor in speech recognition, even with mild hearing losses.

- The speech intelligibility index (SII) weights the acoustic properties of speech and attempts to predict how these properties affect recognition of speech. The SII derives a number from 0.0 (none of the acoustic speech components available) to 1.0 (all of the acoustic speech components available). A clinical version of this approach is called count-the-dots audiogram, where the frequency/intensity components are represented as dots on the audiogram and the weighting is represented by the density of dots at different frequencies. One example of count-the-dots audiogram has 33 dots distributed between 20 and 50 dB at 500, 1000, 2000, and 4000 Hz, where each dot contributes 0.03 to the overall speech recognition (Humes, 1991). When a patient's hearing loss is superimposed with the dots, it gives an indication of how much of the speech spectrum the patient is able to hear (or not hear) and can be a useful counseling or planning tool.

- Suprathreshold speech tests, such as tests for word recognition scores (WRS), are used to actually assess how well a patient recognizes speech when presented at a specified listening level. A WRS test is a routine part of the audiologic evaluation and is used to: (a) estimate how a patient's hearing loss affects speech understanding at different listening levels depending on the question to be answered, (b) compare performance between the two ears, (c) compare performance across time, and (d) provide a more relevant stimulus to assess how a patient performs with a hearing aid.

- WRS testing involves presenting single-syllable phonemically balanced (PB) words, such as the NU-6 word list, and obtaining a percent correct score. Although the NU-6 has several lists of 50 words (full list), most audiologists use a list with 25 words (half list) to save time. Scores can be calculated as whole word scores or phoneme scores (three phonemes per word). Phoneme scoring has the advantage of having more items to score for a limited number of words and this can reduce the variability of the test.

- Supra-threshold presentation levels should be high enough to maximize the patient's score, but be lower than the UCL (e.g., UCL-5 dB). To determine if the WRS is the patient's best performance (PB_{max}), at least two levels should be tested, such as UCL-5 dB and then at a level that is 20 dB lower. If the lower level produces a better WRS, then additional levels (PI–PB function) should be tested to determine if there had been a decline in WRS at the higher test levels, called rollover (possible 8th nerve sign).

- The CASPA is a computer-based speech recognition test that can rapidly obtain a PI–PB function with phoneme scores and shows promise over single presentation methods for WRS testing.

Interpretation of WRS Measures

Audiologists typically report the word recognition scores on the audiogram with some type of limited interpretation, such as, "Speech recognition ability appears to be good (or fair, or poor)." Table 7–2 gives some common categories for generally describing speech impairment based on WRS. For normal hearing listeners and those with conductive hearing losses, the WRS is usually above 90%. For cochlear hearing losses, the scores vary considerably depending on the degree and shape of hearing loss. For 8th nerve pathology such as an acoustic tumor, the WRS can be poorer than one would expect based on the audiometric configuration. Although these categorical descriptors might be useful to provide some simple feedback to the patient, they do not provide any real useful information regarding the significance of the scores relative to what is expected for the degree of hearing loss, or the significance of differences between the two ears or changes that occurred from previous evaluations. To be more meaningful, WRS interpretation must be properly performed based on available data in the literature, which leads to better decisions about the significance of the WRS appropriate for good evidence-based practice. In the following sections, you will learn how to answer some clinical questions regarding interpretation of WRS based on available data.

Table 7–2. Commonly Used Categories to Generally Describe Results of Word Recognition Score (WRS) Testing

WRS (% Correct)	Degree of Impairment	Word Recognition Ability
100–90	None	Excellent/normal
89–75	Slight	Good
74–60	Moderate	Fair
59–50	Poor	Poor
<50	Very poor	Very poor

Critical Differences in WRS Based on Binomial Distribution

Is there a significant difference in WRS between the two ears?

Has there been a significant change in WRS since the previous test?

Is the patient better off with a hearing aid than without one?

Is the WRS significantly better with one hearing aid or another?

The questions listed above involve making decisions about whether or not two word recognition scores are significantly different. The appropriate answers to these questions can be found by referring to established data based on a *binomial distribution*, which was made popular by Thornton and Raffin (1978). The binomial distribution is a statistically derived table of probabilities to describe word recognition scores, and reflects the variability (standard deviation) of word recognition scores as a function of the number of test items and test scores (Gelfand, 2001). The variability of the WRS test decreases as the number of test items increases, and at the extremes of the word recognition scores the variability is lower for a 50-item word list than for a 25-item word list, and is lower at the upper and lower ends of the WRS percent correct continuum. This means that a greater difference in scores is required for a 25-item word list compared with a 50-item word list in order to be significantly different, and a greater difference in scores is required for scores in the middle of the percent correct continuum compared with

the upper and lower extremes in order to be significantly different.

The application of the binomial distribution to WRS data can be used to produce a *critical differences table* that can be used to compare any two word recognition scores. In other words, how different do two scores have to be in order for the difference to be significantly different at the 95% confidence interval? The application of binomial distribution can be used to determine critical difference values for whole word scores or for phoneme scores when properly adjusted.

Table 7–3 shows one example of a critical difference table, based on the binomial distribution, which can be used to compare two word scores or two phoneme scores over different numbers of test items. To use Table 7–3, find the row that represents the lower of the two scores being compared, then find where that row intersects the column that represents the number of words being scored; the number in the intersecting cell is the upper end of the confidence interval (critical value). To be significantly different from the patient's lower score, the patient's higher score must be greater than the intersecting column number. If the second score is less than or equal to the intersecting column number, the two scores cannot be considered significantly different. If the actual second score is less than the amount in the intersecting cell, the two scores cannot be considered significantly different. For example, suppose you obtain word recognition scores using lists of 25 words of 68% and 88% for the right and left ears, respectively. To determine if these scores for the two ears are significantly different from each other, find the row that corresponds to a score of 68%, and then find where that row intersects

Table 7–3. Critical Difference Values for PB Words Based on the Binomial Distribution

95% Confidence		Number of items (phoneme scoring = 2.5 number of words)									
		10	25	50	63			10	25	50	63
The lower of the two scores being compared (in %)	0	33	15	8	6	The lower of the two scores being compared (in %)	50	91	77	70	68
	1	36	17	10	9		51	91	78	71	68
	2	38	20	12	11		52	92	79	71	69
	3	40	22	14	13		53	93	80	72	70
	4	41	23	16	14		54	93	81	73	71
	5	43	25	18	16		55	94	81	74	72
	6	45	27	19	17		56	95	82	75	73
	7	47	29	21	19		57	95	83	76	74
	8	48	30	22	20		58	96	84	77	75
	9	50	32	24	22		59	96	84	78	76
	10	51	33	25	23		60	97	85	78	77
	11	53	35	27	25		61	97	86	79	77
	12	54	36	28	26		62	98	87	80	78
	13	55	38	29	27		63	98	87	81	79
	14	57	39	31	29		64	99	88	82	80
	15	58	40	32	30		65	99	89	83	81
	16	59	42	33	31		66	100	90	83	82
	17	61	43	34	32		67	100	90	84	82
	18	62	44	36	34		68	100	91	85	83
	19	63	45	37	35		69	100	92	86	84
	20	64	47	38	36		70	100	92	87	85
	21	65	48	39	37		71	100	93	87	86
	22	66	49	41	38		72	100	93	88	86
	23	68	50	42	40		73	100	94	89	87
	24	69	51	43	41		74	100	95	89	88
	25	70	53	44	42		75	100	95	90	89
	26	71	54	45	43		76	100	96	91	89
	27	72	55	46	44		77	100	96	92	90
	28	73	56	47	45		78	100	97	92	91
	29	74	57	48	46		79	100	97	93	92
	30	75	58	50	47		80	100	98	94	92
	31	76	59	51	48		81	100	98	94	93
	32	77	60	52	50		82	100	99	95	94
	33	77	61	53	51		83	100	99	95	94
	34	78	62	54	52		84	100	100	96	95
	35	79	63	55	53		85	100	100	97	96
	36	80	64	56	54		86	100	100	97	96
	37	81	65	57	55		87	100	100	98	97
	38	82	66	58	56		88	100	100	98	97
	39	83	67	59	57		89	100	100	99	98
	40	83	68	60	58		90	100	100	99	98
	41	84	69	61	59		91	100	100	100	99
	42	85	70	62	60		92	100	100	100	99
	43	86	71	63	61		93	100	100	100	100
	44	87	72	64	62		94	100	100	100	100
	45	87	73	65	63		95	100	100	100	100
	46	88	74	66	64		96	100	100	100	100
	47	89	75	67	65		97	100	100	100	100
	48	89	75	68	66		98	100	100	100	100
	49	90	76	69	67		99	100	100	100	100

Note: Courtesy of Arthur Boothroyd and Carol Mackersie. Modified with permission. Find where lower score *(row)* intersects number of items scored *(column)*.

the column associated with 25 words; the critical value found in the intersecting cell is 91. That means that scores between 68% and 91% will not be significantly different from each other 95 out of 100 times. For this example, you should report that the word recognition scores between the two ears are not significantly different based on the binomial distribution. The critical differences in Table 7–3 can also be used with phoneme scoring if one multiplies the number of whole words by 2.5 phonemes per word (rather than 3).[2] In other words, if phoneme scoring is used for a list with 25 words, you would use the column labeled 63 items. For example, suppose two phoneme scores being compared are 74% and 92%. The intersecting cell for 74% (row) and 63 items (column) shows a critical value of 88%, which means that the second phoneme score of 92% is significantly different from 74%. Using these binomial confidence values one can report that a patient's performance is significantly different between the two ears, has changed over time, or shows better performance with one hearing aid over another hearing aid.

Differential Diagnosis of Cochlear Versus 8th Nerve

Is the WRS worse than expected for cochlear hearing losses, suggesting an 8th nerve problem?

The use of speech audiometry for differential diagnosis of cochlear versus 8th nerve tumors is not as important as it was 20 years ago. Since that time, audiologists have relied on other tests, like acoustic reflexes and auditory brainstem responses (see Chapter 8), along with tremendous advances in medical imaging techniques that are more sensitive to 8th nerve diagnoses. However, since WRS is obtained as a routine part of the audiologic evaluation, its proper interpretation may signal the need for further evaluation if suspicions of 8th nerve pathology are raised. In general, for an 8th nerve pathology such as an acoustic tumor, the WRS can be disproportionately worse than predicted based on the audiometric configuration and/or

expectations for cochlear hearing losses. In this regard, however, it is important to be sure that the poor score is not just due to an inadequate presentation level as was discussed earlier. Another characteristic of disorders of the 8th nerve is that there can be poorer WRS performance at presentation levels higher than where the PB_{max} was obtained, and this is called *PI–PB rollover*. The following sections will describe three ways to interpret word recognition scores for differential diagnosis of 8th nerve pathology: (a) use of confidence limits, (b) plots of the articulation function, and (c) calculation of a PI–PB rollover ratio.

Confidence Limits for WRS

It would be nice to know with confidence how poor a WRS must be to suggest an 8th nerve problem. Unfortunately, there are very little published data to make that determination. Dubno, Lee, Klein, Mathews, and Lam (1995) reported 95% confidence limits for PB_{max}, for NU-6 word lists, based on cases of confirmed sloping high frequency cochlear hearing losses. Table 7–4 shows the data from Dubno et al. as a function of PTA for 25-item word lists. Based on these data, if the PB_{max} is below the lower confidence limit for cochlear ears, they would be considered disproportionately low and further evaluation for possible 8th nerve problem may be warranted. Dubno et al. also suggested that the lower confidence limit could be used to interpret WRS data for a single presentation level. In other words, if a WRS is within the confidence limits for the appropriate PTA, then additional presentation levels may not be needed. On the other hand, if a WRS is lower than the confidence limit, a PI–PB function should be obtained to determine if the WRS represents the patient's PB_{max} before deciding that the WRS is disproportionately low and suggestive of an 8th nerve problem. Validation of these values with a population of patients with confirmed 8th nerve problems has not been conducted; therefore, audiologists must use this method of interpretation with some caution based on a single study with cochlear hearing losses.

---

[2]Because of the interdependence among the 3 phonemes, a multiplier of 2.5 is used instead of 3 (Boothroyd, personal communication, September 20, 2007).

Table 7–4. Lower 95% Confidence Limits for WRS as a Function of PTA (500, 1000, 2000 Hz) in Ears with Cochlear Hearing Loss.

PTA (dB HL)	Lower 95% Confidence Limit For WRS (percent) based on 25-item NU-6 word lists	PTA (dB HL)	Lower 95% Confidence Limit For WRS (percent) based on 25-item NU-6 word lists
−3.3	100	36.7	68
0.0	100	38.3	64
1.7	100	40.0	64
3.3	96	41.7	60
5.0	96	43.3	56
6.7	96	45.0	56
8.3	96	46.7	52
10.0	96	48.3	52
11.7	92	50.0	48
13.3	92	51.7	48
15.0	92	53.3	44
16.7	88	55.0	44
18.3	88	56.7	40
20.0	88	58.3	40
21.7	84	60.0	36
23.3	84	61.7	36
25.0	80	63.3	32
26.7	80	65.0	32
38.3	76	66.6	32
30.0	76	68.3	28
31.7	72	70.0	28
33.3	72	71.7	34
35.0	68		

Data shown are for 25-item NU-6 word lists.
See Dubno et al. for results using a 50 item word lists.

Source: "Confidence-Limits for Maximum Word-Recognition Scores," by J. R. Dubno, F. S. Lee, A. J. Klein, L. J. Mathews, & C. F. Lam, 1995, *Journal of Speech and Hearing Research, 38.* Copyright 1995 by American Speech-Language-Hearing Association. Adapted with permission.

Differential Diagnosis Using the Speech Intelligibility Index

The SII function can also be used for differential diagnosis of cochlear or 8th nerve problems. Although this approach is an attractive possibility, it is not currently used much in clinical practice. Recall that the articulation function is a relation between how performance (percent correct) for speech materials changes as a function of the SII value. The SII values are related to the amount of acoustic information available to the listener, which will vary as a function of the degree and shape of hearing loss. An estimate of the SII values can be obtained using a count-the-dots audiogram, which could be compared with the expected performance on the word recognition tests for that SII value. The dots representing the speech spectrum can be adjusted to match the level at which the WRS testing was performed, presumably at a level that represents the patient's PB_{max}. If the patient's performance is poorer than the expected range of values from the SII function, it would suggest that the patient's performance is not only related to the acoustic properties of speech as expected for cochlear hearing losses, but a poorer than predicted performance on the speech test would suggest additional speech processing difficulties, which may warrant further evaluation for 8th nerve involvement. For example, if it is established that cochlear losses are expected to achieve a PB_{max} of 80% with an SII = 0.6, and a patient shows a PB_{max} of 55%, could this score be worse than predicted based on the acoustic speech properties? To be applicable to differential diagnosis of 8th nerve disorders, studies need to be done to define the expected SII functions for the NU-6 and W-22 word lists for a population of cochlear and/ or 8th nerve hearing loss patients.

PI–PB Rollover Ratio

Recall that a PI–PB function can be used to obtain a better estimate of a patient's PB_{max}. For normal hearing listeners and those with cochlear hearing losses, once PB_{max} has been reached it remains close to that score for higher presentation levels. Patients with pathologies affecting the 8th nerve, such as acoustic tumors or decline in neural function with age, seem to have an inability to sustain neural activity when the auditory nerve is "stressed" at high intensity levels. For the PI–PB function, patients with 8th nerve problems have been shown to have a decline in WRS at presentation levels above the level where they achieved their PB_{max} (Jerger & Jerger, 1971). Figure 7–13 shows the PI–PB function for a hypothetical patient with an 8th nerve tumor and a patient with a cochlear hearing loss with similar audiograms (mild high frequency sensorineural loss with SRT =

30 dB HL). In the patient with the 8th nerve problem, as the presentation level was increased, the WRS increased until PB_{max} was reached at 60 dB HL, and then worsened at higher presentation levels indicating PI–PB rollover. The lowest score above the PB_{max} is called the PB_{min}.

To completely define the rollover, testing should be completed at as high a presentation level as the patient can tolerate without being uncomfortably loud. Quantification of the rollover is usually done by calculating a *rollover ratio* (or index). The rollover ratio is a simple ratio of the amount of decline relative to the PB_{max}, calculated as follows:

$$Rollover\ ratio = \frac{(PB_{max} - PB_{min})}{PB_{max}}$$

The amount of rollover ratio that is significant for 8th nerve pathologies is dependent on the word list used. For the NU-6 word lists, Bess, Josey, and Humes (1979) reported a cutoff value for the rollover ratio of 0.25, whereas Meyer and Mishler (1985) reported a cutoff value of 0.35. If the rollover ratio is greater than the cutoff value, this should raise the suspicion that there is some 8th nerve involvement.

Speech-in-Noise Tests

The speech measures described above are usually presented in quiet. However, there are many other speech measures that are designed to assess how well a patient can recognize speech in the presence of different levels of background noise, thus obtaining measures of speech recognition that may be more representative of real-world listening situations. A primary complaint for many people with hearing loss is that even though they may hear people talking, they have difficulty understanding what is being said, especially when there is background noise. Some commonly used speech-in-noise tests include the NU-6 with speech spectrum noise or multi-talker babble, the Speech Perception in Noise (SPIN) test, the Synthetic Sentence Identification (SSI) test with a competing

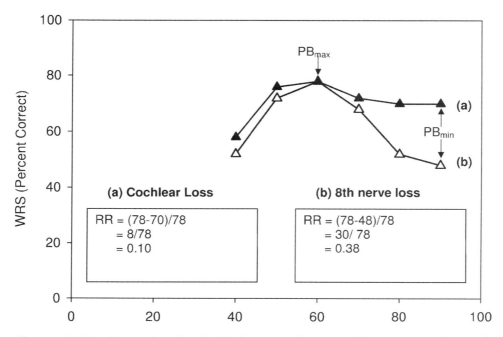

Figure 7–13. Example of a PI–PB function for a cochlear loss and an 8th nerve loss. The rollover ratio (*RR*) is calculated as the PBmax − PB$_{min}$ / PB$_{max}$. Rollover ratios greater than 0.35 may be associated with 8th nerve losses.

story, the Quick Sentence in Noise (QuickSIN) test, and the Hearing in Noise Test (HINT). These tests typically present speech materials as a function of noise level called a speech-to-noise ratio (SNR). For example, if the speech is presented at 50 dB HL and the background noise is presented in the same ear at 45 dB HL, this would be considered a +5 dB SNR (also designated +5 dB S/N). Because the units are decibels, the noise level is subtracted from the speech level instead of divided.

The QuickSIN test was developed by Etymotic Research (Niquette, Gudmundsen, & Killion, 2001) as a clinically useful method of quickly measuring speech identification in noise to evaluate a patient's performance with and without hearing aids. The QuickSIN test embeds key words in unpredictable sentences. The test sentences are presented in background noise that is made up of four people speaking different sentences (four-talker babble) with varying SNRs. Each sentence

has five key words that must be correctly identified. The test is given at 70 dB HL for those with PTA less than 45 dB HL or at MCL for those with PTA greater than 50 dB HL. The test presents one sentence at each SNR, beginning at +25 dB SNR (easiest) and decreasing in 5 dB steps to 0 dB SNR (most difficult). The patient's SNR is compared with SNR expected for normal hearing listeners to get a final score, called SNR loss.

The HINT measures how well a person is able to correctly identify sentences as a function of different speech-to-noise ratios. The HINT has been standardized on a relatively large population (Nilsson, Soli, & Sullivan, 1994). The HINT is available as a computer-based software CD that can work with the audiometer or as a stand-alone unit in which everything is done through the computer. In either situation, the computer presents the sentence material, adjusts the level of the sentences following rules based on how the patient responds (level decreased for correct response and increased for incorrect response), and calculates how the patient performs relative to the standardized database. The typical HINT has the background noise set at 65 dBA,[3] then the sentences are presented at varying levels until a speech-to-noise ratio is obtained that represents the point where 50% correct sentence identification occurs, called the reception threshold for sentences (RTS). The HINT can be used to test the ears binaurally (with sentences and noise presented to both ears at the same time) or with the sentences in one ear and the noise in the other ear. The HINT can be performed under earphones for diagnostic applications or in a sound field for hearing aid applications. The RTS can be used to compare the patient's performance with mean data from normal hearing listeners, or it can be used to determine how much the patient's hearing-in-noise ability is improved with different hearing aids.

Variations with Young Children or Difficult-to-Test Populations

As with pure-tone audiometry, modifications are needed with speech audiometry when testing young children or other difficult-to-test populations. These modifications are usually necessary for children younger than 6 years of age or any patient who is difficult to test using the adult procedures. As a test stimulus, speech is more familiar to children than the more abstract pure-tone stimuli and has an inherently higher reinforcement value. In many cases, audiologists prefer to begin testing young children with speech audiometry in order to make the child more comfortable with the testing situation, and to obtain some information about their hearing abilities in case pure-tone testing cannot be completed. As with pure-tone audiometry, the tester must be enthusiastic, offer lots of positive

reinforcement, and be flexible. Earphones should always be attempted first; however, sound-field testing can be performed when needed. Typically, monitored live voice is used with young children due to the need for flexibility, but recorded materials are available. The primary goal is to obtain a speech recognition threshold and a measure of word recognition ability. The different strategies and speech materials for testing young children are described in the following sections.

Speech Recognition Thresholds (SRT)

As with adults, the SRT requires that the child indicate somehow that he understands the word and/or is able to repeat the word correctly. When this is not possible, then a SDT should be obtained using VRA or conditioned-play techniques if necessary (see earlier section on SDT for interpretation). Obtaining an SRT for a young child is very important because it may be the best indicator of his degree of hearing loss in the speech frequencies and can be a good validation of the pure-tone thresholds.

It is usually better to use words that are familiar to the child, so often the audiologist will use selected items from the adult spondee word list or ask the caregiver which words are in the child's vocabulary. There is also a list of children's spondee words available that is composed of words more likely to be in the child's vocabulary. For those children with a limited expressive vocabulary or reluctance to provide verbal responses, the SRT can be obtained by having the child point to spondee picture cards or objects (lay out four to six cards or objects). With advances in computer-based audiometry, these pictures may be displayed on the computer screen, and when the child touches the correct picture he/she receives some type of visual reward on the screen. Another commonly used strategy is to have the child point to different

---

[3]dBA is a representation of a noise level as measured with a sound level meter with an A-weighted filter network designed to better match the human audibility curve. The A-weighting attenuates frequencies below 700 Hz and above 9000 Hz.

body parts ("Show me your nose."). This can also be done by having the child point to the body parts on an inanimate character, like a doll or clown. This differs from testing adults in that the words may not be spondees and there is a carrier phrase, but these variations are not problematic.

The procedure for finding the lowest level at which the child can respond to the speech stimuli is also less formalized than for adults. Since time is critical when testing children, many audiologists use an up 10, down 20 procedure, where one word is given at each level and the level adjusted up 10 dB if they do not respond correctly and down 20 dB if they do respond correctly. With a cooperative child, the up 5, down 10 method could be used. Another approach is to present four to six words at each presentation level beginning 20 to 30 dB above threshold and decreasing in 5 dB (or 10 dB) steps until he/she misses half of the words. Whatever procedure is used, the goal is to estimate the SRT as the lowest level where the child responds to about half of the words.

Suprathreshold Speech Recognition Scores

Information about a child's ability to recognize speech is performed using procedures similar to those recommended for adults; however, the materials must be within the child's vocabulary. As with adults, the WRS is a percent of words correctly identified. For children 5 to 6 years old, there is a PBK-50 word list (composed of words appropriate for children of kindergarten age) that is commonly used and presented in the same way as the adult PB word lists. When interpreting speech recognition scores for children, it is important to use materials that are standardized for the age being tested and to interpret the findings according to the test's manual. Most of the standardized speech recognition tests for young children involve pointing to the requested picture from a group of four to six items. Examples of tests appropriate for children in the 3- to 6-year-old range include the Word Identification by Picture Identification (WIPI),

Northwestern University Children's Perception of Speech (NU-CHIPS), and the Pediatric Speech Intelligibility (PSI). The WIPI and PSI can be tested with or without background noise. A special version of the HINT is also available for children 6 to 12 years of age.

Masking for Speech Testing

The principles of masking for speech testing are the same as for pure-tone threshold testing (see Chapter 6), and in fact apply to any clinical tests in which the non-test ear (NTE) may be contributing to the signals presented to the test ear (TE). Recall that clinical masking is necessary whenever the interaural attenuation (IA) is exceeded and the signal being presented to the TE can be heard in the NTE by bone conduction (BC). For speech testing, masking would be needed whenever the presentation level of the speech materials in the TE exceeds the IA and cross-hearing in the NTE can occur. The masker used for speech audiometry is a noise that contains a range of frequencies representative of those in the speech spectrum and is called *speech noise masker*. As with narrow-band noise maskers, the speech noise masker is calibrated as effective masking levels so as to effectively raise the air conduction (AC) for the speech materials to the level set on the intensity dial (dB HL). Recall that the masker is always presented to the NTE by AC, but it is the BC threshold that must be tracked to insure that it is not able to hear the speech materials. Since the speech materials have a relatively broad spectrum, any of the bone conduction thresholds in the NTE could provide some contribution; therefore, when making decisions about masking for the speech tests you must compare the presentation level of the speech (by AC) in the TE to the best BC threshold in the NTE. The following should serve as a guiding principle:

Sufficient speech noise must be presented to the NTE by AC in order to elevate the best BC threshold in the NTE so that the speech being presented to the TE can no longer be heard in the NTE.

Of course, the IA will depend on the types of transducer; insert earphones have a greater IA value than supra-aural earphones. Establishing an IA for speech materials is complicated by the variations in the intensity among speech sounds that occur naturally and may be different for different types of materials. Estimates of the IA range from 40 to 45 dB for supra-aural earphones (Yacullo, 1996) and 55 to 65 dB for insert earphones (Sklare & Denneberg, 1987). For speech detection, the IA may be as low as 35 dB HL (Yacullo, 1996). However, for most speech testing it seems reasonable to use 40 dB and 55 dB as the minimums for speech IA for supra-aural earphones and insert earphones, respectively, and these are easy to remember since they are the same as the minimum IA adopted in this text for pure tones.

Masking for SRT

For SRT tests, the decision about the need for masking is the same as for pure-tone threshold testing. Keep in mind, however, that if you mask for pure tones and find that the masked AC pure-tone thresholds were the same as the unmasked thresholds (i.e., no shift in thresholds occurs), then masking is not required for SRT testing. If masking for SRT is needed, then the goal is to deliver enough speech masking noise to the NTE so that you are confident the words are only heard in the TE.

The plateau method of masking for SRT may be more difficult and time-consuming when using one of the recommended SRT procedures (Downs and Minard or ASHA procedures) because each series of words has different rules for varying the presentation level. An alternate approach is to select a single speech masker level that is sufficient to raise the best BC threshold in the NTE to a level that it can no longer hear any of the speech components of the material being presented to the TE. In other words, the level of the masker is chosen so that the difference between the SRT in the TE minus the elevated (by the masker) best BC threshold in the NTE is less than the IA. If you have the pure-tone masked thresholds, then you

can estimate the expected SRT based on the corresponding AC threshold of the best BC threshold or the PTA.

Figure 7–14 shows a typical example of masking for SRT testing using supra-aural earphones and a single selected level of speech noise masker. From the PTA (58 dB HL) for the right ear, you can anticipate that the SRT would be within 10 dB of this level. In addition, you can see that the best BC threshold in the NTE is −5 dB HL at 250 Hz, and there is more than a 40 dB difference between the AC threshold in TE and the BC threshold in the NTE. Therefore, the selected level of masker to the NTE in this example was 35 dB HL. With this level of masker, the best NTE BC (250 Hz) would be elevated to 30 dB HL, so that the difference between the anticipated SRT and the best BC threshold (elevated by masking) in the NTE would be less than 40 dB IA (65 dB HL to 30 dB HL = 35 dB). The actual SRT obtained in the example was 55 dB HL, and the difference between the actual SRT and the best BC threshold (elevated by masking) in the NTE was only 20 dB (55 dB HL to 35 dB HL = 20 dB), well below the minimum IA. Notice that you could have used a speech masker level anywhere between 20 dB HL and 35 dB HL and have the same results. The patient's SRT is recorded in the appropriate box on the audiometric worksheet along with the level of masking noise that was used in the NTE. Notice that in this example, masking would have also been needed if insert earphones had been used.

Masking for WRS Tests

As you can surmise, there are many instances where masking would be needed for WRS (or sentence) testing, since the presentation level of the speech material is at a supra-threshold level and, therefore, is more likely to cross over to the NTE. You have probably realized that if masking is needed for SRT, then it would also be needed for WRS testing. On the other hand, even if masking is not needed for SRT, masking may be needed for WRS testing because WRS testing is always performed at a supra-threshold level. For those

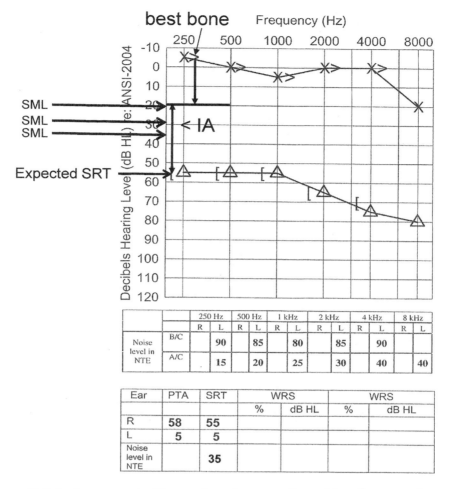

Figure 7–14. An example illustrating the use of masking for speech recognition threshold (*SRT*) testing. In this example, a single level of the speech masker (*SML*) is selected (anywhere between 20 dB HL and 35 dB HL) so that the presentation level of the words at or near threshold, when compared with the masked best bone conduction (*B/C*) threshold in the non-test ear (*NTE*), is less than the interaural attenuation (*IA*) for speech. See text for explanation of masking for SRT. **A/C**, air conduction; **PTA**, pure-tone average; **WRS**, word recognition score.

situations in which masking is needed for WRS testing, a single level of speech masker is used for each WRS level that is tested. As with masking for SRT, the level of the speech masker is selected so that it effectively elevates the best BC threshold so that it cannot hear the speech being presented to the TE. Of course, when performing a PI–PB function, the selected masker level must be appropriately set for each of the speech presentation levels. In all cases, the intent is to be sure that the WRS is representative of the TE.

Figure 7–15 shows an example of masking used for WRS testing using supra-aural earphones. In this example, the presentation level of the NU-6 word list was at 85 dB HL. The difference between the 85 dB HL presentation level in the TE and the

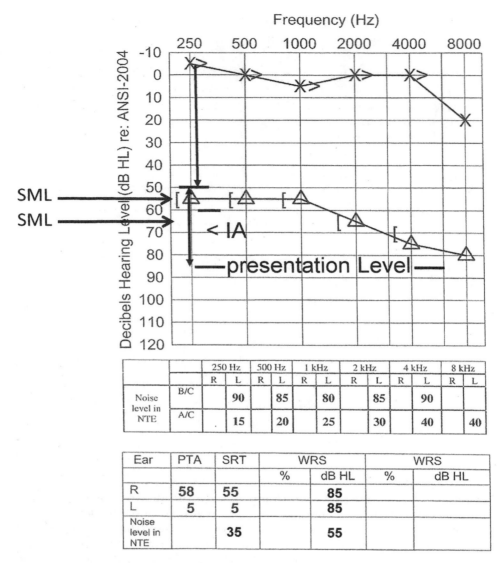

Figure 7–15. An example illustrating the use of masking for word recognition score (*WRS*) testing. In this example, a single presentation level (55 dB HL) of speech noise is an option in order to insure that the 85 dB HL presentation level of the words, when compared with the masked best bone conduction (*B/C*) threshold (50 dB HL) in the non-test ear (*NTE*), is less than the interaural attenuation (*IA*) for speech. An often used rule of thumb for WRS masking is to deliver the speech masker to the NTE at a level that is 20 dB less than the presentation level of the words in the TE. See text for explanation of masking for WRS. **A/C**, air conduction; **PTA**, pure-tone average.

best BC threshold in the NTE (−5 dB HL at 250 Hz) is equal to 90 dB, thus exceeding the minimum speech IA for the supra-aural earphones. For this example, the level of masker selected was 55 dB HL. With this masker level, the AC and BC thresh-olds are elevated (by the masker) to 50 dB HL. At this point, the difference between the presentation level (85 dB HL) and the NTE BC threshold with masking (50 dB HL) is less than the minimum 40 dB IA for speech with supra-aural earphones.

Notice also that a higher level of speech masker (e.g., 65 dB HL) could have been used. A rule of thumb used by many audiologists is to put the speech masker into the NTE at a level 20 dB less than the level of words being presented in the TE. This practice would be appropriate in most situations; however, one must be cautious of over-masking, especially if there is an air–bone gap in the TE. As with pure-tone masking, a masking dilemma may also occur when there is a bilateral conductive hearing loss, because the minimum level of masking could be overmasking. Notice in this example that if WRS testing was done at 85 dB HL, masking would have also been necessary for insert earphones because the 90 dB difference exceeds the minimum 55 dB IA for speech with insert earphones. The masking level used for WRS testing is also included on the audiometric worksheet along with the WRS presentation level and score.

Synopsis 7–3

- The WRS is often categorized in descriptive terms, such as excellent, good, fair, or poor. Patients with normal hearing or conductive hearing losses are expected to have excellent WRS (WRS >90%); those with cochlear hearing losses may vary across all categories in a generally predictable way based on the degree and shape of their hearing loss; those with 8th nerve involvement may have disproportionately poorer WRS than would be predicted from their audiogram.

- It is often useful to evaluate whether the WRS from one ear is different from the other, if there has been a change over time, or if performance is better with one hearing aid than another. To determine whether two scores are significantly different from each other, a binomial distribution table is required (e.g., see Table 7–4) that provides 95% confidence limits when comparing two scores. If two scores are within the 95% confidence values provided by the binomial distribution, then they cannot be considered statistically different from each other.

- WRS testing can also be used for differential diagnosis of cochlear versus 8th nerve pathology, since patients with 8th nerve problems show disproportionately poorer WRS than those with cochlear involvement with the same PTA. Reference to data showing confidence intervals for the NU-6 word lists for cochlear hearing losses as a function PTA are available (e.g., Dubno et al., 1995). If a WRS is outside the confidence interval for cochlear hearing losses, one should determine if the results are consistent with the other diagnostic information to suggest an 8th nerve problem or whether the patient has poor word recognition for other reasons (see Table 6–5).

- A PI–PB function can be used to determine if the WRS shows rollover, a sign of 8th nerve problems. Rollover occurs if the WRS declines at intensity levels higher than where PBmax occurred. A rollover ratio is defined calculated as $PB_{max} - PB_{min} / PB_{max}$.

A rollover ratio for NU-6 word lists which is greater than 0.35 suggests the possibility of 8th nerve involvement, and should be evaluated in context with the other information or results.

- Speech recognition testing in the presence of background noise is also sometimes included in the evaluation to obtain information about how a patient might be performing in more real-world situations. The Hearing in Noise Test (HINT) is one example of a test that has been normed on a relatively large population. The HINT uses sentences presented in quiet and in the presence of a set level of broad spectrum noise. The threshold level of the sentences (where the patient correctly identifies at least 50% of the sentences) is reported as a function of the noise level and this is compared with how normal hearing listeners are expected to perform at the same speech-to-noise ratio. Other speech recognition tests with background noise include the Quick Sentence in Noise (QuickSIN), Speech Perception in Noise (SPIN), and the Synthetic Sentence Identification (SSI).

- For testing children between 3 and 6 years of age, there are special tests available to obtain a measure of supra-threshold speech recognition, most of which include pointing to the correct word from a group of four to six pictures of familiar objects. For SRT, pointing to pictures or to familiar body parts is often used. Speech testing is often done before pure-tone audiometry with young children.

- Masking is needed for speech testing whenever there is the possibility of cross-hearing, as for pure-tone testing. The recommended minimum IA for speech is 40 dB HL and 55 dB for supra-aural and insert earphones, respectively.

- For speech masking, a single level of speech masker is selected for each speech test level, so that the difference between the presentation level of the speech compared with the best BC threshold of the NTE is less that the IA.

References

American National Standards Institute (ANSI). (1997). *Methods for the calculation of the speech intelligibility index.* ANSI S3.5-1997. New York, NY: Author.

American National Standards Institute (ANSI). (2004). *American National Standards for audiometers.* ANSI S3.6 2004. New York, NY: Author.

American Speech-Language-Hearing Association (ASHA). (1988). Guidelines for determining the threshold level for speech. *ASHA, 30,* 85–89.

Bess, F. H., Josey, A. F., & Humes, L. E. (1979). Performance intensity functions in cochlear and eighth nerve disorders. *American Journal of Otolaryngology, 1,* 27–31.

Boothroyd, A. (1999). Computer-assisted speech perception assessment (CASPA) (Version 3.0) [Computer software]. Available from Dr. Boothroyd upon request.

Brandy, W. T. (Ed.). (2002). Speech audiometry. In J. Katz (Ed.), *Handbook of clinical audiology* (5th ed., pp. 96–110). Baltimore, MD: Lippincott Williams & Wilkins.

Chaiklin, J. B., & Ventry, I. M. (1964). Spondee threshold measurement: A comparison of 2- and 5-dB methods. *Journal of Speech and Hearing Disorders, 29,* 47–59.

Downs, D., & Minard, P. (1996). A fast valid method to measure speech-recognition threshold. *Hearing Journal, 49,* 39–44.

Dubno, J. R., Lee, F.-S., Klein, A. J., Mathews, L. J., & Lam, C. F. (1995). Confidence limits for maximum word-recognition scores. *Journal of Speech and Hearing Research, 38,* 490–502.

Fletcher, H. (1950). A method of calculating hearing loss for speech from an audiogram. *Acta Otolaryngologica, 90*(Suppl.), 26–37.

French, N. R., & Steinberg, J. C. (1947). Factors governing the intelligibility of speech sounds. *Journal of the Acoustical Society of America, 19,* 90–119.

Gelfand, S. A. (2001). *Essentials of audiology.* New York, NY: Thieme.

Guthrie, L., & Mackersie, C. M. (2006). *Optimizing presentation level for word recognition testing.* Paper presented at the American Academy of Audiology Conference, Minneapolis, MN.

Humes, L. (1991). Understanding the speech-understanding problems of the hearing impaired. *Journal of the American Academy of Audiology, 2,* 59–69.

Jerger, J., & Jerger, S. (1971). Diagnostic significance of PB word functions. *Archives of Otolaryngology, 93,* 573–580.

Kamm, C., Dirks, D. D., & Mickey, M. R. (1978). Effect of sensorineural hearing loss on loudness discomfort level and most comfortable loudness judgements. *Journal of Speech and Hearing Research, 21,* 668–681.

Mackersie, C. L., Boothroyd, A., & Minniear, D. (2001). Evaluation of the computer-assisted speech perception assessment test (CASPA). *Journal of the American Academy of Audiology, 12,* 390–396.

Maroonroge, S., & Diefendorf, A. O. (1984). Comparing normal hearing and hearing-impaired subjects' performance on the Northwestern Auditory Test number 6, California Consonant Test, and Pascoe's High Frequency Word Test. *Ear and Hearing, 5,* 356–360.

Martin, F. N., Champlin, C. A., & Chambers, J. A. (1998). Seventh survey of audiometric practices in the United States. *Journal of the American Academy of Audiology, 9,* 95–104.

Martin, F. N., & Dowdy, L. K. (1986). A modified spondee threshold procedure. *Journal of Auditory Research, 26,* 115–119.

Meyer, D. H., & Mishler, E. T. (1985). Rollover measurements with Auditec NU-6 word lists. *Journal of Speech and Hearing Disorders, 50,* 356–360.

Mueller, H. G., & Killion, M. C. (1990). An easy method for calculating the articulation index. *Hearing Journal, 43,* 14–17.

Nilsson, M., Soli, S., & Sullivan, J. (1994). Development of the hearing in noise test for the measurement of speech reception thresholds in quiet and noise. *Journal of the Acoustical Society of America, 95,* 1085–1099.

Niquette, P., Gudmundsen, G., & Killion, M. (2001). *QuickSIN Documentation,* Elk Grove, IL: Etymotic Research.

Pavlovic, C. V. (1988). Articulation index predictions of speech intelligibility in hearing aid selection. *American Speech and Hearing Association, 30,* 63–65.

Sklare, D. A., & Denneberg, L. J. (1987). Technical note: Interaural attenuation for tubephone insert earphones. *Ear and Hearing, 8,* 298–300.

Thornton, A. R., & Raffin, M. J. M. (1978). Speech discrimination scores modified as a binomial variable. *Journal of Speech and Hearing Research, 21,* 507–518.

Yacullo, W. S. (1996). *Clinical masking procedures.* Boston, MA: Allyn and Bacon.

8

Physiological Measures

After reading this chapter, you should be able to:

1. Define admittance and describe how the admittance of the middle ear is measured using tympanometry and acoustic reflex threshold tests.
2. Recognize and describe tympanogram shapes (types) and their clinical interpretations.
3. Understand how and when to use high frequency probe-tone tympanometry and acoustic reflex measures; recognize how B and G tympanograms can differentiate mass and stiffness disorders.
4. Describe and interpret measures of wideband middle ear power (reflectance).
5. Interpret acoustic reflex threshold patterns (ipsilateral and contralateral) and acoustic reflex decay measures.
6. Use acoustic reflex threshold criteria for cochlear ears (based on data by Gelfand et al.) to differentiate cochlear, 8th nerve, and functional hearing loss.
7. Describe the measurement of transient evoked otoacoustic emissions (TEOAEs) and distortion product otoacoustic emissions (DPOAEs).
8. Relate the presence and absence of otoacoustic emission (OAE) measures to the degree of hearing loss and differentiation of cochlear and neural disorders.
9. Describe the normal expected auditory brainstem response (ABR) waveform and how it changes with intensity.
10. Interpret ABR results as they relate to hearing thresholds and 8th nerve disorders.

We turn our attention in this chapter to other measures of auditory function that do not require the patient to understand the task or to make any subjective responses. Given the limitations of behavioral tests, like pure-tone and speech audiometry, to differentiate cochlear from neural types of hearing losses, and for testing young infants and other difficult-to-test populations, there has been a long history in the field of audiology directed toward developing reliable physiological measures of the auditory system. These physiological tests require instrumentation that is usually separate from the audiometer. Although these physiological tests are considered objective in nature, they do require the patient to be relatively cooperative or sedated in order to obtain valid responses. It is also important to keep in mind that the monitoring and interpretation of the physiological tests rely, to a certain extent, on the skill and subjective interpretation of the audiologist. Although not an actual complete measure of hearing per se, physiological measures often provide the only information about the function of specific parts of the auditory system. In addition, physiological measures can often provide a cross-check with other results, and/or can provide information that may suggest a particular course of follow-up or treatment. When physiological measures are combined with audiometric results and/or medical imaging, a more complete picture of the patient's problem can be determined.

Today, there are several physiological measures that are established in clinical audiology, including tympanometry, acoustic reflexes, otoacoustic emissions (OAEs), and auditory brainstem responses (ABRs). Tympanometry and acoustic reflexes are tests that are included in *immittance audiometry*, and are of such importance that they are routinely included in the basic audiological evaluation, along with pure-tone and speech audiometry. Immittance tests provide a look at how well sound energy is able to be transmitted through the outer ear and middle ear. The OAE and ABR tests are part of what is called *auditory evoked (electroacoustic or electroneural) responses*, and are widely used as part of newborn "hearing" screening programs and/or when behavioral tests are unsuccessful. Auditory evoked responses may also be useful for providing some

helpful information relative to the diagnosis of possible 8th nerve or central auditory system disorders. The OAE tests measure electro-acoustic "echoes" within the ear canal that are emitted as part of the normal physiological activity of the cochlea, thought to be primarily related to outer hair cell (OHC) activity. The ABR test measures the underlying neural activity of the brainstem (neuro-electric potentials) from disk electrodes placed on the surface of the scalp. The ABR test can evaluate different types and degrees of peripheral auditory disorders by monitoring how the neural activity emanating from the cochlea is affected by conductive or cochlear disorders. The ABR test can also be used to identify disorders in the 8th nerve and low brainstem pathways. The following sections provide an introductory look at the instrumentation, procedures, and interpretations of physiological tests as they are commonly used in clinical audiology.

Immittance

Immittance audiometry infers the extent to which sound energy is transferred through the outer and middle ear systems. If we apply a known sound source to the ear, the acoustic and mechanical properties of the outer and middle ear provide a certain amount of opposition to the flow of energy. The opposition to the flow of energy is called *impedance*, such that a high impedance system has a greater opposition to the flow of energy. The reciprocal of impedance is called *admittance*, which is a measure of how much of the applied energy flows through the system, such that a high admittance system has a greater flow of energy. A high admittance system has a low impedance, and vice versa. If either impedance or admittance is known, the other can be determined by a relatively simple calculation, since they are reciprocals. Impedance is usually designated as Z and measured in units of *ohms* (e.g., $Z = X$ ohms); admittance is usually designated as Y and measured in units of *millimhos* (e.g., $Y = X$ mmhos). They are related such that $Y = 1/Z$ or $Z = 1/Y$. The term *immittance* is used to encompass the concepts

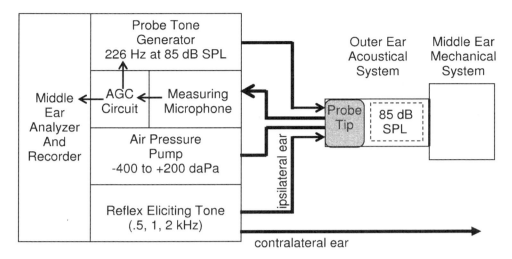

Figure 8–1. Block diagram showing the key components of an admittance instrument or middle ear analyzer. The air pressure pump is used to apply air pressure during tympanometry. The reflex eliciting tones (ipsilateral and contralateral) are used for acoustic reflex testing. See text for an explanation on how the probe tone is used to measure the admittance of the outer and middle ear. *AGC,* automatic gain circuit

of both admittance and impedance. However, today's immittance instruments are designed to measure the admittance characteristics of the auditory system.

The instrument used in immittance audiometry goes by a variety of names, such as an "immittance instrument," "admittance instrument," or "middle ear analyzer." A variety of immittance instruments are commercially available from different manufacturers. Figure 8–1 shows the basic components of an admittance instrument. To obtain a measure of admittance, an 85 dB SPL pure tone (usually 226 Hz), called the *probe tone,* is presented to the ear through a probe assembly placed at the entrance to the ear canal. A microphone, which is also part of the probe assembly, is used to monitor the level of the probe tone in the ear canal. For infants younger than 6 months, conventional tympanometry with a 226 Hz probe tone is not a valid measure, and other probe-tone frequencies are recommended (as described later in this chapter).

For a normal outer and middle ear system, there is an expected admittance associated with a given probe tone. Modern instruments use an *automatic gain control* (AGC) circuit to automatically adjust the output of the probe tone to maintain the probe tone at 85 dB SPL in the ear canal. The change in dB SPL needed by the AGC circuit is a reflection of how much energy is admitted by the system, and is used to calculate the admittance.

The measured admittance is compared with the admittance characteristics of known cavity sizes. For example, for a 226 Hz probe tone, 1.0 mmho is approximately equal to the admittance associated with a 1.0 cubic centimeter (cm^3) or 1.0 milliliter (mL) volume of air at sea level. Although the mmho is the more preferable unit, some instruments plot the admittance in units of cm^3 or ml. This simple relationship of admittance to volume is one of the reasons why 226 Hz is used as the probe tone. Figure 8–2 shows that, as cavity size increases,[1] the admittance of

---

[1]Acoustic immittance (Y_a) is equal to volume velocity (U) divided by the pressure (P). As cavity size increases (larger U), the admittance increases for a constant pressure. Likewise, as admittance increases, the cavity size increases for a constant pressure.

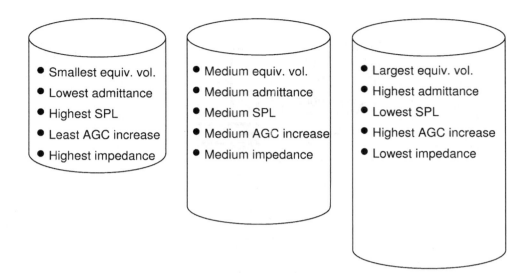

- Smallest equiv. vol.
- Lowest admittance
- Highest SPL
- Least AGC increase
- Highest impedance

- Medium equiv. vol.
- Medium admittance
- Medium SPL
- Medium AGC increase
- Medium impedance

- Largest equiv. vol.
- Highest admittance
- Lowest SPL
- Highest AGC increase
- Lowest impedance

Figure 8–2. Illustration of the relationship between the volume of a cavity and measures of admittance or impedance. As cavity size increases, the admittance increases due to a reduced sound pressure level (*SPL*) of the probe tone, and more gain is required by the automatic gain circuit (*AGC*) to maintain the 85 dB SPL probe-tone level in the ear canal. Clinically, admittance measures are related to the admittance of cavities of known volumes and compared with the expected admittance for normal ears.

an acoustic system increases and, therefore, the AGC circuit must increase the SPL to maintain the 226 Hz probe tone at 85 dB SPL. Because of the relation of admittance to cavity size, the clinical measures of admittance are calibrated to be equivalent to different cavity sizes that approximate the range of admittance characteristics found in the ear. Clinically, the admittance values obtained from a patient are compared with what is expected from a normal ear. When admittance is lower than normal, it is equivalent to the admittance of a smaller cavity and indicates that less energy is flowing into the ear. When admittance is higher than normal, it is equivalent to the admittance of a larger cavity and indicates that more energy is flowing into the ear. The clinical immittance tests monitor how the dB SPL of the probe tone is affected by changes that occur in the transmission of sound in the outer and middle ear. The different types of immittance tests are described in the following sections.

Tympanometry

Tympanometry measures how the admittance changes as a function of applied air pressure and how this function is affected by different conditions of the middle ear. Figure 8–3 shows a typical graph used for tympanometry, a *tympanogram*. The admittance scale (*y*-axis) is in units of mmhos or ml calibrated to known cavity sizes. The pressure range (*x*-axis) represents pressures above and below atmospheric pressure, which is represented by 0 decaPascals (daPa). The air pressure is delivered by the air pressure pump of the immittance instrument through the probe assembly (see Figure 8–1). For tympanometry, it is important to have the probe assembly make an airtight seal at the entrance to the ear canal by selecting the appropriate-size rubber probe tip so that the air pressure can be applied. Getting an airtight seal may take some practice; it is usually helpful

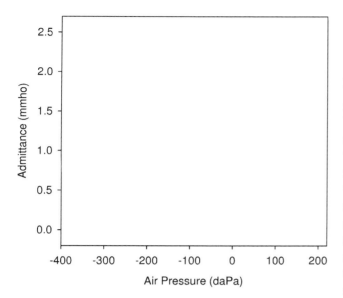

Figure 8–3. A typical graph that is used to display tympanograms. The admittance instrument is used to measure the admittance in millimhos (mmhos) along the *y*-axis, as a function of applied air pressure in decaPascals (daPa) along the *x*-axis. The 0 daPa value represents the atmospheric pressure, and the other daPa values are above (+) or below (–) atmospheric pressure.

to select a probe tip that is slightly larger than the ear canal and to pull up and back on the auricle to straighten the cartilaginous portion of the ear canal as the probe is inserted.

Tympanometry provides a means of separating the admittance related to the ear canal from the admittance related to the middle ear. This is performed by first applying maximum positive air pressure (+200 daPa), which effectively reduces the ability of the tympanic membrane to vibrate: The admittance recorded at +200 daPa is a relatively low admittance that is a reflection of the admittance of the ear canal only. This would be equivalent to the admittance of a smaller cavity because the middle ear is not functional and, therefore, does not allow as much sound energy to be admitted. Once the admittance of the ear canal is obtained at +200 daPa, the air pressure is swept through the range of pressures (usually

done automatically) from +200 to −400 daPa. For a normal functioning middle ear, there should be a maximum admittance at 0 daPa (atmospheric pressure) because that is where the air pressure in the external ear canal is equal to the air pressure in the middle ear, and allows the tympanic membrane to vibrate most effectively. The maximum admittance measured at 0 daPa is equivalent to the volume of a larger cavity and is a reflection of the function of both the outer ear and middle ear in the transmission of the probe tone. As the applied air pressure becomes negative, the admittance decreases again (equivalent to the volume of a smaller cavity) because the tympanic membrane does not vibrate as efficiently. Figure 8–4 illustrates the principles of recording a tympanogram at three different pressure points. The admittance of the middle ear is represented by the difference between the admittance obtained at +200 daPa and the admittance obtained at 0 daPa (or the point of maximum admittance).

Figure 8–5 shows a normal tympanogram, conventionally called a *Type A tympanogram*. The shape of the normal (Type A) tympanogram has the peak admittance occurring at 0 daPa and a systematic reduction in admittance at the higher and lower pressures. The pressure where the tympanogram peak occurs is called the *tympanometric peak pressure* (TPP). The admittance at +200 is related to the *equivalent volume of the ear canal* (V_{ec}). The overall peak of the tympanogram (Peak Y) may include the admittance of both the outer ear and the middle ear; therefore, the actual *admittance of the middle ear* (Y_{tm}), as calculated at the tympanic membrane, is the difference in admittance between Peak Y and V_{ec}. The manner in which the tympanogram is displayed in Figure 8–5 is called a *non-compensated tympanogram*, which means that the graph displays the admittance value for the ear canal (V_{ec} at +200 daPa) and the additional admittance that is related to the middle ear (Y_{tm} at 0 daPa). Today's immittance instruments can also display the tympanogram as a *compensated tympanogram,* which is shown in Figure 8-6. A compensated tympanogram automatically removes the admittance due to the ear canal (at +200 daPa) and graphically displays

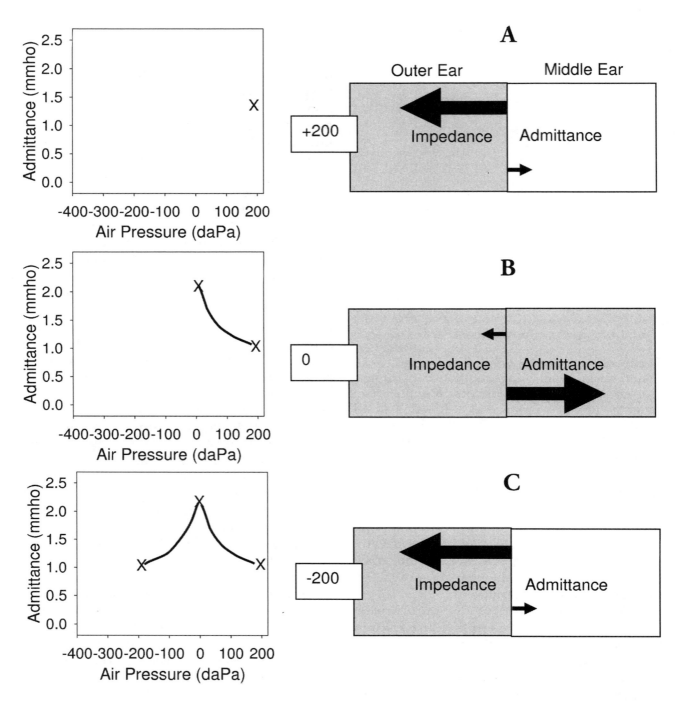

Figure 8–4. A–C. Illustration of how a normal tympanogram is generated. In **A**, the applied air pressure is at +200 daPa above atmospheric pressure and results in a minimum admittance that is equivalent to a relatively small cavity. This small admittance represents the admittance of only the outer ear because the tympanic membrane is not able to vibrate normally. In **B**, when the applied air pressure is lowered to 0 daPa (atmospheric pressure), the admittance reaches a maximum because the tympanic membrane can now vibrate most effectively. In this case, the admittance is equivalent to a larger cavity that represents the admittance of the outer and middle ear. In **C**, when the applied air pressure is at –200 daPa, the tympanic membrane does not vibrate effectively and the admittance is again equivalent to a small cavity that represents the admittance of only the outer ear. The actual admittance of the middle ear itself is represented by the difference between the maximum admittance and the admittance at +200 daPa.

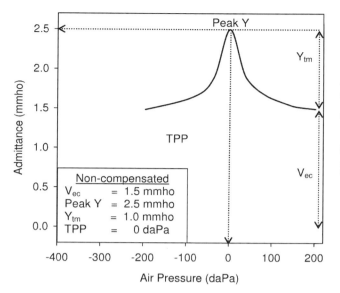

Figure 8–5. A normal *non-compensated* tympanogram. The admittance of the outer ear (V_{ec}) is first obtained at +200 daPa and is then subtracted from the overall admittance (*Peak Y*) to obtain the admittance of the middle ear (Y_{tm}). The air pressure where the peak of the tympanogram occurs is called the tympanometric peak pressure (*TPP*).

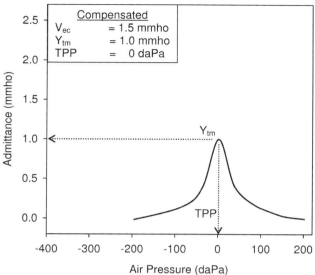

Figure 8–6. A normal *compensated* tympanogram. The admittance of the outer ear (V_{ec}) is first obtained at +200 daPa but is not displayed on the graph; instead the tympanogram is automatically displaced downward by the amount of the V_{ec} so that the peak admittance is a direct reflection of the admittance of the middle ear (Y_{tm}). The V_{ec} is only displayed as a numerical value. The air pressure where the peak of the tympanogram occurs is called the tympanometric peak pressure (*TPP*).

only the admittance of the middle ear. The compensated tympanogram begins at +200 daPa with an admittance of 0 mmhos. With a compensated tympanogram, the admittance of the ear canal (V_{ec}) is provided on the printout in numerical format. Compensated tympanograms are popular because the admittance on the *y*-axis is a direct measure of the middle ear admittance (Y_{tm}). Most of the tympanograms in this text will be displayed in the compensated format.

The ranges of normative values for the different tympanometric measures vary across studies and are dependent on a variety of parameters, including age, gender, pump speed, and direction of pressure change. Some normative values for the different tympanometric measures are shown in Table 8–1 (American Speech-Language-Hearing Association Audiologic Assessment Panel, 1997; Margolis & Hunter, 2000; Roush, Bryant, Mundy,

Zeisel, & Roberts, 1995). As you can see, the normal admittance values have a relatively wide range; however, when a measure is outside these norms, there is a good correlation with an abnormal middle ear condition.

Ear Canal Equivalent Volume

The *ear canal equivalent volume* (V_{ec}), as estimated from the admittance obtained at +200 daPa, can provide some diagnostic information about the condition of the tympanic membrane or ear canal. For a normal ear canal and tympanic membrane, the admittance at +200 should be within the normal range of ear canal volumes (see Table 8–1).

Table 8–1. Sample Normative (90%) Ranges for Tympanometric Measures of Static Acoustic Admittance of the Middle Ear (Y_{tm}), Equivalent Volume of Ear Canal (V_{ec}), Tympanometric Width (*TW*), and Tympanometric Peak Pressure (*TPP*)

	Y_{tm} (mmhos)	V_{ec} (ml)	TW (daPa)	TPP (daPa)
Adults (≥18 years)[a]	0.30–1.70	0.6–2.0	51–114	−100 to 50
Children (3 to 10 years)[a]	0.25–1.05	0.3–0.9	80–159	−100 to 50
Infants and toddlers (6 to 30 months)[b]	0.20–0.70	NA	102–204	−174 to 18
ASHA screen fail criteria[c]	<0.3	>1.0	>200	Not used

[a]Data from Margolis and Hunter (2000).
[b]Data from Roush et al. (1995).
[c]Data from ASHA Audiologic Assessment Panel (1997).

Figure 8–7 illustrates how the V_{ec} can be used to determine the status of the tympanic membrane or the ear canal for different conditions. In Figure 8-7A, the tympanic membrane is intact and the V_{ec} is within the normal range. In Figure 8-7B, the tympanic membrane has a perforation or a pressure equalization (PE) tube surgically inserted for the treatment of a chronic ear infection, resulting in a V_{ec} that is larger than the normal range because it now is equivalent to a larger cavity that includes the outer ear and middle ear. Alternately, as shown in Figure 8-7C, if the V_{ec} is lower than the expected normal range, this may be an indication that the external ear canal is obstructed by a foreign object or has impacted cerumen. For either of these abnormal V_{ec} conditions, the tympanogram will not show any changes in admittance as the applied air pressure is varied and appears as a flat line. As cautionary notes, a small V_{ec} may also be caused by a plugged probe assembly, or the probe assembly is pushed up against the ear canal wall. It is also possible that an ear with a perforation could show a normal V_{ec} if there is thick fluid or other tissue mass that is filling the middle ear.

In some patients, you may not be able to obtain an adequate seal of the probe tip because the applied positive air pressure or a swallow by the patient may open up the eustachian tube and release the air pressure. In those cases, it is useful to set the tympanogram to measure V_{ec} at −200 daPa

(which can hold the eustachian tube in its naturally closed position) and ask the patient not to breathe while performing the tympanogram by sweeping the air pressure from negative to positive.

Tympanometric Width

Another way to quantify a tympanogram's shape is to measure the width of the tympanogram, *tympanometric width* (TW), at a defined point. Tympanometric width is defined as the absolute value of the pressure range, in daPa, that corresponds to the width of the tympanogram at half the height of the peak of the tympanogram. Figure 8-8 illustrates how TW is calculated. First establish the point that is half of the height of the Y_{tm}; then draw a horizontal line at this half-height point to intersect the positive and negative sides of the tympanogram. At each of the two intersection points, drop a vertical line down to the two corresponding pressure points along the *x*-axis: The TW is the difference between these two pressure points and is expressed in daPa. Most modern instruments automatically calculate and display the value of TW. Figure 8-9 shows examples of abnormally wide tympanograms. An abnormal TW is usually associated with middle ear fluid that is either accumulating or resolving; and as the condition of the middle ear changes, the tympanogram

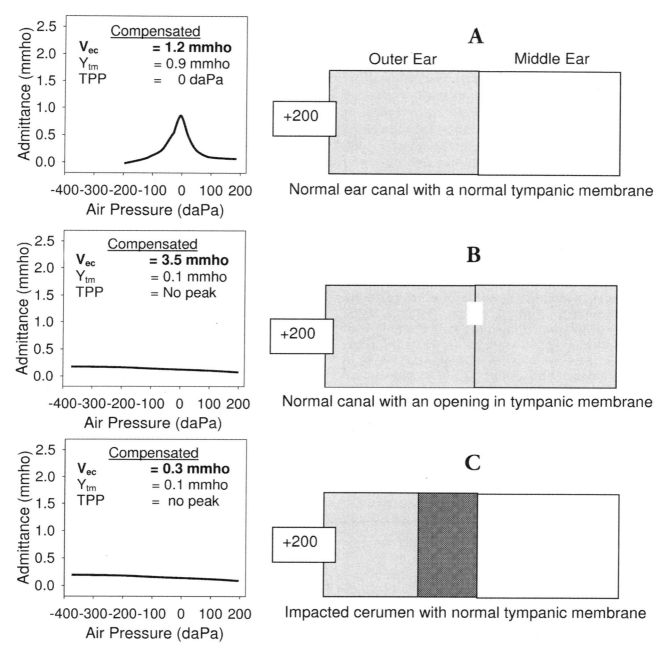

Figure 8–7. A–C. Illustration of how admittance of the outer ear (V_{ec}) is used clinically. In **A**, the tympanic membrane is intact, as evidenced by a normal-shaped tympanogram and a normal V_{ec}. In **B**, the tympanic membrane has a perforation, as evidenced by the flat tympanogram and larger than normal V_{ec}. In **C**, the ear canal is impacted with earwax (cerumen), as evidenced by a flat tympanogram and a smaller than normal V_{ec}. Y_{tm}, admittance of the middle ear; *TPP*, tympanometric peak pressure.

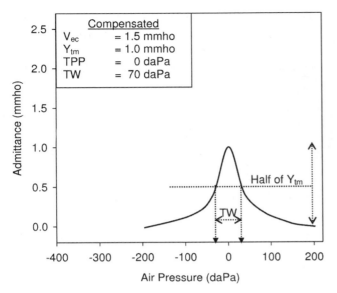

Figure 8–8. Illustration of how to calculate tympanometric width (*TW*). First, find the value on the *y*-axis that represents half the height of the admittance of the middle ear (Y_{tm}) and draw a horizontal line so that it intersects the tympanogram on both sides. Then draw vertical lines down from the two intersecting points to the air pressure scale. The TW is the absolute value of the difference between the two pressure points. Most admittance instruments can automatically calculate the TW. V_{ec} admittance of the outer ear; *TPP*, tympanometric peak pressure.

may become a flat line or may become normal. Refer to Table 8–1 for normal ranges of TW based on several studies. For example, a TW >159 daPa would be abnormal for children 3 to 12 years old based on data by Margolis and Hunter (2000).

Sensitivity and Specificity of Tympanometric Measures

The selection of a criterion value for the tympanometric measures, such as those found in Table 8–1, will have an associated level of *sensitivity* that estimates how good the criterion value correctly identifies ears with middle ear fluid, as well as a *specificity* that estimates how good the criterion value correctly identifies normal ears. Although it would be nice to have a criterion that results in 100% sensitivity and 100% specificity, most tests are not that good. It is important to select a criterion value that identifies those you want to identify but minimizes the number of patients who do not have the problem, also referred to as the *false positive rate*. For most tests, there is a trade-off between the sensitivity and specificity. For example, one could select a low TW criterion that would increase the sensitivity, but this would also increase the false positive rate, and you would

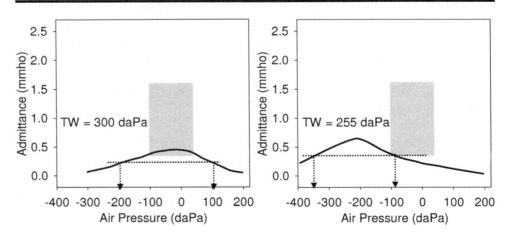

Figure 8–9. Two examples in which the tympanic width (*TW*) is abnormally wide. The normal range for TW is indicated by the *shaded box*. Calculation of TW is independent of the tympanic peak pressure (TPP).

end up over-referring for treatment patients who do not have middle ear fluid. You could select a larger value of TW in order to reduce the false positive rate, but this would also reduce the sensitivity. The trick for any test is to pick a criterion value that gives you the highest sensitivity, but also a reasonably low false-positive rate.

Figure 8-10 shows how the sensitivity and specificity (or false positive rate) change for different values of TW and Y_{tm} (Nozza, Bluestone, Kardatzke, & Brackman, 1994). The ideal test

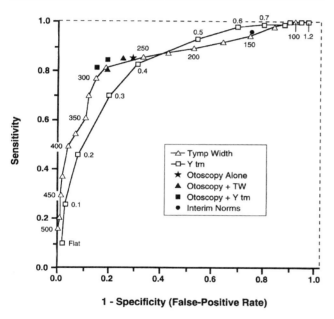

Figure 8-10. Data from Nozza et al. (1994) which show how the sensitivity and specificity can change for different values of tympanometric width (*TW*) and peak admittance of the middle ear (Y_{tm}). See text for a more complete explanation. For TW, a width criterion greater than 275 daPa would result in the highest sensitivity and lowest false positive rate. For Y_{tm}, an admittance criterion less than 0.3 mmhos would result in the highest sensitivity and lowest false positive rate. Different criterion values could be selected if one wanted to increase the sensitivity; however, this would result in more false positives. Likewise, false positives could be decreased, but this would result in decreased sensitivity. From Nozza et al. 1994, p. 315. Copyright 1994 by Williams & Wilkins.

would be represented by the left corner of the graph where the sensitivity is 1.0 and the false positive rate is zero. The data points that are closest to the left corner will have the best trade-off between the highest sensitivity and the lowest false positive rate. For the data shown, the best criterion value for TW would be about 275 daPa. Likewise, the best criterion value for Y_{tm} would be about 0.3 mmhos. By having data like those in Figure 8-10, you could even choose different criterion values depending on whether it was more desirable to increase sensitivity (but increase false positive rate) or to reduce false positive rate (but decrease sensitivity). If you compare the data from Figure 8-10 with the normal ranges given in Table 8-1, you can see that the lower value for Y_{tm} in Table 8-1 (0.25 mmhos) agrees fairly well with the best criterion shown for the data in Figure 8-10 (0.3 mmhos). However, the upper values for TW, shown in Table 8-1 for each age group, are less than the best TW shown in Figure 8-10 (275 daPa). This means that there are relatively high false positive rates associated with the values in Table 8-1. You can see the increase in false positives by plotting the different criterion points for TW from Table 8-1 onto Figure 8-10.

Types of Tympanograms

A commonly used scheme to describe tympanograms is based on the types described by Jerger (1970). As already described, the normal tympanogram is referred to as a Type A tympanogram (see Figure 8-6). Abnormal tympanograms, as illustrated in Figure 8-11, are labeled *Type A_s*, *Type A_d*, *Type B*, and *Type C* tympanograms. While Jerger's classification scheme is widely used, not everyone reading an audiology report will know what the types mean. A more useful approach is to describe the actual characteristics of the tympanogram, for example, "a flat tympanogram" or "a normal-shaped tympanogram with the peak admittance occurring at −300 daPa." The different types of tympanograms and their descriptions are briefly described below.

Normal admittance (Type A) tympanogram has a characteristic peak shape with the Y_{tm} and the

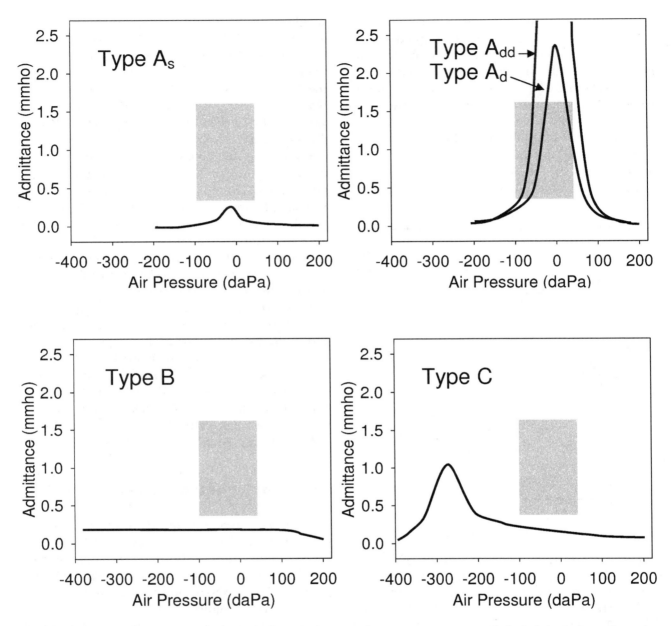

Figure 8–11. Examples of commonly found abnormal tympanograms and their labels based on the Jerger (1970) classification scheme. See text for descriptions of these tympanogram types and their associated pathologies.

TPP within the normal range. A normal (Type A) tympanogram occurs in normal functioning middle ears, but can also be found in some ears with otosclerosis (a fixation of the stapes in the oval window) or disarticulation (disruption) of the ossicular chain. A patient with a normal (Type A) will not have an air–bone gap if the patient has a normal functioning middle ear; however, a patient may have a normal (Type A) tympanogram and an air–bone gap (conductive loss) on the audiogram if she has an ossicular chain abnormality like otosclerosis or disarticulation.

Reduced admittance (Type A$_s$) tympanogram has a characteristic peak shape with the TPP in the normal range as for Type A; however, the Y$_{tm}$ is lower than the lower end of the normal range. This type of tympanogram is sometimes referred to as "shallow." A reduced (Type A$_s$) tympanogram suggests reduced movement of the tympanic membrane, which may be seen in some cases of otosclerosis and in some cases of otitis media (fluid in the middle ear). A patient with a reduced (Type A$_s$) tympanogram is likely to have some air–bone gaps (conductive loss) on the audiogram.

High admittance (Type A$_d$ or Type A$_{dd}$) tympanogram has a characteristic peak shape with the TPP in the normal range as for Type A; however, the Y$_{tm}$ is higher than the upper end of the normal range. A high admittance (Type A$_d$) tympanogram suggests a highly mobile tympanic membrane, which may be seen in some cases of disarticulation of the ossicular chain or cases of thinned tympanic membranes resulting from previous middle ear infections. A high admittance (Type A$_{dd}$) tympanogram has an extremely high-value Y$_{tm}$; in fact, the admittance may go off the chart. These high admittance types (Type A$_d$ or Type A$_{dd}$) are highly suggestive of a disarticulation of the ossicular chain and will usually have an air–bone gap (conductive loss) on their audiogram.

Flat (Type B) tympanogram does not have the characteristic peak shape seen for Type A, but instead appears as a relatively flat tracing across the pressure range. A flat (Type B) tympanogram is quite common in cases of otitis media with effusion (fluid in the middle ear). A flat (Type B) tympanogram will also occur when there is a perforation in the tympanic membrane or if a pressure equalization (PE) tube has been put into the tympanic membrane as a treatment for otitis media; however, perforations or PE tubes can be differentiated from otitis media by a larger than normal V$_{ec}$. A flat (Type B) tympanogram can also occur with impacted cerumen, a clogged probe assembly, or with the probe pushed against the ear canal wall; however, these conditions will be accompanied by a lower than normal V$_{ec}$. The audiologist must be sure that a flat (Type B) tympanogram is not due to poor placement or poor operation of the probe assembly. The patient with a flat (Type B) tympanogram may or may not have air–bone gaps on the audiogram depending on the reason for the flat tracing: A flat (Type B) tympanogram with a normal V$_{ec}$ is expected to have air–bone gaps on the audiogram; a flat (Type B) tympanogram with a large V$_{ec}$, due to a small perforation or PE tube, most likely will not have air–bone gaps on the audiogram; a flat (Type B) tympanogram with a low V$_{ec}$, due to a foreign object or impacted cerumen, may have small air–bone gaps on the audiogram.

Negative pressure (Type C) tympanogram has a characteristic peak shape as seen with Type A; however, the TPP is shifted to a more negative pressure point. A negative pressure (Type C) tympanogram indicates that the pressure in the middle ear space is not equalized to the atmospheric pressure. Some negative pressure is common in ears as a temporary condition due to sniffling or subsequent to a recent airplane flight. These situations are generally not of much clinical significance, and in many cases once the pressure is equalized by opening the eustachian tube by swallowing or "popping" the ears, the negative pressure (Type C) tympanogram will change to a normal (Type A) tympanogram. However, when the TPP is outside the normal ranges and a negative pressure (Type C) tympanogram persists for an extended period of time, it may suggest poor eustachian tube function due to allergy or a cold. Poor eustachian tube function can lead to fluid in the ear, at which point the tympanogram will change to flat (Type B). A patient with a negative pressure (Type C) tympanogram will usually not have air–bone gaps on the audiogram unless the Type C tympanogram is also accompanied by a reduced Y$_{tm}$ or an abnormal TW.

In summary, an abnormal tympanogram is a good indication of some middle ear involvement that affects the admittance characteristics of the middle ear. However, the tympanogram is not a predictor of the amount (if any) of conductive hearing loss and is most useful when used in conjunction with the pure-tone audiogram or other information about the patient. It is important to keep in mind also that the shape of the tympanogram does not always define the precise pathology, since some of the shapes can occur for different middle ear conditions. For example, when a normal, Type A, tympanogram is obtained you should not assume that the middle ear is normal because this can be found in some cases of otosclerosis or disarticulations; however, patients with these disorders should have air–bone gaps on their audiograms (see Chapter 9). A normal (Type A) tympanogram without any air–bone gaps on the audiogram rules out middle ear involvement, however, if there is an air–bone gap on the audiogram it suggests some involvement of the ossicular chain, but rules out fluid in the middle ear (which should have a flat type B tympanogram).

In addition, a normal (Type A) tympanogram rules out a perforation in the tympanic membrane, obstruction of the ear canal, and fluid in the middle ear. Tympanometry is a valuable tool and is routinely included as part of the basic audiological test battery. In some cases, especially with children or other difficult-to-test populations in which the pure-tone audiogram is not obtainable or is incomplete, tympanometric data can be helpful as long as you keep in mind the limitations of interpretation and use the information with other relevant patient information.

Synopsis 8–1

- Physiological tests such as tympanometry, acoustic reflex thresholds, and otoacoustic emissions are routinely included in the basic hearing evaluation. When used in conjunction with the history, pure-tone audiometry, and/or speech audiometry, physiological measures can help differentiate or confirm different types of hearing disorders.

- Immittance is a term that refers to measures of impedance or admittance. Admittance is the ease with which the energy flows through a system. Impedance is the opposition to the flow of energy through a system.

- Most clinical instruments measure the admittance using a probe assembly sealed at the entrance to the ear canal. The probe assembly has a miniature speaker to deliver a probe tone (usually 226 Hz at 85 dB SPL) and a microphone to monitor the dB SPL of the probe tone. The admittance is determined by measuring how the SPL of the probe tone changes with applied pressure (tympanometry) or due to the middle ear reflex in response to a reflex eliciting tone (acoustic reflexes).

- In tympanometry, air pressure is applied over a range of +200 to −400 daPa relative to atmospheric pressure (0 daPa) and the change in admittance as a function of air-pressure is graphed on a tympanogram. At the extreme positive and negative applied pressures, the admittance is reduced due to the immobility of the tympanic membrane caused by the applied air pressure. The positive pressure point allows for the estimation of the ear canal volume (V_{ec}) that is subtracted from the overall admittance in order to provide a measure of the middle ear admittance (Y_{tm}). A larger than normal V_{ec} can indicate a tympanic membrane perforation or pressure equalization tube. A smaller than normal V_{ec} can indicate a cerumen-impacted ear canal or blocked probe.

Other tympanogram measures include the pressure where peak admittance occurs (TPP) or the width of the tympanogram at half its maximum height (TW). Tympanograms have conventional types and descriptions as follows:

- Normal (Type A) tympanogram: Peak shape with a normal Y_{tm} occurring with a TPP around 0 daPa. Suggestive of normal functioning middle ears and some cases with otosclerosis or ossicular disarticulation.

- Reduced admittance (Type A_s) tympanogram: Peak shape with a reduced (shallow) Y_{tm} occurring with a TPP around 0 daPa. Suggestive of otosclerosis or otitis media.

- High admittance (Type A_d or A_{dd}) tympanogram: Peak shape with a higher than normal Y_{tm} occurring with a TPP around 0 daPa. Suggestive of ossicular disarticulation or highly mobile/flaccid tympanic membrane.

- Flat (Type B) tympanogram: Low admittance and flat tracings (no change in Y_{tm} across the pressure range). Suggestive of otitis media with effusion. Also occurs with a tympanic membrane perforation or pressure equalization tube; however, these can be identified by the V_{ec}.

- Negative pressure (Type C) tympanogram: Peak shape with a normal or reduced Y_{tm} occurring with a TPP in the negative pressure range. Suggestive of temporary eustachian tube dysfunction and/or resolving or developing stages of otitis media with effusion.

- See Table 8–1 and Figure 8–10 for normative tympanometric values.

Multicomponent and Multifrequency Tympanometry

In the previous section, the tympanometric measures were described for recordings made with a conventional low frequency (226 Hz) probe tone. The use of the low frequency probe tone may be justified when evaluating middle ear pathologies that predominantly affect the stiffness component of the middle ear system. However, there are some middle ear pathologies that are dominated by the mass component of the middle ear system, and these are better assessed using higher frequency probe tones (e.g., 678 or 1000 Hz). Mass dominant pathologies might include those that add mass to the system, such as scar tissue on the tympanic membrane or adhesions on the middle ear ossicles, or a break in the ossicular chain (disarticulation) that becomes mass dominant due to the reduction of the stiffness component. In addition, research has shown that infants younger than 4 months of age are better assessed with higher frequency (1000 Hz) probe tones due to developmental differences in outer and/or middle ear systems, and residual mesenchyme in the middle ear for a short period after birth (Hall & Swanepoel, 2010; Shanks & Shohet, 2009). Tympanometry using higher frequency probe tones can more readily differentiate between stiffness and mass dominant pathologies. For example knowledge about the relative contributions of the stiffness and mass components provide differential diagnosis of pathologies due to fixation of the ossicular chain (otosclerosis) or disarticulation, both of which show up as a conductive hearing loss on the audiogram, and may even have relatively normal appearing tympanograms to low frequency probe tones.

The admittance of the middle ear system is affected by the friction, mass, and stiffness of the structures. The admittance related to the frictional component is called *conductance* (G), the admittance related to the mass is called *mass susceptance* (B_m), and the admittance related to the stiffness is called *stiffness susceptance* (B_s).[2] These three components are related to each other in a complex manner. The easiest way to visualize the relationship of these components is through vectors as shown in Figure 8–12. Each component has a different relationship between an applied sinusoidal force and the resulting motion (velocity). The conductance component is in phase with the applied force, which means that when the force is at a minimum, the motion is at a minimum, and when the force is at a maximum, the motion is at a maximum. In the vector plot, the conductance (in-phase component) is represented as a horizontal line. On the other hand, the susceptance components are out of phase with the applied force such that when the force is at a maximum, the motion is at a minimum, and when the force is at a minimum, the motion is at a maximum. The easiest way to visualize this is to think of the mass as having inertia that needs to be overcome by the applied force before it is set into motion; it takes maximum force to get the object moving, and once the inertia is overcome the object moves with minimal additional outside force. Likewise, the stiffness susceptance acts like a spring: When the applied force is at a maximum, the motion is at a minimum, and when the applied force is at a minimum, the motion is at a maximum. These relations make the susceptance components 90° out of phase with the conductance component. However, it should be noted that the mass susceptance and the stiffness susceptance are 180° out of phase with each other, and are plotted in opposite directions of the vector plot.

If one were to only evaluate the absolute value of the admittance (/Y/), as is done using conventional low frequency immittance measures, you can see that the magnitude of this immittance vector could occur anywhere along the semicircle and would not provide any information about the relative contributions of the stiffness and mass. To determine the precise location where the admittance vector lies along the semicircle requires knowing the total susceptance (B_t) and the conductance (G) for a particular ear. The total susceptance (B_t) is equal to the difference between B_s and B_m, and this will be determined by the relative contributions from these two susceptance components for a particular ear. The complex relation of the admittance components is mathematically extrapolated from the vector plot based on the Pythagorean theorem:

$$Y^2 = G^2 + B_t^2$$
$$Y = \sqrt{G^2 + B_t^2}.$$

Most clinical immittance instruments have the option of measuring the B and G components. This approach is called *multiple-component tympanometry*. Looking at the vector plot in Figure 8–12A, you can see that when the admittance of a middle ear system is dominated by the stiffness susceptance (B_s), the overall admittance of the middle ear would be in the top half of the plot (stiffness controlled). As Figure 8–12B shows, if the admittance of the middle ear system is dominated by the mass component (–B_m), the overall admittance of the middle ear would be in the bottom half of the plot (mass controlled). When the stiffness susceptance and the mass susceptance are equal to each other, the ear is controlled only by the conductance component since the two susceptance components cancel each other out; when this occurs, the admittance would be represented along the horizontal axis and represents the resonant frequency of the middle ear.

---

[2]Alternatively, for admittance measures, the stiffness susceptance is described as compliance susceptance. In this text, the term stiffness susceptance is used to simplify the clinical explanations differentiating between otosclerosis and disarticulation.

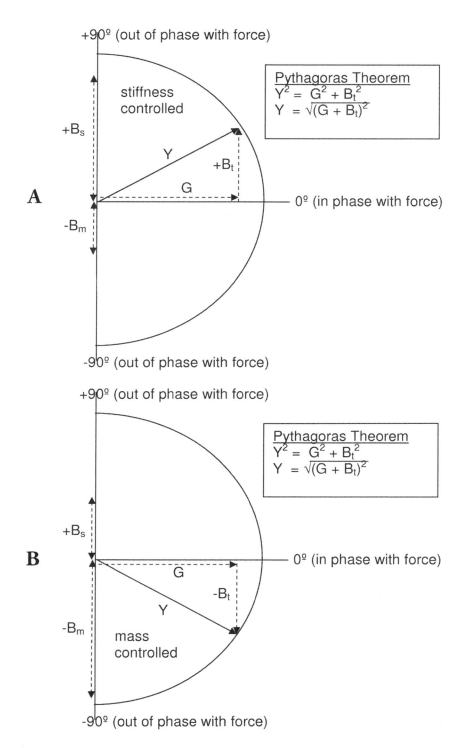

Figure 8–12. A and B. A vector diagram illustrating how stiffness susceptance (B_s), mass suscep-tance ($-B_m$), and conductance (G) interact to define the overall admittance (Y). The *top portion* of the figure shows these components for a stiffness controlled middle ear, and the *bottom portion* of the figure shows these components for a mass controlled middle ear. The conductance is in phase with the applied force, while the mass susceptance and stiffness susceptance are 90° out of phase with the applied force, but are 180° out of phase with each other. The overall susceptance (B_t) is equal to the sum of B_s and B_m. In a stiffness controlled middle ear, the B_t is positive; in a mass controlled middle ear, the B_t is negative.

239

So, how does frequency enter into this? The more complete equation for admittance can be written as:

$$Y = \sqrt{G^2 + \left(s / 2\pi f - 2\pi fm\right)^2}$$

(where f = frequency; m = mass; s = stiffness; Y = admittance; G = conductance).

Inserting a higher frequency into this equation makes the mass susceptance of a normal ear larger and the stiffness susceptance smaller. Inserting a lower frequency into this equation makes the mass susceptance smaller and the stiffness susceptance larger. As you can see, for low frequency probe tones the admittance is mostly dominated by the stiffness component and the vector is in the top half of the vector plot. As the probe-tone frequency increases, the admittance reflects more and more contributions of the mass component. When the probe-tone frequency is at the middle ear's resonance frequency, which is normally between 800 and 1200 Hz, the mass and stiffness components are equal (resonant frequency) and the vector is along the conductance line. When probe tones

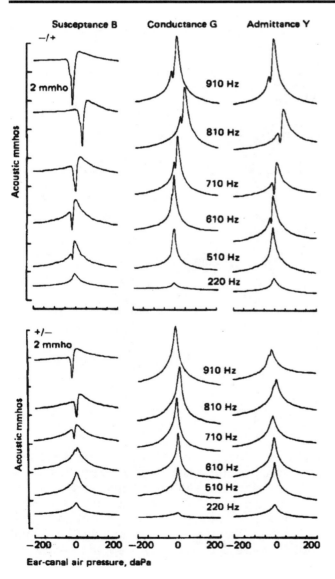

Figure 8–13. Multiple-component tympanograms as a function of probe-tone frequency for a normal middle ear. As frequency increases, the susceptance component (B) first begins to show notching around the peak of the tympanogram. The appearance of the notch begins as the mass susceptance (B) starts to become more relevant, but the admittance vector (Y) would still be in the positive portion of the vector (see also Figure 8–12A). When the depth of the notch is equal to the value at the beginning of the tympanogram (+200), often called the "tail," the middle ear is in resonance. The resonance point occurs when the mass susceptance is equal to the stiffness susceptance and the ear's admittance is controlled only by the conductance component. When the notch is lower than the tail, the mass component is more dominant than the stiffness component, and the overall susceptance (B) would be in the negative portion of the vector (see also Figure 8–12B). From Margolis et al., 1985, p. 47. Copyright 1985 by Karger.

are above the resonant frequency, the vector will be in the bottom half of the vector plot. In clinical recordings of multiple-component tympanometry, the probe tone is usually 678 or 1000 Hz because this gives some information on both stiffness and mass affects.

The actual tympanograms recorded using higher frequency probe tones have predictable variations in normal middle ears, and the results for patients are compared with what is expected for normal middle ears. Figure 8–13 shows how the tympanogram shape changes with increasing probe-tone frequency (Margolis, Van Camp, Wilson, & Creten, 1985). The most notable variation seen with high frequency probe tones is a characteristic notch that appears on the susceptance tympanogram at the location where the peak of the tympanogram would occur (at TPP). The notch begins to appear in the susceptance tympanogram when the mass components are beginning to be more relevant. The deeper the notch, the more dominant is the mass component. When the notch

is equal to the "tail" (the beginning part of the tympanogram at +200 daPa), it is considered to be at the middle ear resonant frequency, and mass and stiffness cancel each other out. When the notch is below the tail, the ear is considered to be mass dominant. Vanhuyse, Creten, and Van Camp (1975) described some normal variations of tympanograms for a 678 Hz probe tone. According to the Vanhuyse et al. classification scheme, recordings of the B and G tympanograms can show any of the following types in normal middle ears:

1B1G = 1 peak on the B and 1 peak on the G tympanograms

3B1G = 3 peaks on the B and 1 peak on the G tympanograms

3B3G = 3 peaks on the B and 3 peaks on the G tympanograms

5B3G = 5 peaks on the B and 3 peaks on the G tympanograms.

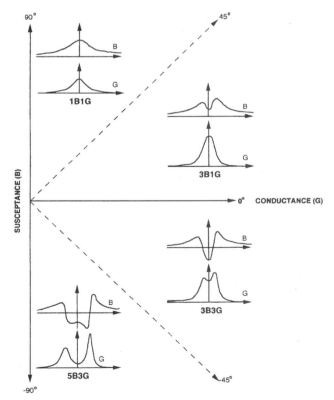

Figure 8–14. Different patterns of susceptance (B) and conductance (G) tympanograms that can occur from normal middle ears for a 678 Hz probe tone based on the Vanhuyse classification scheme. Most normal middle ears would show a 1B1G or 3B1G pattern. These patterns would occur in the positive half of the vector plot. However, there are some normal variations that show greater effects of mass susceptance, which results in a 3B3G or 5B3G pattern. These patterns would usually occur in the negative half of the vector plot. From Fowler & Shanks, 2002, p.191. Copyright 2002 by Lippincott Williams & Wilkins.

These types of normal tympanograms are shown in Figure 8–14 (Fowler & Shanks, 2002). Most normal middle ears show a 1B1G or 3B1G, which reflect ears that are stiffness controlled, and are shown in the upper half of the vector plot. Some normal ears have a greater influence of the mass (or less influence of the stiffness) as reflected in a 3B3G or 5B3G trace, and are shown in the lower half of the vector plot. When recording with a 678 Hz probe tone, one can assume an ear is abnormally mass controlled if it does not follow criteria for normal tympanograms based on the Vanhuyse et al. scheme:

- No more than 5 peaks on the B and 3 peaks on the G tympanograms.
- The width of the outer B peaks is less than the width of the outer G peaks.
- The width of the outermost peaks on the 3B trace is less than 75 daPa.
- The width of the outermost peaks on the 5B trace is less than 100 daPa.

If the 678 Hz tympanogram does not satisfy the above criteria, the patient most likely has a mass dominant pathology.

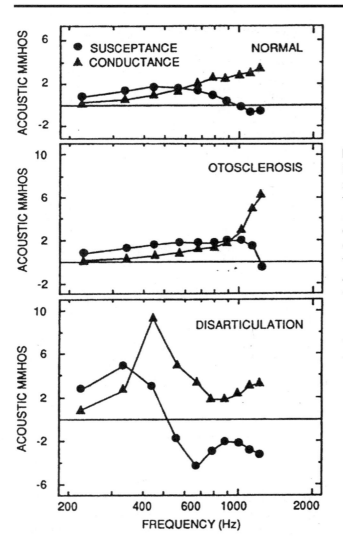

Figure 8–15. Multiple-frequency option from immittance recording instrument showing the susceptance (B) and conductance (G), taken from the tympanograms at their tympanic peak pressure (TPP), as a function of probe-tone frequency. The point where the susceptance curve (B) crosses the 0 mmho line is an estimate of the person's middle ear resonant frequency. Abnormally high stiffness pathologies, like otosclerosis (fixation of the stapes), show resonant frequencies that are higher than a normal middle ear. Abnormally low stiffness pathologies, like a disarticulation of the ossicles (which acts like an abnormally high mass pathology), show lower than normal resonant frequencies. From Shanks & Shelton, 1991, p. 322. Copyright 1991 by Elsevier.

An additional option available in most immittance instruments is to automatically make recordings over a range of probe-tone frequencies (226 to 2000 Hz), called *multiple-frequency tympanometry*. Multiple-frequency tympanometry can be used to provide an estimate of the patient's resonance frequency, that is, the point where the mass susceptance is equal to stiffness susceptance (0° on the vector plot). The resonant frequency will be lower than the normal range for an ear with a mass controlled pathology, such as a disarticulation, and will be higher than the normal range for a stiffness controlled pathology, such as otosclerosis (Shanks & Shelton, 1991). Figure 8–15 shows the susceptance and conductance values as a function of probe-tone frequency. The resonant frequency is determined at the point where the susceptance crosses 0 mmho, representing the point where stiffness and mass components cancel each other out.

Wideband Middle Ear Power (WMEP) Measures

Another, relatively new, method for measurement of middle ear properties is called *wideband middle ear power* (WMEP), *wideband reflectometry*, or *middle ear reflectometry* (Feeney, Grant, & Marryott, 2003; Hunter, Tubaugh, Jackson, & Prospes, 2008; Hall & Swanepoel, 2010). Similar to multifrequency tympanometry, WMEP measures the stimulus power that is reflected from the tympanic membrane (not admitted into the middle ear) for a variety of applied frequencies, but without the need of a complete airtight seal of the probe and without changing air pressure. Measures of WMEP are faster than multifrequency tympanometry and may become more established as a clinical test, especially now that instruments that perform WMEP are becoming commercially available, and are combined with otoacoustic emission testing (see below for description of otoacoustic emissions). Figure 8–16 shows some normal and clinical measurement data for WMEP. The amount of power reflected (*y*-axis) as a function of frequency

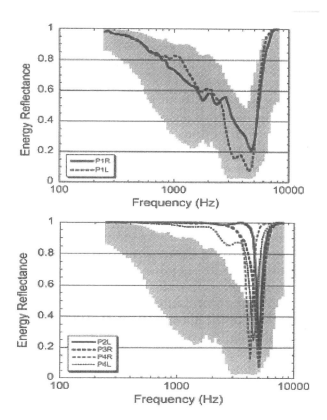

Figure 8–16. Examples of wideband middle ear power (WMEP) measures, showing how the reflected energy changes as a function of stimulus frequency. The *shaded portion* represents normal ranges, which are characterized by a dip (less energy reflected) in the region where the ear is most sensitive (resonance). In the *top panel* are examples of WMEP measures from ears with sensorineural losses, and can be seen to lie within the normal range as expected due to normal middle ear function. In the *bottom panel* are examples of WMEP measures from ears with middle ear fluid (otitis media), and are characterized by much higher reflected energy in the lower frequencies as expected with these types of conductive hearing losses. From Feeney et al., 2003, p. 906. Copyright 2003 by American Speech-Language-Hearing Association

(*x*-axis) shows that, for a normal ear, there is a dip (less energy reflected) representing the least amount of reflected energy around the ear's resonance frequency, and there is a systematic increase in the amount of reflected energy in the frequency ranges above and below the most sensitive region. In the bottom panel of Figure 8-16, the WMEP measures from some ears with fluid (otitis media) show a sharper dip, which is primarily a result of greater than normal reflected energy for frequencies lower than the resonant frequency, as would be expected for these types of conductive hearing losses.

Acoustic Reflex Thresholds

Another part of the immittance evaluation is the *acoustic reflex threshold* (ART) test. The ART is done with the same immittance instrument, and is usually performed right after obtaining a tympanogram. As you recall from Chapter 3, the ear has an involuntary middle ear reflex in response to loud sounds that causes a contraction of the stapedius muscles. The acoustic reflex pathway is

shown again in Figure 8-17 so that you can refer to it when interpreting results from ART testing.

It is important to remember that the acoustic reflex is a bilateral response. A loud tone delivered to one ear will result in contraction of the stapedius muscle in both ears. The contraction of the stapedius muscle alters the transmission of sound through the ossicular chain. The clinical utility of measuring ARTs extends beyond just the assessment of outer and middle ear pathologies. As you can see from Figure 8-17, abnormalities of the cochlea, 8th cranial nerve, lower brainstem, and/or the 7th cranial nerve may also influence the ability to record an acoustic reflex.

Recording Principles

Acoustic reflex testing monitors the changes in admittance that should occur when the middle ear muscle (stapedius) contracts in response to a loud tone, the *reflex eliciting tone*, that is presented to

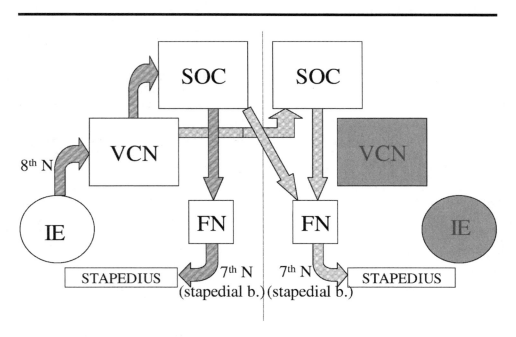

Figure 8-17. Block diagram of the acoustic reflex pathway for stimulation of one ear. Notice that there is an ipsilateral and contralateral pathway that results in bilateral contraction of the stapedius muscles. See Chapter 3 for more details. **SOC,** superior olivary complex; **VCN,** ventral cochlear nucleus; **FN,** facial nucleus; **IE,** inner ear.

the ear. Typically, 500, 1000, and 2000 Hz tones are used as reflex eliciting tones when testing for ARTs. The contraction of the stapedius muscle is measured with the immittance instrument as a reduction in admittance of the probe tone (226 Hz) due to the stiffening of the ossicular chain that is in response to the reflex eliciting tone (e.g., 1000 Hz). Referring back to Figure 8-1, you can see that the immittance instrument has a second tone generator that has capability of delivering the reflex eliciting tones (500, 1000, and 2000 Hz) to either ear. When the reflex eliciting tone is presented to the same ear where the admittance is being measured, it is called an *ipsilateral acoustic reflex* ("ipsi"). When the reflex eliciting tone is presented to the opposite ear from where the admittance is being measured, it is called a *contralateral acoustic reflex* ("contra"). The reflex eliciting tone used for ART testing is usually about 1 s in duration. The reflex eliciting tone is usually presented at 1000 Hz, but some audiologists also include testing at 500 and 2000 Hz. The acoustic reflex measures are performed at a single pressure, usually at the point of tympanometric peak pressure (TPP).

For the ART test, the immittance instrument monitors the admittance of the probe tone (226 Hz, 85 dB SPL) to see if it shows an abrupt decrease during the presentation of the reflex eliciting tone. For most reflex eliciting tones, the tone level must be at least 70 dB HL in order to produce a measurable reflex. Some normative ART data are shown in Table 8-2 (Wiley, Oviatt, & Block, 1987). To account for the variability, in clinical situations the normal range for ART is generally considered to be 70 to 95 dB HL (mean = 85 dB HL). The ART for broadband noise is about 20 dB lower than for tones.

Figure 8-18 illustrates a series of acoustic reflex measures for different levels of a reflex eliciting tone. The ART is established by manually changing the level of the reflex eliciting tone until the minimum dB HL is found that produces a criterion change in admittance. The ART is commonly defined as the lowest dB HL of the reflex eliciting tone that produces a repeatable admittance change of at least 0.02 mmhos (or 0.02 ml). When the dB HL of the reflex eliciting tone is below the stapedius reflex threshold there is no measurable change in admittance; however, when the dB HL of the reflex eliciting tone is high enough to cause the stapedius to contract, the admittance decreases during the presentation of the reflex eliciting tone. A decrease in admittance is observed as a downward deflection in the recording. As the dB HL of the reflex eliciting tone increases above the ART, there is a range in which the stapedius contraction strengthens and the size (amplitude) of the downward deflection of the acoustic reflex increases with increasing dB HL. To have more confidence in establishing the ART, it is recommended that testing be done at a level 5 dB higher than what is being considered as the threshold to see if there is the expected increase in amplitude of the deflection. In clinical situations, the acoustic reflex recordings from some patients can be contaminated with movement artifacts, swallowing, and/or clenching of teeth, which the tester must recognize and try to resolve in order to obtain valid ARTs. Testing at a level lower than 70 dB HL is a good strategy to determine if any deflections are present due to artifacts.

The equipment's maximum level for the reflex eliciting tones is typically 115 dB HL. Although relatively rare, it has been reported that some patients have experienced some tinnitus or additional hearing loss as a result of testing acoustic reflexes above 105 dB HL (Hunter, Ries, Schlauch, Levine, & Ward, 1999), and it is important to exercise caution when testing at levels higher than 105 dB HL.

Table 8–2. Mean Acoustic Reflex Thresholds (in dB HL) with Standard Deviation in Parentheses for Normal Hearing Ears

	500 Hz	1000 Hz	2000 Hz	Broadband Noise
Contralateral Stimulus	84.6 (6.3)	85.9 (5.2)	84.4 (5.7)	66.3 (8.8)
Ipsilateral Stimulus	79.9 (5.0)	82.0 (5.2)	86.2 (5.9)	64.6 (6.9)

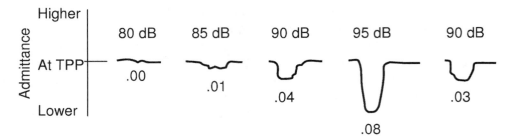

Figure 8–18. Illustration of acoustic reflex measures for different levels of the reflex eliciting tone. The acoustic reflex threshold is defined as the lowest level of the reflex eliciting tone that produces a downward deflection (reduced admittance) ≥ 0.02 mmhos. In this example, the acoustic reflex threshold is 90 dB HL. However, in order to help differentiate the acoustic reflex from possible artifact (see text), it is good practice to demonstrate that there is no deflection at the level 5 dB below the selected threshold level (see 85 dB HL in this example), and that the deflection should get larger in amplitude at the level 5 dB above the selected threshold level (see 95 dB HL in this example). In addition, it is good practice to show a repeatable deflection at the selected threshold level (see the two similar deflections at 90 dB HL in this example).

The ARTs are typically recorded for both ipsilateral and contralateral conditions for each ear. It is conventional to describe contralateral ART testing as it relates to the ear receiving the reflex eliciting tone. For example, a right contralateral ART means that the reflex eliciting tone was presented to the right ear and the probe assembly was in the left ear. However, many immittance instruments plot the ARTs relative to the ear with the probe assembly. To be unambiguous, it is recommended that the contralateral ARTs be recorded in a manner which clearly indicates which ear the reflex eliciting tone was in ("stim ear") and which ear the probe was in (probe ear); for example, "Stim R/Probe L." The ART for each frequency and recording condition is usually recorded on the audiometric data sheet along with the audiogram, tympanogram, and speech test results.

Clinical Interpretations of Acoustic Reflex Thresholds

The clinical interpretations of ARTs involve looking at the patterns of results for both ipsilateral

and contralateral recording conditions for each ear. The pattern of results will depend on the location of the problem in the acoustic reflex pathway. While certain characteristic patterns for ARTs can be established, they are much more useful when used in conjunction with the tympanogram, audiogram, and/or patient complaints/history. Learning how to interpret ARTs can be facilitated by considering the following three general conditions, all of which are necessary in order to elicit an acoustic reflex:

1. ***The ear with the probe assembly must not have any outer or middle ear pathology.*** If there is evidence of a conductive hearing problem with any degree of an air–bone gap on the audiogram and/or an abnormal tympanogram, the immittance instrument will not be able to record a change in admittance (even though the stapedius is activated). In this situation, the acoustic reflex is usually reported as absent. Acoustic reflexes will also be absent when the ear with the probe assembly has a perforation or a pressure equalization tube in the tympanic membrane, even

though there may not be an air-bone gap on the audiogram. Acoustic reflexes will also be absent when the ear canal is impacted with cerumen.

2. ***The ear with the reflex eliciting tone must receive a tone that is loud enough.*** Assuming that condition 1 (see above) is met, this second condition can be affected in different ways depending on the type of hearing loss. For a conductive hearing loss in the ear receiving the reflex eliciting tone, using contralateral test condition, an air-bone gap acts to reduce (attenuate) the level of the reflex eliciting tone reaching the cochlea. To offset this, the tester would increase the dB HL of the reflex eliciting tone to see if a reflex can be obtained before the upper limit of the equipment (usually 115 dB HL) is reached. If one assumes an average ART of 85 dB HL, then the level of the reflex eliciting tone can only be increased by 30 dB HL before the equipment limit is reached. Therefore, if the amount of air-bone gap in the stimulus ear is greater than 30 dB HL, the acoustic reflex will usually be absent because the reflex eliciting tone cannot be increased enough before the equipment limit is reached to offset the amount of conductive hearing loss. On the other hand, if the air-bone gap is less than or equal to 30 dB HL the acoustic reflex should be observed, but the level of the reflex eliciting tone needed to produce the ART will be elevated outside the normal expected range, that is, the ART would be expected between 100 and 115 dB HL.

For a cochlear hearing loss, there is an entirely different expectation. It is well established that loudness is not affected in the same way as for conductive hearing losses. Instead of the loudness of the reflex eliciting tone being attenuated, as occurs for a conductive hearing loss, the loudness of the reflex eliciting tone for a sensorineural hearing loss of cochlear origin is similar to that of a normal ear at these higher stimulus levels. This is related to a process called *recruitment*, in which there is an abnormal growth of loudness in an ear with a cochlear hearing loss.

In an ear with recruitment, as the intensity of a tone is increased above the behavioral threshold, the perceived loudness increases at a faster rate than for normal hearing ears; and when the tone reaches moderately high intensity levels, the perceived loudness level is similar to that perceived by a normal ear. This loudness recruitment phenomenon is seen in the ARTs for cochlear hearing losses as well. In fact, a cochlear hearing loss up to about 70 dB HL can be expected to have a measurable acoustic reflex. Interpretation of ART as a function of degree of cochlear hearing loss is based on data by Gelfand, Schwander, and Silman (1990). Figure 8–19 shows an example of the Gelfand et al. data for contralateral ARTs obtained at 1000 Hz for different degrees of known cochlear hearing loss (Gelfand, 2001). The data show the 90th, 50th, and 10th percentiles of ARTs. For clinical interpretation, it is generally recommended that the upper (90th percentile) end of the range be used as the upper cutoff for the expected ARTs as a function of degree of cochlear hearing loss. For example, one would expect the ART to be less than or equal to 95 dB HL for a cochlear hearing loss up to 45 dB HL (same as expected for a normal hearing ear). For a cochlear hearing loss between 50 and 70 dB HL, the 90th percentile expected value increases from 100 to 115 dB HL. As you can also see in Figure 8–19, even 50% of persons would be expected to have an acoustic reflex with a cochlear hearing loss as great as 80 dB HL. Although some audiologists may describe the ARTs in the 100 to 115 dB range as "elevated," a better description would be that "The ARTs are within the expected range for cochlear hearing losses based on the 90th percentile data of Gelfand et al. (1990)." The benefit of using the latter description will be apparent after describing, in the next section, the expectations for ARTs (also elevated) when the sensorineural hearing loss is due to a problem in the 8th nerve.

Table 8–3 lists the 90th percentile values for cochlear hearing losses that should

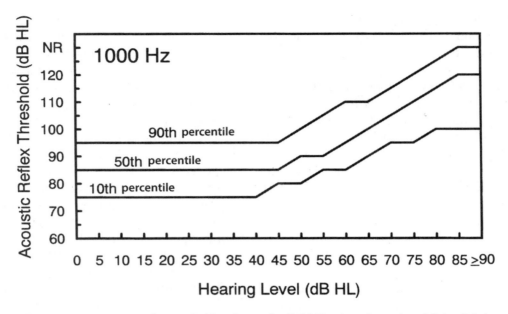

Figure 8–19. Data from Gelfand et al. (1990) showing the 90th, 50th, and 10th percentiles for acoustic reflex thresholds in ears with cochlear losses. Acoustic reflex thresholds above the 90th percentile curve should raise suspicion of possible 8th nerve disorder. See also Table 8–3 for 90th percentile values for 500, 1000, and 2000 Hz. From Gelfand et al., 1990, p. 245. Copyright 1990 by American Speech-Language-Hearing Association.

be considered when interpreting ARTs from patients with sensorineural hearing loss. The Gelfand et al. (1990) data are for contralateral ART testing, but similar patterns are found for ipsilateral ART testing (Cohen & Prasher, 1992) if the probe ear is free of any middle or outer ear pathology. The Gelfand et al. (1990) data are for 226 Hz probe tones and can be applicable up to the 115 dB HL limit of today's equipment. If adopting 105 dB HL as a safer limit for the reflex eliciting tones, as recommended by Hunter et al. (1999), the use of Gelfand's 90% criteria would be more limited at the higher degrees of hearing loss. However, one could use Gelfand's 50% criterion values as the most expected results, but this would alter the sensitivity and specificity of ARTs. Remember, the Gelfand et al. (1990) data only apply if there is no outer ear or middle ear pathology in the ear with the probe

assembly and there is no air–bone gap in the ear with the reflex eliciting tone.

3. ***The neural pathway must be adequate to activate the contraction of the stapedius.*** The acoustic reflex pathway includes both the 8th (sensory) and 7th (motor) cranial nerves, therefore, one would expect different patterns depending on the type and extent of neural dysfunction. For 8th cranial nerve disorders (e.g., acoustic neuroma), there is a compromise in the neural impulses from the stimulus ear that affects the activation of the ipsilateral and contralateral acoustic reflex pathways. It does not take very much of a disruption in neural activity to eliminate the acoustic reflex when the stimulus is presented to the ear with the 8th cranial nerve disorder. Therefore, the most expected result for an ear with an 8th cranial nerve disorder is that the ipsilateral and contralateral ARTs will

Table 8–3. 90th Percentile Values for Acoustic Reflex Thresholds (*ART*) for Contralateral Recordings

Hearing Threshold (dB HL)	ART at 500 Hz (dB HL)	ART at 1000 Hz (dB HL)	ART at 2000 Hz (dB HL)
0	95	95	95
5	95	95	95
10	95	95	95
15	95	95	95
20	95	95	95
25	95	95	95
30	95	95	100
35	95	95	100
40	95	95	100
45	95	95	105
50	100	100	105
55	105	105	110
60	105	110	115
65	110	110	115
70	115	115	120
75	120	120	125
80	120	125	NR
85	NR	NR	NR
>90	NR	NR	NR

Based on Data from Gelfand et al. (1990).

be absent most of the time when the reflex eliciting stimulus is in the affected ear, even with a mild degree of hearing loss. Since 8th cranial nerve disorders are usually only present in one ear, the ARTs for stimulation of the non-involved ear will be normal unless some other pathology is also present. There are, however, some patients with an 8th nerve disorder in which an acoustic reflex can be obtained between 100 and 115 dB HL. In these cases, the same data from Gelfand et al. (1990; see Figure 8-19) can be used to differentiate an 8th cranial nerve disorder from a cochlear disorder. For example, if the ART is outside

(higher than) the 90th percentile for cochlear ears for a specific degree of hearing loss, this would suggest the possibility of an 8th cranial nerve disorder because very few cochlear ears would be expected to have acoustic reflexes at those levels. A recommended clinical description might be "The ART is outside the expected 90th percentile range for cochlear ears with that degree of hearing loss and suggests possible 8th nerve involvement." As you can see, the use of the description "elevated" in reference to ARTs in the 100 to 115 dB range does not adequately differentiate a cochlear disorder from an 8th cranial nerve disorder, and elevated ARTs are also seen in conductive losses with air–bone gaps less than or equal to 30 dB HL.

For 7th cranial nerve involvement (e.g., Bell palsy), the acoustic reflex test is useful to differentiate whether the problem in the 7th cranial nerve is located *proximal* (more central) or *distal* (more peripheral) to the stapedial branch of the nerve (see the diagram of the 7th cranial nerve shown in Figure 3-3). A hearing loss must also be ruled out prior to interpreting the acoustic reflex thresholds relative to 7th cranial nerve function. When the immittance probe is in the ear on the same side as the 7th cranial nerve problem, the ARTs will be absent if the problem is proximal to the stapedial branch and present when the problem is distal to the stapedial branch. Stated differently, if the ARTs are normal with the probe assembly in the ear on the affected side, the 7th cranial nerve problem is distal to the stapedial branch; and if the ARTs are absent, the problem is proximal to the stapedial branch. For 7th cranial nerve problems that are proximal to the stapedial branch, monitoring of the ARTs over time may be useful to determine recovery of function.

The ART can also be affected by pontine level brainstem disorders, although these cases are quite rare. For example, when there is a problem in the pathways that cross from one side of the brainstem to the other at the level of the superior olivary complex (SOC), referred to as an *intra-axial* lesion, the ARTs may be present for ipsilateral testing from each ear and absent for contralateral testing from each ear. In this case, the 8th and 7th cranial nerve pathways are intact on each ipsilateral side; however, the neural information is not carried across the brainstem to the 7th cranial nerve on the other side due to some lesion in the midline of the pontine region of the brainstem.

Clinical Examples of ART Interpretations

The expectations for ARTs in different types of pathologic conditions are summarized in Table 8–4. Use this summary as you work through the hypothetical cases shown in Table 8–5. For each of the cases in Table 8–5, ask yourself whether or not each of the three previously described conditions for eliciting a reflex have been met or not for ipsilateral and contralateral recordings. All conditions must be met in order to be able to record an acoustic reflex. It is a good idea to look first for any outer or middle ear pathology in either ear. If outer or middle ear pathology is ruled out, then look at the stimulus ear for interpretation. The following explanations are for the examples shown in Table 8–5. For these examples, it was assumed that testing could be performed up to 115 dB HL.

Example 1: Reflexes are absent when the probe is in the right ear (R Ipsi and Stim L/Probe R) because the right ear has a pathology in the conductive pathway. When the reflex eliciting tone is in the right ear (Stim R/Probe L), the reflex is elevated because the degree of conductive loss is less than 30 dB and the level of the reflex eliciting tone can be increased (up to 115 dB limit) to overcome the attenuation. The reflex is normal when the probe and the reflex eliciting tone are in the left ear (L Ipsi).

Example 2: Reflexes are absent for all recording conditions because both ears have a conductive pathology. Note that any pathology or degree of conductive loss in the ear with the probe assembly will override the ability to increase the level of the reflex eliciting tone to offset the degree of conductive loss in that ear during ipsilateral recording.

Example 3: The interpretation of reflexes should focus on the ear with the reflex eliciting tone because the ear with the probe does not have any outer or middle ear pathology. Reflexes are expected to be present for all conditions because both ears have cochlear hearing losses and, therefore, recruitment of loudness is expected. The expected ARTs would be expected to be less than or equal to the 90th percentile data from Gelfand et al. (1990; see Table 8–4). In this case, the ART is less than or equal to 95 dB HL for the 45 dB cochlear loss (R Ipsi and Stim R/Probe L), and the ART is less than or equal to 110 dB HL for the 65 dB cochlear loss (L Ipsi and Stim L/Probe R).

Example 4: Reflexes are absent when the probe is in the right ear (R Ipsi and Stim L/Probe R) because the right ear has a pathology in the conductive pathway. In this case, there is no conductive hearing loss; however, there is a perforation in the tympanic membrane that precludes the measurement of a reflex. The R Ipsi reflex is normal when the probe is in the left ear because the left ear has normal hearing and no outer or middle ear pathology. For the right contralateral condition (Stim R/Probe L), the reflex is normal because the right ear does not have any hearing loss, so the level of the reflex eliciting tone in the right ear should be normal; the reflex should be measurable in the left ear because the left ear does not have any outer or middle ear pathology.

Example 5: Reflexes are most likely to be absent when the reflex eliciting tone is presented to the right ear (R Ipsi and Stim R/Probe L) because the 8th nerve tumor does not allow adequate neural activity to activate the reflex even with the mild sensorineural hearing loss. Reflexes are normal when the reflex eliciting tone is presented to the left ear (L Ipsi and Stim L/Probe R) because there is no hearing loss in the left ear and neither ear has any outer or middle ear pathology.

Table 8–4. Summary of the Most Expected Acoustic Reflex Thresholds for the Different Types of Pathologies

Pathology	Contra recording with probe in the affected ear	Contra recording with stimulus in the affected ear	Ipsi recording with probe and stimulus in the affected ear	Corollary
Conductive	▪ If any ABG, then ART = *absent* ▪ If perforation, PE tube, or impacted cerumen, then ART = *absent*	▪ If ABG ≤30 dB, then ART = *elevated* ▪ If ABG >30 dB, then ART = *absent*	▪ If any ABG, then ART = *absent* ▪ If perforation, PE tube, or impacted cerumen, then ART = *absent*	▪ If you get a reflex in the normal range, there should not be any OE/ME path in the probe ear.
Cochlear	Not relevant (dependent on stimulus in the affected ear)	▪ If hearing loss is ≤45 dB HL, then ART = *normal* ▪ If hearing loss is 50–70 dB, then ART = *elevated* and ≤ 90th percentiles of Gelfand et al. ▪ If hearing loss is 70–80 dB HL, then ART may be *absent* or *elevated* and ≤ 90th percentiles of Gelfand et al.	▪ If hearing loss is ≤45 dB HL, then ART = *normal* ▪ If hearing loss is 50–70 dB, then ART = *elevated* and ≤ 90th percentiles of Gelfand et al. ▪ If hearing loss is 70–80 dB HL, then ART may be *absent* or *elevated* and ≤ 90th percentiles of Gelfand et al.	▪ Expect an acoustic reflex for most cochlear losses ▪ A normal reflex does not rule out cochlear hearing loss, nor does it define the degree of cochlear loss
8th nerve	Not relevant (dependent on stimulus in the affected ear)	▪ ART = *absent* is the most expected result ▪ ART >90th percentile for degree of hearing loss ▪ Abnormal acoustic reflex decay	▪ ART = *absent* is the most expected result ▪ ART >90th percentile for degree of hearing loss ▪ Abnormal acoustic reflex decay	▪ If ART is absent with normal or hearing losses ≤70 dB = "red flag" for 8th nerve pathology ▪ If ART >90th percentile, this is a "red flag" for possible 8th nerve pathology
7th nerve	▪ If 7th nerve problem is distal to stapedial branch, then ART = *normal* ▪ If 7th nerve problem is proximal to stapedial branch, then ART = *absent*	Not relevant (dependent on probe in the affected ear)	▪ If 7th nerve problem is distal to stapedial branch, then ART = *normal* ▪ If 7th nerve problem is proximal to stapedial branch, then ART = *absent*	
Functional	Not relevant (dependent on stimulus in the affected ear)	▪ ART <10th percentile for degree of loss	▪ ART <10th percentile for degree of loss	▪ If ART is not consistent with type or degree of hearing loss, then suspect functional loss

Contra, contralateral acoustic reflex; *Ipsi*, ipsilateral acoustic reflex; *ABG*, air-bone gape; *ART*, acoustic reflex threshold; *PE*, pressure equalization; *OE*, outer ear; *ME*, middle ear.

Based on using a 1000 Hz reflex eliciting tone with 115 dB HL upper limit. Gelfand et al. data are based only on contralateral recordings; however, those data are also used in this table for ipsilateral recordings. The 90th percentiles from Gelfand et al. are beyond normal equipment limits (115 dB HL) and many will have absent reflexes; however, the reflexes can be present based on the lower percentiles, for example, the 50th percentile extends to 80 dB HL. Contralateral recordings should be done when suspicion of 8th nerve involvement because the output level goes higher than for ipsilateral recordings and the Gelfand et al. data are based on contralateral recordings, but have been applied here to ipsilateral recordings (Gelfand et al., 1990).

Table 8–5. Hypothetical Examples of Expected Acoustic Reflex Threshold (*ART*) Patterns.

		Expected ART (dB HL)			
Example	Hypothetical Conditions	R Ipsi	L Ipsi	Stim R Probe L	Stim L Probe R
1	RE: 20 dB conductive loss LE: normal hearing and function	Absent	≤95	100–115	Absent
2	RE: 20 dB conductive loss LE: 20 dB conductive loss	Absent	Absent	Absent	Absent
3	RE: 45 dB cochlear loss LE: 65 dB cochlear loss	≤95	≤110	≤95	≤110
4	RE: normal hearing with perforation LE: normal hearing and function	Absent	≤95	≤95	Absent
5	RE: 8th nerve tumor, mild SN loss LE: normal hearing and function	Absent or 100–115	≤95	Absent or 100–115	≤95
6	RE: 20 dB conductive loss LE: 7th nerve lesion distal to stapedius	Absent	≤95	100–115	Absent

RE, right ear; *LE*, left ear; *Ipsi*, ipsilateral acoustic reflex; *Stim*, stimulus.

Example 6: Reflexes are absent when the probe is in the right ear (R Ipsi and Stim L/Probe R) because the right ear has a pathology in the conductive components. The reflex is expected to be present when the probe is on the left ear (L Ipsi) because the left-sided 7th cranial nerve lesion is distal (more peripheral) to the stapedial branch of the 7th cranial nerve; however, because there is also a 20 dB conductive hearing loss in the right ear, the reflex is elevated for Stim R/Probe L.

It is also important to keep in mind the following caveats regarding interpretations of ARTs:

■ Normal ARTs do not mean normal hearing.
■ Abnormal reflexes can result from different pathologies.
■ When differentiating cochlear versus 8th cranial nerve pathology, be sure to rule out any outer or middle ear pathology.
■ Ears may have multiple pathologies; failure of any rule can cause abnormal ARTs.

Acoustic Reflex Decay

Acoustic reflex decay is an additional measure of the acoustic reflex activity to provide evidence of possible 8th cranial nerve pathology. The acoustic reflex decay is measured using a reflex eliciting tone that is presented for 10 s at a level that is 10 dB above the acoustic reflex threshold. Figure 8–20 shows what happens during stimulation and recording of acoustic reflex decay. For a normal functioning ear, the response to the reflex eliciting tone is displayed as a well-defined deflection (reduced admittance) at the initiation of the reflex eliciting tone that continues at generally the same amplitude for the entire 10 s. However, if the amplitude of the deflection decreases (drifts back toward baseline) by more than 50% within 5 s, it is considered positive acoustic reflex decay and is a positive sign for abnormal 8th cranial nerve involvement (e.g., an acoustic neuroma). The abnormal acoustic reflex decay is related to the inability of the 8th cranial nerve fibers to sustain adequate neural information, also called abnormal

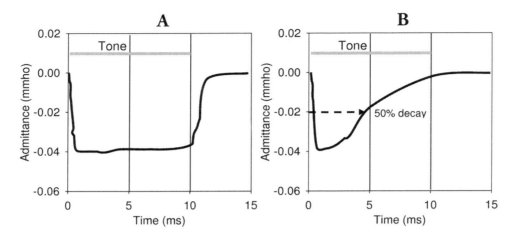

Figure 8–20. A and B. Illustration of acoustic reflex decay measures. For acoustic reflex decay testing, a reflex eliciting tone is presented at a level of 10 dB above the acoustic reflex threshold, and is presented for 10 ms (illustrated by the *tone bar*). During stimulation, there is an expected decrease in admittance (downward deflection) due to the contraction of the stapedius muscle, which should be sustained for the duration of the tone. In **A**, the amplitude of the deflection remained fairly constant for the duration of the 10 s tone; however, in **B**, the amplitude of the deflection returned toward baseline (referred to as decay) by 50% within the first 5 s of stimulation. Clinically, if acoustic reflex decay is more than 50%, it is considered positive acoustic reflex decay and suggestive of an 8th nerve disorder; otherwise, it is considered negative acoustic reflex decay.

adaptation, which is not sufficient to maintain the acoustic reflex during prolonged stimulation by the reflex eliciting tone.

It is recommended that acoustic reflex decay testing be done with 500 and/or 1000 Hz reflex eliciting tone using a contralateral recording condition. Higher frequency tones are not useful because a large number of normal hearing ears show positive acoustic reflex decay above 1000 Hz. Testing for acoustic reflex decay requires that the acoustic reflex threshold be established first and that the acoustic reflex thresholds occur within a range that allows an additional 10 dB to be added. Assuming equipment limits of 115 dB HL, the acoustic reflex threshold must be less than or equal to 105 dB HL in order to be able to test for acoustic reflex decay. If one adopts the recommended safe level of 105 dB HL (Hunter et al., 1999), the acoustic reflex threshold must be less than or equal to 95 dB HL in order to test for acoustic reflex decay

and may limit the cases in which acoustic reflex decay testing can be used to differentiate cochlear from 8th nerve disorders. Keep in mind also that most patients with 8th cranial nerve disorders will not have acoustic reflexes and, therefore, acoustic reflex decay testing cannot be performed. In some cases, a patient may have normal hearing thresholds and normal acoustic reflex thresholds, but shows abnormal acoustic reflex decay, and this may be the only suspicious sign of a possible 8th cranial nerve tumor. The acoustic reflex decay test is often routinely included in the immittance test battery because it does not take much more additional time and it is important not to miss a patient that may have an 8th cranial nerve tumor. It is recommended that acoustic reflex decay testing be included in the test battery whenever you are suspicious of an 8th cranial nerve problem, especially when there is an asymmetric high frequency hearing loss.

Synopsis 8–2

- Tympanometry with higher frequency probe tones (1000 Hz) is more appropriate for better differentiating stiffness dominant pathologies from mass dominant pathologies than tympanometry with the more conventional low frequency probe tone (226 Hz).

- Admittance (Y) is a complex combination of mass susceptance

- (-B_m), stiffness susceptance (B_s), and conductance (G), which in a vector plot can be described using the Pythagorean theorem:

$$Y = \sqrt{G^2 + \left(B_s - B_m\right)^2}$$

- Stiffness dominant pathologies (e.g., otosclerosis) are characterized by minimal notching on the B tympanogram and higher than normal resonance frequency, whereas mass dominant pathologies (e.g., disarticulation) are characterized by deep notching and multiple peaks on the B tympanogram and lower than normal resonance frequency using a sweep of probe-tone frequencies.

- Wideband middle ear power (WMEP) measures are becoming more commonplace as another means of describing middle ear function. WBEP measures the amount of sound power that is reflected off the tympanic membrane as a function of frequency. Normal functioning middle ears show a trace that reflects the ear's sensitivity to frequency and has the least amount of sound energy reflected around the most sensitive (resonance) area. Ears with middle ear fluid (otitis media) show a greater amount of sound energy being reflected in the lower frequencies.

- The immittance instrument can be used to monitor the contraction of the stapedius muscle by briefly stimulating the ear with a loud reflex eliciting tone (500, 1000, and/or 2000 Hz) and measuring any changes in the admittance of the 226 Hz probe tone. A reduction in admittance ($\geq$0.02 mmhos) during stimulation indicates that the stapedius muscle contracted, assuming artifacts have been ruled out.

- The acoustic reflex is a bilateral response to tones; therefore, recordings can be made for stimulation of one ear while recording the admittance with the probe in the other ear (contralateral reflex) or in the same ear as the stimulation (ipsilateral reflex).

- The normal range for the acoustic reflex threshold to tones is 70 to 95 dB HL. Acoustic reflex thresholds are reported as "absent" if not measurable at the upper range of testing.

- Clinical interpretation of acoustic reflex threshold testing is guided by the following:
  - Any outer or middle ear pathology (with or without air–bone gaps) in the ear with the probe (probe ear) will result in an absent acoustic reflex.

- An air–bone gap greater than 30 dB in the ear with the reflex eliciting tone (stim ear) will result in an absent acoustic reflex because the tone cannot be made loud enough before reaching equipment limits. For air–bone gaps less than or equal to 30 dB HL in the ear with the reflex eliciting tone, the acoustic reflex threshold should be measurable between 100 and 115 dB HL.

- For cochlear hearing losses, loudness recruitment causes acoustic reflexes to be measurable for hearing losses as high as 70 to 80 dB HL in the ear receiving the reflex eliciting tone. Gelfand et al. (1990) data should be consulted to determine the 90% criterion for acoustic reflex thresholds for different degrees of cochlear hearing loss. For example, at 1000 Hz, the acoustic reflex threshold is expected to be less than or equal to 95 dB HL in 90% of cochlear ears with hearing losses up to 45 dB HL and 100 to 115 in 90% of ears with hearing losses from 50 to 70 dB, respectively. See Table 8–3.

- For 8th cranial nerve pathologies, the neural activity of the 8th cranial nerve from the ear receiving the reflex eliciting tone (stim ear) is not adequate to produce a measurable acoustic reflex. The acoustic reflex threshold data can be used to differentiate cochlear versus 8th cranial nerve pathologies by referring to the Gelfand et al. data. For example, an 8th cranial nerve disorder is suspected if the acoustic reflex threshold is greater than 90% criterion value for a specific degree of sensorineural hearing loss. For most 8th cranial nerve pathologies, the acoustic reflex is absent even with relatively good pure-tone audiometric thresholds. Positive acoustic reflex decay is also an 8th cranial nerve sign.

- For 7th cranial nerve pathologies, the activation of the stapedius can be assessed relative to the probe ear. The acoustic reflex threshold will be absent if the 7th cranial nerve pathology is proximal to the stapedial branch of the 7th cranial nerve and present if the pathology is distal to the stapedial branch.

Otoacoustic Emissions (OAEs)

Otoacoustic emissions (OAEs) are low-intensity acoustic vibrations measured in the ear canal with a sensitive microphone. As discussed in Chapter 3, the discovery of OAEs by Kemp (1978) went hand in hand with new discoveries about the active processes in the cochlea, especially the motility of the OHCs (Brownell, 1983). The emissions originate in a normally functioning cochlea, predominantly as a result of the movement of the OHCs enhancing the vibrations on the basilar membrane. The emissions travel outward along the basilar membrane, through the middle ear ossicles, and vibrate the tympanic membrane to produce the OAEs in the ear canal. The OAEs are on the order of −10 to 20 dB SPL (Glattke & Robinette, 2007; Lonsbury-Martin, Martin, & Whitehead, 2007; Probst & Harris, 1993). The OAEs can be recorded with a sensitive microphone in the ear canal when coupled to a specialized computer that enhances the low-level OAEs and reduces the unwanted signals, such as background noise, in a process called signal averaging. Because the active process of the OHCs is operational only at low to moderate intensity levels, a cochlear hearing loss in the mild to moderate range due to a loss of OHC function is sufficient to eliminate OAEs.

Measurements of OAEs can be done in a couple of minutes for each ear, which has made them very popular for routine clinical use. In just a few minutes of testing, the function of the OHCs can be determined. During the 1990s, measurement of OAEs became widely adopted as an efficient and effective audiological procedure. Over the next decade, there was widespread implementation of mass newborn hearing screening programs using OAEs. Newborns who do not pass the OAE screening are referred for further audiologic follow-up (see also Chapter 10).

Many audiologists include OAE testing as part of the basic audiologic evaluation of all patients because OAEs can provide a good cross-check with audiometric information. Because OAEs reflect preneural events, they can also be used to determine if a sensorineural hearing loss is due to a problem in the cochlea or in the neural pathway. For example, if a patient has a sensorineural hearing loss and has normal OAEs, this would suggest that the cochlea is functioning normally and the problem lies in the 8th cranial nerve or central auditory pathway. It is important to keep in mind that OAEs are a screening procedure that can only determine whether the OHCs are functioning normally or not. OAEs do not provide a measure of how much hearing loss a patient may have, nor can they quantify the amount of cochlear dysfunction; OAEs will be absent for a mild to moderate degree of hearing loss, as well as for a profound hearing loss. When evaluating OAE results, it is also important to determine if there is any conductive hearing loss, because a problem with the outer or middle ear can interfere with the outward transmission of the cochlear-generated OAEs. OAEs can usually be recorded in ears with negative middle ear pressure (see tympanometry above)

when done at the TPP (Hof, Anteunis, Chenault, & van Dijk, 2005). In addition, ears with functioning pressure equalization tubes should not preclude OAEs from being recorded (Dahr & Hall, 2012) . The clinical utility of OAE measures lies in its integration with other audiological tests. However, the presence of OAEs argues for normal auditory function in the outer ear, middle ear, and cochlear OHCs of the auditory system.

There are two main types of evoked[3] OAEs that are in clinical use, those evoked by transients, called *transient evoked otoacoustic emissions*, and those evoked by two closely spaced pure tones that create additional tones in the cochlea, called *distortion product otoacoustic emissions*. Only a brief description of each of these OAEs is provided in this introductory text. For further information on the instrumentation and recording parameters, see other resources (e.g., Gorga, et al., 1997; Hall, 2000; Robinette & Glattke, 2007).

Transient Evoked Otoacoustic Emissions (TEOAEs)

Transient evoked otoacoustic emissions (TEOAEs) are evoked by the presentation of a series of brief transients (clicks). Because of the brief duration, the clicks have a broad frequency spectrum and, therefore, stimulate a wide portion of the basilar membrane. With TEOAEs, the emissions are recorded during the short silent intervals between the successive clicks and occur with a characteristic time delay after each click, called latency. Figure 8–16 illustrates the basic instrumentation and recording of TEOAEs in a normal ear. In the main part of the screen is the actual time-domain waveform of the TEOAEs recorded in the ear canal. The expected latency period of the TEOAE components is between 5 and 15 ms.

If you look carefully at the waveform in Figure 8–21, you should be able to see that the periods of the peaks at the beginning (shorter latency)

---

[3]Evoked OAEs are produced by an externally applied stimulus and found in nearly all normal functioning cochleae. Spontaneous OAEs are another class of cochlear emissions that can also be recorded in the ear canal, but which occur in the absence of any externally applied stimulus. Spontaneous OAEs are only found in about half of normally functioning cochleae, and thus are not well suited for clinical use.

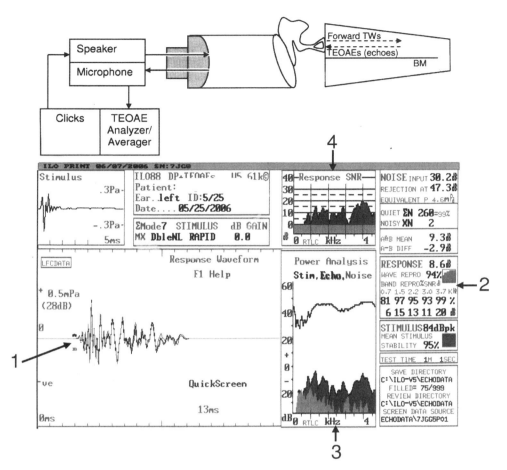

Figure 8–21. The *upper part* illustrates the principles of TEOAE generation and recording. The *lower part* shows an example of a typical recording of TEOAEs from a normal hearing ear. The area labeled (*1*) shows the
OAE waveforms from two superimposed tracings obtained from the two
separate memory files. The TEOAEs from the higher frequencies occur near
the beginning of the waveforms (shorter latency), while the TEOAEs from
the lower frequencies occur with a longer latency. The amount of correlation between these two tracings at the different frequencies, called reproducibility (REPRO), is quantified in the area labeled (*2*). The amplitude of
the TEOAE and the background noise are shown in the area labeled (*3*). The
amplitude of the TEOAE relative to the noise, called signal-to-noise ratio
(SNR), is shown in the area labeled (*4*).

part of the waveform are shorter, and thus higher
in frequency and reflective of the activity at the
basal regions of the cochlea. The periods of the
peaks later in the waveform are longer, and thus
lower in frequency and reflective of the activity
at the more apical regions of the cochlea. The
TEOAEs that are recorded in the ear canal reflect

the broad frequency range activated along the basilar membrane; however, the frequencies of the
TEOAE are distributed over a latency period that
reflects the time course of the traveling wave (forward and reverse) along the basilar membrane. In
other words, the higher frequency (basal) portion
of the basilar membrane has a shorter latency and

the lower frequency (apex) portion of the basilar membrane has a slightly longer latency. From the recorded waveform, the OAE instrument performs a FFT analysis to calculate the spectrum of the OAE response as well as the noise that is present in the recording. Due to recording constraints, the TEOAEs can only be measured between 1000 and 4000 Hz.

The interpretation of TEOAE involves looking at which frequencies show an acceptable emission, usually 3 to 6 dB above the noise, called the *signal-to-noise ratio* (SNR). In addition, the OAE measurement instrument calculates a *reproducibility value* for each of the frequency regions. To do this, the instrument stores OAE responses to half of the stimuli into one memory file and the other half into a second memory file. The two memory files are displayed on top of each other to provide a visual look at the reproducibility. The reproducibility (correlation between the two recordings) is calculated for different frequency components and displayed as a percentage for each frequency band. The higher the reproducibility, the more confidence you have that there is a true response. Reproducibility should be at least 50% at each of the frequency regions (Kemp, Ryan, & Bray, 1990), and a higher reproducibility criterion (e.g., 75%) may be more appropriate for clinical applications. Failure to have a reproducible response that is at least 3 dB above the noise for any of the frequency regions would indicate that the OHCs from those frequency regions are not functioning normally. The amplitude of the TEOAEs varies considerably across people and ages (they are much larger in infants than adults); therefore, amplitudes are not very useful for estimating an OAE threshold or for predicting degree of hearing loss. In fact, TEOAEs are only measured at a moderately high intensity level in order to maximize the opportunity to obtain a response above the noise.

TEOAEs are well suited for auditory screening because they provide a quick estimate of the integrity of the peripheral auditory function over the 1000 to 4000 Hz frequency range. It is generally accepted that TEOAEs will most likely be absent if hearing loss is greater than 30 to 35 dB HL. According to Robinette, Cevette, and Probst (2007), TEOAEs are expected to be present in 99%

of ears when all pure-tone thresholds are better than 20 dB HL, always absent when all pure-tone thresholds are greater than 40 dB HL, and may or not be present with pure-tone thresholds between 25 and 35 dB HL. TEOAEs effectively separate those with normal function from those who need further follow-up evaluations. The presence of TEOAEs indicates cochlear function no worse than 35 dB HL and no outer and middle ear involvement. If the patient has more than a mild sensorineural hearing loss and TEOAEs are present, then the hearing problem lies in the neural portions of the auditory system. TEOAEs are widely used in newborn hearing screenings. Studies have shown that a fair number (10 to 15%) of newborns fail the initial TEOAE screening, most likely due to some transient middle/outer ear condition; however, upon rescreening the majority of those will pass (Prieve, 2007).

Distortion Product Otoacoustic Emissions (DPOAEs)

The cochlea is a non-linear system, which means that there are additional tones, called distortion products, which can be generated in the cochlea that were not externally presented. Figure 8–22 illustrates how DPOAEs are generated and recorded. When two pure tones (where f1 is lower than f2) are simultaneously presented to a human ear, the most prominent distortion product occurs at a frequency equal to 2f1-f2, the *cubic difference tone*. The externally presented pure tones are called the *primary tones*, and the 2f1-f2 is the distortion product tone that is generated in the cochlea. For example, if the primary tones are 1000 and 1200 Hz, the 2f1-f2 = 800 Hz. The 2f1-f2 distortion product is at least 50 dB lower than the level of f1. The 2f1-f2 DPOAE is largest when the ratio of f1/f2 is equal to about 1.22 and the intensities of f1 and f2 are 65 and 50 dB SPL, respectively (Gaskill & Brown, 1990; Whitehead, Stagner, Lonsbury-Martin, & Martin, 1995). The DPOAE recording instrument filters out the frequencies of the primary tones and focuses its measurement only on the distortion product frequency. Unlike

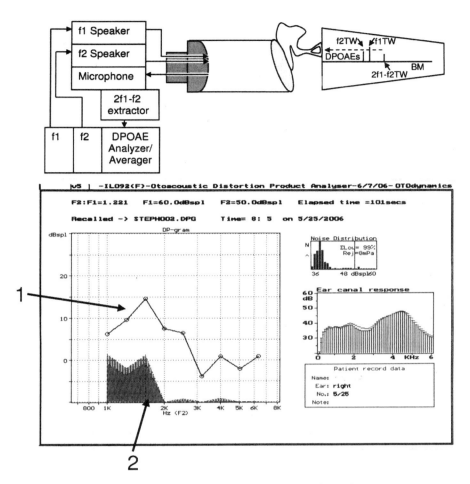

Figure 8–22. The *upper part* illustrates the principles of DPOAE generation and recording. The DPOAE analyzer extracts the 2f1–f2 distortion products that are generated in the cochlea from the different pairs of primary tones, f1 and f2, as they are swept across the frequency range. The *lower part* shows an example of a typical recording of DPOAEs from a normal hearing ear. The area labeled (*1*) shows the amplitude of the DPOAEs as a function of the f2 primary tone. The *shaded area*, labeled (*2*), shows the noise level.

TEOAEs, where the responses are recorded *after* each stimulus, the DPOAE method measures the responses *during* cochlear activation; however, it is not clear whether the different types of stimulation have any clinical significance. By changing the frequencies of the two primary tones (maintaining the 1.22 ratio), distortion products can be generated from different frequency regions in the cochlea. The DPOAEs are recorded for different pairs of primary tones, which are typically swept across the frequency range from 1000 to 6000 Hz. The frequency sweep is repeated and responses recorded with signal averaging until the background noise is sufficiently reduced and the DPOAE is enhanced. Generally, it takes about four or five sweeps across the frequency range to establish an acceptable DPOAE above the noise (called *noise floor*). Although the instrument is measuring the 2f1–f2 DPOAE, it is the place along the basilar membrane where the two primary tones are interacting that must also be functioning normally in order to generate the distortion product. The typical DPOAE results are plotted as a function of f2, or the geometric mean of f2 and f1, because the OHC function within the corresponding region is primarily responsible for the distortion product that is generated. It should be pointed out that while the DPOAE plot has the appearance of an audiogram, it not a representation of audiometric thresholds. The analysis of the DPOAE recording typically involves looking at the absolute amplitude of the DPOAE and/or the ratio of the DPOAE relative to the noise floor with the primaries at standard intensity levels (e.g., 65 and 50 dB SPL for f1 and f2, respectively). Generally, the DPOAE amplitude should be at least 5 to 6 dB above the noise floor. DPOAEs can also be measured as a function of stimulus level. In this procedure, an *input–output function* is generated by varying the level of f1 or f2 separately, or both f1 and f2 together, to obtain an estimate of the DPOAE threshold. The use of DPOAE input–output functions is not yet in widespread clinical use.

As with TEOAEs, it is generally accepted that DPOAEs are present in normal ears and absent in ears with cochlear hearing loss. The degree of cochlear hearing loss that is sufficient to eliminate DPOAEs is not firmly established. DPOAEs are expected to be present with pure-tone thresholds better than 25 dB HL and absent for hearing losses greater than 40 dB using moderate level primary tones; however, they may also be present with reduced amplitudes, for hearing loss as high as 50 to 60 dB HL, especially when higher level primary tones are used (Gorga, Neely, Johnson, Dierking, & Garner, 2007). This would make the DPOAEs less attractive as a newborn screening tool than TEOAEs because some infants who have a mild cochlear hearing loss may pass the DPOAE screening. More research is needed to determine if decreased amplitudes of DPOAEs can provide information regarding the degree of hearing loss. It has also been suggested that DPOAEs are somewhat better than TEOAEs in assessing the higher frequencies, but somewhat worse than TEOAEs at the lower frequencies (Gorga et al., 2007), and DPOAEs would be better for monitoring changes in hearing loss, especially in the higher frequencies (Robinette et al.,

2007). The DPOAEs are also reduced or eliminated by the presence of any conductive involvement as they are transmitted through the middle ear; therefore, any conductive loss must be considered when DPOAEs are absent. The presence of normal DPOAEs is evidence of good peripheral auditory function. As with TEOAEs, if DPOAEs are present in a patient with a moderate sensorineural hearing loss, this would suggest that the hearing loss may be due to a problem in the neural portions of the auditory system.

Auditory Brainstem Response

The *auditory brainstem response* (ABR)[4] is one of a series of auditory evoked responses that can be measured from the neural pathways of the auditory system using small disk electrodes placed on the surface of the head. The electrodes are connected to a specialized computer (called a *signal-averaging computer*) that averages the synchronous neural responses, which are generated as electrical potentials that can be measured on the scalp, much like an electroencephalogram (EEG). The observation of an ABR is dependent on *neural synchrony*, which is due to a relatively large number of auditory neurons firing simultaneously. To achieve neural synchrony, the ABR requires the use of brief acoustic signals with rapid onset times, called *transients* (*clicks*) or tone bursts. Clicks have a broadband spectrum, whereas tone bursts have a more restricted spectra. The computer measures the electrical activity picked up by the electrodes for a short time period after each stimulus, referred to as *time-locked*. A typical ABR requires about 2,000 stimuli presented at a rate of about 33 to 57/s. When the ABR recording is averaged over a large number of stimuli (e.g., 2,000) the synchronous ABR response is enhanced and the random background electrical activity (EEG) or other noise is reduced. Because the responses are quite small, successful recording requires that the patient be still or preferably asleep (natural or sedated). The clinical utility of ABRs is enhanced

---

[4]Sometimes, the ABR is called the brainstem evoked response (BSER) or the brainstem auditory evoked response (BAER).

by the fact that they are unaffected by level of attention, sleep state, or drugs, and can be reliably recorded across all ages, including premature infants.

The ABR is not part of the basic audiometric test battery, but is briefly described in this chapter because it is a very useful physiological measure that is routinely performed by audiologists for special populations, including: (a) testing young children or other difficult-to-test patients whose behavioral thresholds are not able to be obtained or are questionable, (b) evaluation of patients suspected of 8th cranial nerve disorders, (c) as a screening test for newborn auditory sensitivity, and (d) as a follow-up for infants who fail an OAE screening. The interested reader is referred to other references (e.g. Atcherson & Stoody, 2012; Burkard, Don, & Eggermont, 2007; Hood, 1998) for more detailed information on the ABR and other evoked electrical potentials.

The ABR was first identified in the late 1960s and early 1970s (Jewett, Romano, & Williston, 1970;

Sohmer & Feinmesser, 1967) and became a well-established special clinical test by the late 1970s, before the discovery of OAEs. The ABR occurs very early in time (called *latency*) after the onset of the transient. The latency of the normal ABR is within 2 to 10 ms after stimulation by a click stimulus. Other transient evoked auditory, such as the *middle latency response* (10 to 50 ms after stimulation) and the *late latency response* (50 to 250 ms after stimulation), were discovered prior to the ABR, and although the MLR and LLR have some clinical utility, they are not used as routinely as ABR, especially for testing young children.

The ABR is characterized by a series of six to seven waves (peaks) as shown in Figure 8–23. To improve interpretation, each recording condition is replicated and typically plotted on top of each other. The earliest positive wave is called *wave I* and is a reflection of the synchronous discharge of neurons in the distal portion of the auditory portion of the 8th cranial nerve as it is leaving the cochlea. The subsequent waves are generated by the

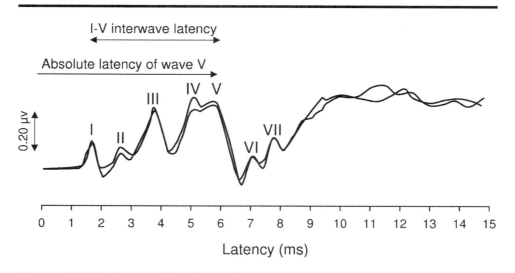

Figure 8–23. A normal auditory brainstem response (ABR) waveform at a relatively high intensity level showing the waves (positive peaks) labeled *I–VII*. The latency (time) of each wave is called the absolute latency, which is relative to the onset of the brief stimulus (at 0 ms). An example of absolute latency is shown for wave V, which is usually the most prominent wave. The latency difference between any two waves is called the interwave latency difference. The I–V interwave latency difference is the one most often used clinically. Waves II, IV, VI, and VII are often difficult to discern and are not used clinically.

synchronous neural activity in the proximal part of the 8th cranial nerve (wave II), cochlear nucleus (wave III), superior olivary complex (wave IV), lateral lemniscus, and input to the inferior colliculus (wave V) (Møller, 1994).

Although the neural generators for the different ABR waves are in the 8th cranial nerve and brainstem, their latencies and thresholds are characteristically affected by peripheral hearing disorders. *Wave V* is the most prominent wave in the ABR waveform and is the wave most often used for clinical assessment of ABR threshold because it is the only wave present near threshold. The ABR can also be used for neurological evaluations by looking at the latency differences between the various waves, especially the wave I to wave V latency difference. Abnormal I–V latency differences suggest an abnormality in the brainstem. The presence of the various waves, the overall shape of the waveform (*morphology*), the absolute latencies of the different waves, especially wave V, and the interwave latency differences between waves I and V are the most often evaluated components of the ABR for clinical purposes. The absolute amplitudes of the ABR waves are too variable be used clinically.

ABR and Auditory Sensitivity

In a clinical evaluation of auditory sensitivity, the ABR is recorded as a function of stimulus intensity to determine the lowest level in which a wave V is observed, called the ABR threshold. Conductive hearing losses and cochlear hearing losses will alter the response of the neural output; thus, the ABR is a useful tool for assessing peripheral hearing disorders. The ABR in a normal hearing ear shows characteristic changes as the stimulus intensity changes.

Figure 8–24 shows a series of ABR waveforms to click stimuli as a function of intensity for a normal hearing ear. Notice how wave V remains the most visible waveform as intensity decreases and is characterized by a systematic increase in latency. At low intensities, the ABR wave V latency to click stimuli reflects the synchronous neural activity from around the 2000 Hz region, which

has better auditory sensitivity than other frequencies. For a normal ear, as intensity is increased, the wave V latencies shorten to reflect the activity from neurons in the higher frequency basal regions of the cochlea, which are stimulated first and where the faster traveling wave velocity produces greater neural synchrony. The ABR threshold recorded from clicks is used as an estimate (within 10 to 15 dB) of the degree of hearing loss in the 2000 to 4000 Hz region (Bauch & Olsen, 1986).

In addition, the wave V latency is often plotted as a *latency-intensity function* (L-I function, as shown in Figure 8–25). The shape of the L-I function is often helpful in identifying the type of hearing loss. A patient with a flat conductive hearing loss will have an L-I function that parallels the normal L-I function due to the reduction in stimulus intensity at each recording level resulting from the conductive hearing loss. A patient with a sloping or relatively flat high frequency cochlear hearing loss will have an elevated threshold, but may also have a steeper than normal L-I function. The steeper L-I function begins with a delayed wave latency near threshold due to the hearing loss in the mid to high frequencies. As the stimulus intensity is increased, it crosses the threshold in the higher frequencies where the latency is a reflection of these more basal responding regions that produce the more synchronous response dominating the waveform. At the highest intensities, the cochlear hearing loss has wave V latency within the normal expected range, and the waveform is indistinguishable from a normal ear. In cases with a very steep or severe high frequency hearing loss, the L-I function may not end within the normal latency region at the higher intensities because there are not enough high frequency neurons to stimulate. It is also important to realize that ABR to clicks becomes problematic in identifying cases in which there is a low frequency hearing loss with better high frequency hearing. In these cases, the ABR will reflect only the more synchronously responding higher frequency regions once the stimulus is high enough to exceed their thresholds. Therefore, whenever there is good high frequency hearing, the ABR to clicks may not be effective and the L-I function will be entirely within the

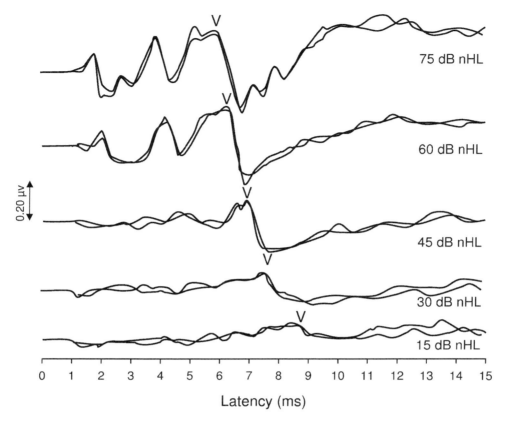

Figure 8–24. Example of auditory brainstem response (ABR) recordings as a function of stimulus (click) intensity level for a normal hearing ear. The click intensity levels are referenced to normal behavioral threshold to the clicks, and are labeled *dB nHL* in order to differentiate from dB HL used for audiometric stimuli. Notice that at lower intensities wave V is the only wave that is observable, and it is usually present down to levels of 15 to 20 dB nHL in quiet recording conditions. Wave V latency systematically increases as intensity decreases.

normal range due to the dominance by the normally functioning mid to high frequencies that produce a normal ABR. In these situations, ABR to clicks can be more frequency specific by using different high-pass maskers to eliminate the more synchronously responding high frequency regions (Kramer & Teas, 1979).

The ABR can also be recorded for short-duration tonal stimuli (called *tone bursts*) at frequencies between 500 and 4000 Hz, and these tone bursts can provide a more frequency-specific response than the broadband clicks. However, the ABR cannot evaluate frequencies less than 500 Hz (and sometimes 500 Hz is difficult) because there is not enough neural synchrony in those lower frequency regions. For tone-burst stimuli at 500 and 1000 Hz, the waveform morphology usually shows only a broadened wave V peak, and the wave V latency is increased as one would predict because the neural response is originating at the more apical regions of the cochlea (longer traveling wave time). However, as with clicks, at higher intensities the 500 and 1000 Hz tone bursts are not frequency specific because they will stimulate

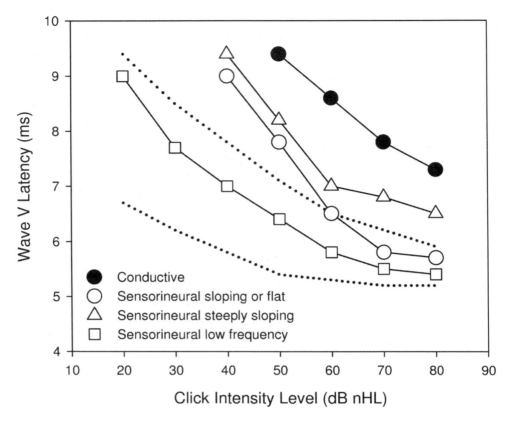

Figure 8–25. Examples of click-generated wave V latency-intensity (L-I) functions for different types of hearing losses. The *dotted curves* represent two standard deviations of the normal expected L-I function.

the higher frequency regions of the cochlea once the stimulus is above their thresholds. Again, it is important to realize that a patient with a low frequency hearing loss may have a normal ABR if the stimulus (click or tone burst) is capable of stimulating the higher frequency regions. However, the techniques of *high-pass masking* and *notched-noise masking* can provide better frequency-specific information, especially when the response is being dominated by the better responding high frequency regions. In this technique, the high-pass or notched-noise masking *desynchronizes* the higher frequency regions and produces a response that is reflective of the lower frequency regions or region within the notched noise (Don & Eggermont, 1978; Kramer & Teas, 1979). For tone-burst recordings performed in notched noise, frequency-specific ABR thresholds can be within

10 to 20 dB of behavioral thresholds (Stapells, Picton, Durieux-Smith, Edwards, & Moran, 1990).

Although there is generally good correspondence between ABR thresholds and pure-tone behavioral thresholds, it is important to keep in mind that the ABR only represents the neural function reflecting cochlear output and neural conduction along the lower brainstem pathway and, therefore, is not a measure of conscious hearing. Hearing loss can still be present in a patient with a normal ABR, and in those cases a more central involvement or functional component must be considered.

ABR and 8th Nerve Pathologies

The ABR can also be used to identify possible 8th nerve pathologies by evaluating how the neural

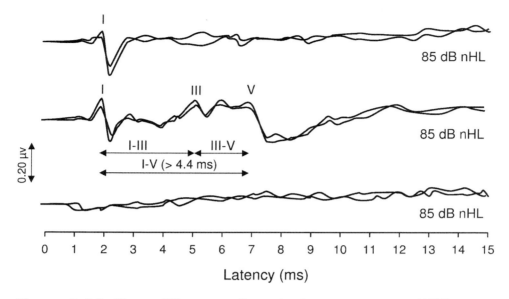

Figure 8–26. Three different auditory brainstem response (ABR) waveforms illustrating the different abnormal recordings that are associated with 8th nerve disorders. For neurological evaluations, it is best to make the recordings at a high intensity in order to try to obtain waves I, III, and V. See Figure 8–24 for definition of dB nHL.

activity is conducted through the 8th nerve. For example, an acoustic neuroma (tumor on the 8th nerve) that affects the proximal portion of the 8th nerve may show a normal wave I, but the later waves would be affected. When evaluating 8th nerve or brainstem function, the ABR is recorded at a relatively high stimulus level in an attempt to record waves I, III, and V. The ABR for a patient with an 8th nerve pathology may show: (a) wave I present with poorly defined or absent later waves, (b) wave I, III, and V present, but the interwave intervals (I–III and/or I–V) are delayed more than two standard deviations from the normal interwave intervals, (c) a difference in wave V latency between the two ears (interaural latency difference) that is more than two standard deviations from the normal interaural latency difference, or (d) no discernible waves even though there is sufficient hearing to expect normal wave latencies. Figure 8–26 shows the ABR recording from three different patients illustrating the abnormal responses associated with an 8th nerve pathology.

Auditory Steady-State Response (ASSR)

Another objective test (i.e., no subjective responses required of patient) that is becoming more widely used clinically, especially for estimating thresholds for mid to lower frequencies in infants, is the *auditory steady state response* (ASSR) (Rance, Rickards, Cohen, De Vidi, & Clark, 1995). The ASSRs are periodic responses evoked by periodic (modulated) stimuli. The stimuli can be amplitude modulated or frequency modulated at different rates (modulation frequencies), either simultaneously or sequentially (Hall & Swanepoel, 2010; Rance, 2008; Stapells, 2008). The various modulation frequencies (e.g., 1000 Hz carrier tone amplitude modulation at 80 Hz) will be processed at their appropriate tonotopic places along the basilar membrane and these modulations are carried up the auditory neural pathways to the brain, where they can be recorded with surface electrodes similar to other evoked potential measures. The ASSR is a reflection of how different levels of the brain react to the modulation frequencies of the stimuli. The carrier frequency determines where on the basilar membrane the stimulation is taking place, and the modulation rate determines the periodicity of the neural response in a normal hearing person. The ASSR is analyzed by measuring the spectrum of the response to determine if it is producing activity at the modulation rate and, hence, determine the extent to which the patient is able to process the carrier frequency. The filter settings of the recording instrument should be set to maximize the modulation frequencies and not the carrier frequencies, for example, 30 to 300 Hz. With today's clinical instruments, the spectra are automatically subjected to statistical rules to determine if a steady-state response is significantly above the noise floor. Modulation frequencies in the range 70 to 110 Hz produce steady-state responses that are not affected by levels of sleep or maturation, and most likely represent activity arising primarily at the level of the brainstem. To estimate thresholds, a regression analysis based on normative ASSR data or a correction factor analysis is performed by the recording instrument (Hall & Swanepoel, 2010). It is also possible, and clinically useful, to simultaneously present stimuli at different carrier frequencies (to one or both ears), each with a different modulation rate, to get a more rapid analysis of the patient's auditory function across a broader frequency range. For more details on ASSR, the interested reader should consult other sources (e.g., Hall & Swanepoel, 2010; Rance, 2008).

Synopsis 8–3

- In response to sound, the normal cochlea produces additional mechanical energy due to the motility of the OHCs, and these vibrations are transmitted out of the ear where they are recorded as OAEs in the ear canal. OAEs are preneural events but can be affected by hearing loss in the cochlea, middle ear, or ear canal.

- Because OAEs are preneural, their presence would suggest normal cochlear function, and lead one to suspect that a sensorineural hearing loss was due to a neural (8th nerve or central) disorder, or that they may be feigning a hearing loss.

- A normal TEOAE should be at least 3 dB above the noise floor at each of the measurable frequencies (1000, 2000, 3000, 4000 Hz) and show a reproducibility of more than 75%. TEOAEs are not reliable for frequencies below 1000 Hz or above 4000 Hz.

- DPOAEs are recordings of cochlear generated distortion product frequencies, which occur for different pairs of primary tones, called f1 and f2 (where f1/f2 = 1.22, f1 = 65 dB SPL, and f2 = 50 dB SPL). DPOAEs are plotted as a function of f2 frequency, which is varied between 1000 and 6000 Hz. A normal DPOAE should show a response that is at least 5 to 6 dB above the noise floor at each f2 frequency.

- TEOAEs are typically absent with cochlear hearing losses greater than 30 dB HL, which makes them ideal for newborn hearing screening. Neither TEOAEs nor DPOAEs are able to quantify the degree of hearing loss because they would be absent for peripheral hearing losses ranging from mild to profound. Disorders of the middle ear and outer ear can eliminate OAEs and confound the interpretation of OAEs in newborn hearing screenings.

■ The ABR is characterized by a series of wave peaks that occur within 2 to 10 ms following a brief click or tone burst and are recorded with electrodes taped to the head. The ABR is a reflection of the synchronous neural activity that occurs only with rapid onset stimuli (transients). Wave I originates from the peripheral portion of the 8th nerve and the later waves from lower brainstem pathways. Each of these waves is affected by the peripheral auditory system, as well as the neural conduction through the 8th nerve and low brainstem pathways. The most prominent peak is called wave V. Wave V is typically recordable in a normal ear to within 10 dB of behavioral threshold.

■ A latency-intensity function may be useful in characterizing possible hearing loss. A conductive hearing loss shows an elevated threshold and delayed wave V latency at each intensity level. A cochlear hearing loss shows an elevated threshold with a longer wave V latency near threshold, but at high intensities wave V latency occurs within the normal range when there are enough higher frequency neurons that are stimulated. A very steep high frequency cochlear hearing loss shows wave V latency flattens out before reaching the normal latency range. Noise masking can be used to eliminate the higher frequency regions and improve frequency specificity, especially in cases where there is a mid-frequency hearing loss with better high frequency sensitivity.

■ For neural assessment, the absence or abnormal delay of the peaks after wave I is evaluated. For example, an 8th nerve tumor could have a wave I, but the later waves may be absent or the latency interval between waves I and V could be prolonged.

■ Auditory steady-state response (ASSR) produces responses that reflect the rates of modulation (e.g., 70 to 110 Hz) for different carrier frequencies, and show promise for estimating frequency-specific auditory thresholds, including the lower frequencies. ASSRs are subjected to a spectral analysis to determine which frequency regions are producing/following the modulation rate for the applied frequencies. A statistical analysis is done to determine if a steady-state response is significantly above the noise floor.

References

American Speech-Language-Hearing Association Audio-logic Assessment Panel 1996. (1997). *Guidelines for audiologic screening.* Rockville, MD: Author.

Atcherson, S. R., & Stoody, T. M. (2012). *Auditory electrophysiology.* New York, NY: Thieme.

Bauch, C. D., & Olsen, W. (1986). The effect of 2000–4000 Hz hearing sensitivity on ABR results. *Ear and Hearing, 7,* 314–317.

Brownell, W. E. (1983). Observations on a motile response in isolated outer hair cells. In W. R. Webster & L. Aitken (Eds.), *Mechanisms of hearing* (pp. 5–10). Clayton, Australia: Monash University Press.

Burkard, R. F., Don, M., & Eggermont, J. J. (2007). *Auditory evoked potentials.* Baltimore, MD: Wolters Kluwer, Lippincott Williams, & Wilkins.

Cohen, M., & Prasher, D. (1992). Defining the relationship between cochlear hearing loss and acoustic reflex thresholds. *Scandinavian Audiology, 21,* 225–238.

Dahr, S., & Hall, J. W. (2012). *Otoacoustic emissions.* San Diego, CA: Plural Publishing.

Don, M., & Eggermont, J. (1978). Analysis of the click-evoked brainstem potentials in man using high-pass noise masking. *Journal of the Acoustical Society of America, 63,* 1084–1092.

Feeney, M. P., Grant, I. L., & Marryott, L. P. (2003). Wideband energy reflectance measurements in adults with middle-ear disorders. *Journal of Speech, Language, and Hearing Research, 46,* 901–911.

Fowler, C. G., & Shanks, J. E. (2002). Tympanometry. In J. Katz (Ed.), *Handbook of clinical audiology* (5th ed., pp. 175–204). Baltimore, MD: Lippincott Williams & Wilkins.

Gaskill, S. A., & Brown, A. M. (1990). The behavior of the acoustic distortion product, 2 f1–f 2, from the human ear and its relation to auditory sensitivity. *Journal of the Acoustical Society of America, 88,* 821–839.

Gelfand, S. A. (2001). *Essentials of audiology.* New York, NY: Thieme.

Gelfand, S. A., Schwander, T., & Silman, S. (1990). Acoustic reflex thresholds in normal and cochlear-impaired ears: Effects of no-response rates on 90th percentiles in a large sample. *Journal of Speech and Hearing Disorders, 55,* 198–205.

Glattke, T. J., & Robinette, M. S. (2007). Transient evoked otoacoustic emissions in populations with normal hearing sensitivity. In M. S. Robinette & T. J. Glattke (Eds.), *Otoacoustic emissions: Clinical applications* (3rd ed., pp. 87–106). New York, NY: Thieme.

Gorga, M. P., Neely, S. T., Johnson, T. A., Dierking, D. M., & Garner, C. A. (2007). Distortion product otoacoustic emissions in relation to hearing loss. In M. S. Robinette & T. J. Glattke (Eds.), *Otoacoustic emissions: Clinical applications* (3rd ed. pp. 197–226). New York, NY: Thieme.

Gorga, M. P., Neely, S. T., Ohlrich, B., Hoover, B., Redner, J., & Peters, J. (1997). From laboratory to clinic: A large scale study of distortion product otoacoustic emissions in ears with normal hearing and ears with hearing loss. *Ear and Hearing, 18,* 440–455.

Hall, J. W. III. (2000). *Handbook of otoacoustic emissions.* San Diego, CA: Singular.

Hall, J. W. III, & Swanepoel, D. W. (2010). *Objective assessment of hearing.* San Diego, CA: Plural Publishing.

Hof, J. R., Anteunis, L. J., Chenault, M. N., & van Dijk, P. (2005). Otoacoustic emissions at compensated middle ear pressure in children. *International Journal of Audiology, 44,* 317–320.

Hood, L. J. (1998). *Clinical applications of the auditory brainstem response.* San Diego, CA: Singular.

Hunter, L. L., Ries, D., Schlauch, R., Levine, S., & Ward, W. (1999). Safety and clinical performance of acoustic reflex tests. *Ear and Hearing, 20,* 506–514.

Hunter, L. L., Tubaugh, L., Jackson, A., & Prospes, S. (2008). Wideband middle ear power measurements in infants and children. *Journal of the American Academy of Audiology, 19,* 309–324.

Jerger, J. (1970). Clinical experience with impedance audiometry. *Archives of Otolaryngology, 92,* 311–324.

Jewett, D., Romano, M., & Williston, J. (1970). Human auditory evoked potentials: Possible brainstem components detected on the scalp. *Science, 167,* 1517–1518.

Kemp, D. T. (1978). Stimulated acoustic emissions from within the human auditory system. *Journal of the Acoustical Society of America, 64,* 1386–1391.

Kemp, D. T., Ryan, S., & Bray, P. (1990). A guide to the effective use of otoacoustic emissions. *Ear and Hearing, 11,* 93–105.

Kramer, S. J., & Teas, D. C. (1979). BSR (wave V) and N1 latencies in response to acoustic stimuli with different bandwidths. *Journal of the Acoustical Society of America, 66,* 446–455.

Lonsbury-Martin, B., Martin, G., & Whitehead (2007). Distortion product otoacoustic emissions in populations with normal hearing sensitivity. In M. Robinette & T. Glattke (Eds.), *Otoacoustic emissions: Clinical applications* (3rd ed., pp. 107–130). New York, NY: Thieme.

Margolis, R. H., & Hunter, L. L. (2000). Acoustic immittance measurements. In R. J. Roeser, M. Valente, & H. Hosford-Dunn (Eds.), *Audiology diagnosis* (pp 381–423). New York, NY: Thieme.

Margolis, R. H., Van Camp, K. J., Wilson, W. R., & Creten, W. L. (1985). Multifrequency tympanometry in normal ears. *Audiology, 24,* 44–53.

Møller, A. R. (1994). Neural generators of auditory evoked potentials. In J. T. Jacobson (Ed.), *Principles and applications in auditory evoked potentials.* Boston, MA: Allyn & Bacon.

Nozza, R. J., Bluestone, C. D., Kardatzke, D., & Brackman, R. N. (1994). Identification of middle ear effusion by aural acoustic admittance and otoscopy. *Ear and Hearing, 15,* 310–323.

Prieve, B. A. (2007). Otoacoustic emissions in neonatal hearing screening. In M. S. Robinette & T. J. Glattke (Eds.), *Otoacoustic emission: Clinical applications* (3rd ed., pp. 365–402). New York, NY: Thieme.

Probst, R., & Harris, F. (1993). Transiently evoked and distortion-product otoacoustic emissions: Comparison of results from normally hearing and hearing-impaired human ears. *Archives of Otolaryngology-Head and Neck Surgery, 119,* 858–860.

Rance, G. (2008). *Auditory steady-state response: Generation, recording, and clinical applications.* San Diego, CA: Plural Publishing.

Rance, G., Rickards, F. W., Cohen, L. T., De Vidi, S., & Clark, G. M. (1995). The automated prediction of hearing thresholds in sleeping subjects using auditory steady-state evoked potentials. *Ear and Hearing, 16,* 499–507.

Robinette, M. S., Cevette, M. J., & Probst, R. (2007). Otoacoustic emissions and audiometric outcomes across cochlear and retrocochlear pathology. In M. S. Robinette & T. J. Glattke (Eds.), *Otoacoustic emission: Clinical applications* (3rd ed., pp. 227–272). New York, NY: Thieme.

Robinette, M. S., & Glattke, T. J. (Eds.). (2007). *Otoacoustic emission: Clinical applications* (3rd ed.). New York, NY: Thieme.

Roush, J., Bryant, K., Mundy, M., Zeisel, S., & Roberts, J. (1995). Developmental changes in static admittance and tympanometric width in infants and toddlers. *Journal of the American Academy of Audiology, 6,* 334–338.

Shanks, J. E., & Shelton, C. (1991). Basic principles and clinical applications of tympanometry. *Otolaryngology Clinics of North America, 24,* 299–328.

Shanks, J. E., & Shohet, J. (2009). Tympanometry in clinical practice. In J. Katz (Ed.), *Handbook of clinical audiology* (6th ed., pp. 157–188). Baltimore, MD: Lippincott Williams & Wilkins.

Sohmer, H., & Feinmesser, M. (1967). Sources of electrocochleographic responses as studied in patients with brain damage. *Annals of Otology, Rhinology, and Laryngology, 76,* 427–435.

Stapells, D. R. (2008). The 80 Hz auditory steady-state response compared with other auditory evoked potentials. In G. Rance (Ed.), *The auditory steady-state response* (pp. 149–160). San Diego, CA: Plural Publishing.

Stapells, D. R., Picton, T. W., Durieux-Smith, A., Edwards, C. G., & Moran, L. M. (1990). Thresholds for short-latency auditory evoked potentials to tones in notched noise in normal and hearing-impaired subjects. *Audiology, 29,* 262–274.

Vanhuyse, V. J., Creten, W. L., & Van Camp, K. J. (1975). On the w-notching of tympanograms. *Scandinavian Audiology, 4,* 45–50.

Whitehead, M. L., Stagner, B. B., Lonsbury-Martin, B. L., & Martin, G. K. (1995). Effects of ear-canal standing waves on measurements of distortion-product otoacoustic emissions. *Journal of the Acoustical Society of America, 98,* 3200–3214.

Wiley, T. L., Oviatt, D. L., & Block, M. G. (1987). Acoustic-immittance measures in normal ears. *Journal of Speech and Hearing Research, 30,* 161–170.

9

Selected Disorders of the Auditory System

After reading this chapter, you should be able to:

1. Define terminology used to describe the time of onset and duration of hearing disorders.
2. Understand how audiometric results can help provide differential diagnoses of common auditory disorders.
3. Become familiar with common ear pathologies, including their physical characteristics, patient complaints, effects on ability to hear, and treatment options.
4. Identify disorders associated with the outer ear and middle ear and how they affect hearing.
5. Identify disorders associated with the inner ear and how they affect hearing.
6. Identify disorders associated with the 8th nerve and how they affect hearing.
7. Match hearing disorders to their types of hearing loss, for example, normal, conductive, or sensorineural.
8. Create representative audiograms for different pathologies.
9. Demonstrate an awareness of the possibility of functional hearing loss and patient characteristics that make one suspicious of it. Describe some common strategies for audiometric testing of patients suspected of functional hearing loss. Describe and interpret the Stenger test.
10. Understand the differences between subjective and objective tinnitus. Recognize when to make medical referrals for tinnitus. Describe three methods for treating subjective tinnitus.

This chapter provides general descriptions of some selected auditory disorders and their associated pathologies. The auditory disorders are separated into those that affect the different parts of the auditory system, the outer ear, middle ear, cochlea, 8th nerve, and central pathways. Keep in mind, however, that some auditory disorders, such as head trauma or otosclerosis, can affect more than one part of the ear. A patient may also have more than one type of auditory disorder from different causes, such as a sensorineural hearing loss from noise trauma affecting the cochlea and a conductive hearing loss from an ear infection in the middle ear. This chapter also briefly covers nonorganic (functional) hearing losses, where the patient may be exaggerating or feigning a hearing loss. At the end of the chapter, there is a discussion of tinnitus (internally generated sounds), a common symptom of many hearing disorders. As you will see, not all auditory disorders have associated hearing losses, and many types of hearing losses are not outwardly visible. Where appropriate, the disorders covered in this chapter are highlighted by characteristic results from audiologic tests that were described in earlier chapters, as well as descriptions of symptoms, underlying causes, and treatments. Familiarity with auditory pathologies is important for audiologists and speech-language pathologists in making decisions about appropriate referrals to medical practitioners and in selecting and interpreting audiological tests.

Describing Auditory Disorders

Before getting into the specific disorders, some associated concepts and terminology need to be addressed. One important component in describing auditory disorders is to define which part or parts of the ear are affected, called *differential diagnosis*. One of the most important pieces of information that can help in a differential diagnosis is a patient's case history. Information about the patient's primary complaints or symptoms are important, as well as some directed questions about when the problem began, whether it has worsened, any hearing or communication problems and their severity, whether symptoms came

on suddenly or gradually, any associated dizziness, any associated circumstances or activities, medications taken, family history, previous hearing tests and/or surgeries, and use of hearing aids. Based on the patient's answers to these questions and/or information from other sources, additional questions may be appropriate. Audiologic test results are also important to help differentially diagnose auditory pathologies by determining if there is any hearing loss and, if so, determine whether it is conductive, mixed, sensorineural, or unilateral and/or bilateral. In many cases, a more precise location of the problem can be determined from the audiological tests. For example, audiologic test results may help localize the disorder to a possible perforation of the tympanic membrane or suggest that there may be pathology of the 8th nerve. It is important to keep in mind that a medical diagnosis can only be determined by a physician, who conducts a thorough medical examination and may order lab work, imaging studies, or other diagnostic tests. All medically related auditory disorders must be referred by hearing health care professionals to a physician for evaluation and ongoing care. In cases where an adult has a sensorineural hearing loss, with no apparent medical or neural involvement, the audiologist may provide appropriate services without the need for medical evaluation; however, any hearing loss in a child should be referred to a physician for evaluation, and if hearing aids are warranted, medical approval from the physician must be obtained.

In addition to differential diagnosis and documentation of any hearing loss, there are many other terms that provide additional information about auditory disorders. A *genetic hearing loss* (also called *hereditary hearing loss* or *familial hearing loss*) is due to differences in the genes that are passed on through a hereditary source. The recent Human Genome Project, which is attempting to identify and map all of the genes in human DNA, has led to an abundance of new knowledge regarding genes that are associated with hearing loss and deafness. Hearing loss may be the only consequence of a genetic condition, such as that caused by a genetic protein mutation known as *connexin-26*, which is the most common genetic cause of hearing loss, and which may be expressed at birth or at a later prelinguistic stage (Nance & Dodson, 2007). Although most genetic hearing losses are not related to other syndromes, many genetic hearing losses are associated with known genetic and/or hereditary syndromes (having multiple disorders), including those that affect the outer and/or middle ear, such as Treacher Collins, DeGeorge, Goldenhar, Paget, and Apert; those that affect the cochlea, such as Usher, Jervell and Lange-Nielsen, Herrmann, Alport, Klippel-Feil, and Waardenburg; and those that can affect either or both the conductive and sensorineural portions, such as Down, CHARGE association, Crouzon, Hunter, and Möbius. According to Nance and Dodson (2007), there have been more than 150 genes identified that are associated with hearing loss. A *congenital hearing loss* is one that is present at birth, resulting from prenatal (prior to birth) factors or the perinatal (during birth) factors. A congenital hearing loss can be due to genetic factors or other pathologic causes. A genetic hearing disorder may also produce a hearing loss after birth and is called either an *early-onset genetic hearing loss* (during infant–toddler stage) or a *late-onset genetic hearing loss* (during childhood or adult stages). Genetic hearing losses do not always have a hereditary link, and can occur spontaneously during development. A list of factors known to have a high association with congenital or developmental hearing losses is known as the *high-risk register* (Joint Committee on Infant Hearing, 2000). The interested reader is referred to other textbooks (Shprintzen, 2001; Toriello, Reardon, & Gorlin, 2004) for additional information on genetic and other congenital hearing disorders.

A hearing loss that is not of genetic or congenital origin is called an *acquired hearing loss*, which is a hearing loss that occurs after birth and usually caused by disease, trauma, drugs, or aging. Hearing losses can also be described in terms of their time course: An *acute disorder* is one that is in its initial phase and lasts a relatively short duration; a *chronic disorder* is a condition that is persistent over a relatively long period of time; an *intermittent disorder* is a condition that comes and goes or reoccurs often. Other terms or conditions that are associated with auditory disorders include *otorrhea*, which refers to fluid (usually infected) that is draining into the external auditory canal from the middle ear, *aural fullness*, which is a sense of pressure in the ear reported by patients

and can be a sign of fluid in the middle ear or some types of sensorineural hearing loss, and *otalgia*, which means pain in the ear and often comes from different cranial nerves innervating the ear, face, teeth, temporomandibular joint, or throat (Jordan & Roland, 2000). In many cases, the cause of a hearing loss is *idiopathic* if of unknown cause, especially when referring to a *sudden hearing loss*.

Outer Ear Disorders

Disorders of the outer ear can occur in the auricle or external ear canal. Outer ear disorders are usually visible with the eye and/or with an otoscope. Outer ear disorders require medical evaluation, and in most cases can be medically or surgically treated. Outer ear disorders can result from embryological developmental abnormalities causing anatomical defects, or can be acquired due to infections, cancer, trauma, tumors, or obstructions. Many outer ear disorders do not have any associated hearing loss related to the outer ear condition, but some abnormalities may suggest a hearing loss in other parts of the auditory system, especially those related to congenital disorders.

Disorders of the Auricle

Auricular (pertaining to the auricle) pathologies generally do not have any associated hearing loss. Congenital auricular abnormalities result from alterations of the embryologic developmental events at various stages or cell location. These events may lead to structural variations of the auricle that range from slight variations in the structure, size, location, angle, or differences between the two ears, to complete absence of one or both of the auricles, called *anotia*. An abnormally small and malformed auricle is called *microtia*. Even bilateral microtia and anotia do not result in any appreciable hearing loss or communication problems. In cases of anotia or microtia, it is important to determine if there are other abnormalities, especially of the outer ear canal or middle ear (Roland & Rohn, 1997). Other auricular developmental anomalies include a small dimple just anterior to the tragus, called *preauricular pit* or *sinus*, or a small skin growth, called *preauricular appendage* or *tag*. Treatment for congenital auricular abnormalities is for cosmetic reasons generally in later childhood, and involves surgical correction or attachment of a realistic looking plastic ear. Surgical decisions must take into account problems in other parts of the auditory system, whether the problem is unilateral or bilateral, and an assessment of hearing abilities.

Acquired auricular disorders are usually due to some form of trauma that results in some cosmetic damage. Sources of trauma include physical blows to the auricle, frostbite or burns, penetrating object, bites, abrasions, or pulling on an earring. Trauma due to blunt forces can produce *auricular hematoma*, which is internal bleeding within the auricle, and this may lead to damage to the cartilage (Kinney, Kinney, & Vidimos, 1997). In most cases, the acute damage to the auricle heals itself, but the cartilage may remain misshapen. Patients may elect to have cosmetic surgery to repair the damage or appearance.

Acquired auricular disorders may also occur from disease, infections, or cancer. Infections may be bacterial, such as impetigo due to *Staphylococcus* infection. Infections may also be viral, such as herpes zoster (Ramsay Hunt syndrome) that produces severe pain, vesicles, and facial nerve problems, or herpes simplex (Kinney et al., 1997). Antibiotics may be prescribed to treat infections that occur in auricular disorders. Neoplasms, which are abnormal tissue growth or tumors, can also invade the auricle. Some neoplasms are benign cysts; however, others may be cancerous, including squamous cell carcinoma, basal cell carcinoma, or melanoma, and surgical treatment is typically required.

Disorders of the External Ear Canal

Disorders of the external canal may or may not have associated hearing loss, depending on the extent and type of disorder. Congenital embryological abnormalities of the external ear canal can occur in isolation or with some auricular evidence and/or involvement in other parts of the auditory system, including the middle ear or the cochlea.

Atresia (atretic ear) is the absence of an external auditory canal due to embryologic events, and may be unilateral or bilateral. The absence of the ear canal may be due to the failure of the canal to form an opening in the temporal bone, or it may be due to the canal being filled with tissue. Atresia will cause a maximum conductive hearing loss of around 50 to 60 dB HL, due to the blockage of sound through the outer ear to the middle ear. If the atresia is bilateral, there most likely will be a masking dilemma (see Chapter 6) that makes it difficult to determine the extent of hearing loss in each ear or whether there is any sensorineural hearing loss in one of the ears. Figure 9–1 summarizes the background and audiologic profile for a young child with atresia. Treatment for bilateral atresia is surgery in one of the ears, but this decision is dependent on the type and degree of hearing loss in each ear. Unilateral atresia is usually not surgically corrected; the patient may do quite well as a unilateral listener. An audiologic treatment option is to fit the patient with a bone conducting type of hearing aid (see Chapter 11).

Impacted cerumen is an acquired disorder of the external auditory canal that occurs when there is an over-accumulation of cerumen that becomes impacted somewhere along the canal. Although cerumen has a natural migration out of the ear canal, it can occasionally become trapped, especially with the use of cotton swabbed cleaning tips that have a tendency to push some of the cerumen deeper into the ear canal where it is more difficult to migrate out of the ear. Over time, this trapped cerumen completely blocks off a part of the ear canal and can cause a mild conductive hearing loss. The hearing will return to normal following removal of the cerumen. Cerumen impaction is usually unilateral but can occur in both ears if the patient continues the action that causes the cerumen accumulation and delays seeking medical treatment. Figure 9–2 summarizes the background and audiological profile for a case with impacted cerumen. Medical treatment for cerumen impaction is to have the cerumen removed by a trained health care provider who uses special instruments to scoop it out, or by irrigating the ear canal with

ATRESIA (UNILATERAL)

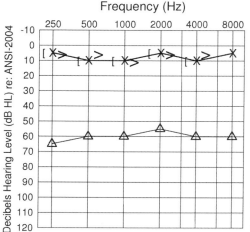

Location: Outer ear canal

Causes: Congenital absence of external ear canal due to failure to form during embryologic development.

Complaints: None as infant; may have classroom difficulties as child.

Physical Signs: Atretic ear canal on affected side. May have microtia.

Audio: Moderately severe conductive loss in affected ear. May also be bilateral.

Treatments: Elective surgery; CROS or BAHA hearing aid. Preferential seating in classroom.

Figure 9–1. Profile of a typical case with unilateral atresia.

IMPACTED CERUMEN (UNILATERAL)

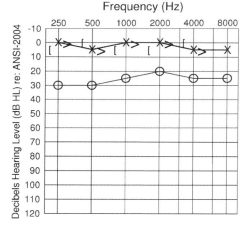

Location: Outer ear canal

Causes: Cleaning ears with cotton swabs

Complaints: Difficulty hearing on affected side

Physical Signs: Cerumen plug; unable to visualize tympanic membrane

Audio: Mild conductive loss on affected side

Treatments: Removal of cerumen by health service provider; over-the-counter softening agents; instruct patient to not clean canals with cotton swabs.

Figure 9–2. Profile of a typical case with unilateral impacted cerumen.

a forced flow of water. Over-the-counter cerumen-softening agents are also available and may be an effective treatment in mild cases. An accumulation of cerumen that comes in contact with the tympanic membrane, even without being impacted, can affect the movement of the tympanic membrane due to a greater mass, and may produce a mild conductive hearing loss in the higher frequencies only.

Foreign objects can find their way into the ear canal, especially with young children. Some examples of foreign objects that find their way into the ear include cotton swabs, sand, insects, earrings, clay, food, beads, pen caps, small batteries, and pieces of glass. Hearing loss from foreign objects depends on whether or not they block off a part of the ear canal, in which case there may be a mild conductive hearing loss (similar to cerumen impaction). Objects in the ear canal may be uncomfortable, painful, or can cause lacerations, abrasions, cerumen impaction, or infections. Treatment for foreign objects is to have the object removed by a trained medical health care provider.

Stenosis (stenotic ear) is an abnormal narrowing of the external auditory canal, usually due to developmental anomalies. According to Roland and Rohn (1997), if an ear canal is less that 4 mm in diameter it should be considered a stenotic ear. Stenosis does not result in any conductive hearing loss, as long as there is some amount of opening that can allow sounds to strike the tympanic membrane; however, the patient may be more prone to ear infections or to hearing loss from impacted cerumen or foreign objects because of the narrower opening.

Exostosis (*exostoses*), often referred to as *surfer's ear*, is a condition of bony outgrowths, covered with skin, that occur in the external ear canal. These bony outgrowths result from irritation of the ear canal due to repeated and prolonged exposure to cold water, typical of surfers; however, the precise cause of these benign bony growths is not known. Exostosis is characterized by multiple bumps and is usually bilateral. Exostosis is painless and generally nonproblematic, unless the bumps create enough of a narrowing of the ear canal to cause cerumen impaction or trap debris and moisture that lead to infections, or impinge on the tympanic membrane. In problem cases, the exostoses can be surgically removed, but will likely reoccur with continued exposure to cold water. An *oste-oma* is also a rounded bony growth, typically pearl shaped, that can also occur in the ear canal. An osteoma is a benign tumor that occurs spontaneously and usually does not cause any problems; therefore, surgical treatment is generally not required. An osteoma may be confused with exostosis; however, an osteoma is usually a single bump and occurs unilaterally. Hearing loss does not occur from exostosis or osteoma, unless it leads to a secondary problem.

Otitis externa is an infection of the tissues lining the external ear canal. These infections are usually caused by bacteria or fungus; however, the herpes zoster virus (Ramsay Hunt syndrome) can also produce lesions in the external ear canal. Otitis externa is sometimes called *swimmer's ear* when it is caused by bacterial infections from improperly maintained swimming pools. The most common bacteria causing otitis externa is *Pseudomonas*, which is quite common in the environment. *Pseudomonas* is usually prevented from multiplying because of the acidity of cerumen; however, when the cerumen is washed out by swimming, the protection is gone and there is an increased risk of developing otitis externa, especially problematic in the summer months when swimming is popular (Jordan & Roland, 2000). Otitis externa is often painful and may be accompanied by swelling and/or a fluid discharge. Hearing loss usually does not accompany otitis externa. Treatment for otitis externa is with topical or oral antibiotics, depending on the severity. Wearing earplugs when swimming may also help prevent otitis externa.

Synopsis 9–1

- Audiologic results can help in the differential diagnosis of ear disorders by documenting any hearing loss and determining if it is related to the conductive or sensorineural parts of the auditory system.

- Audiologists must recognize medically related hearing disorders and make appropriate referrals for medical evaluation and treatment decisions.

- Hearing loss at birth is referred to as a congenital hearing loss. These may be due to hereditary links, genetic mutations during development, or infections or trauma during the prenatal and perinatal periods. Acquired hearing disorders are those that occur later in life from noncongenital factors.

- Hereditary (genetic) hearing losses can manifest as congenital hearing losses or can develop as early- or late-onset hearing losses that can occur during childhood or even in the adult years.

- Hearing disorders can be described relative to their time of onset and/or duration; acute = initial phase; chronic = persisting over a period of time; intermittent = resolves and reoccurs.

- Some common terms associated with ear disorders include otorrhea (ear drainage), otalgia (ear pain), aural fullness (pressure feeling in ear), and idiopathic (of unknown cause).

- Outer ear disorders are usually visible with the eye or otoscope, and many do not have any associated hearing loss.

- Table 9–1 summarizes the disorders of the outer ear covered in this chapter.

Table 9–1. Summary of Outer Ear Disorders

Disorder	Description	Type of Hearing Problem
Anotia/microtia	Absent or misshapen auricle; congenital pathology, genetic origin	None, unless accompanied by atresia
Atresia	Absence of external ear canal	Maximum (50 to 60 dB HL) conductive loss
Exostosis (Surfer's ear)	Mounds of bony growth in ear canal; acquired from repeated exposure to cold water	No hearing loss; may lead to secondary problems (impacted cerumen, infections)
Foreign object	Variety of objects that find their way into the ear	No hearing loss unless completely blocks off canal or causes blockage of cerumen; may be painful or lead to infection; needs to be removed by physician
Hematoma	Bleeding under skin of auricle; acquired pathology from trauma	No hearing loss; needs medical attention
Impacted cerumen	Accumulation of cerumen that blocks off ear canal; often from cleaning ears with cotton swabs	Mild conductive hearing loss

Table 9–1. (*Continued*)

Disorder	Description	Type of Hearing Problem
Osteoma	Benign pearl-shaped bony tumor in ear canal; spontaneous origin	No hearing loss; usually does not cause any medical problem
Otitis externa (Swimmer's ear)	Bacterial, fungal, or viral (Herpes zoster) infections of the ear canal	No hearing loss; can be painful; needs medical attention
Pits or tags	Indentations or skin tags anterior to auricle; congenital pathology, genetic origin	None, unless genetic disorder affects other parts of the ear
Stenosis	Small diameter ear canal; usually congenital disorder; genetic origin	No hearing loss; may lead to secondary problems (impacted cerumen, infections)

Middle Ear Disorders

Otitis Media

Otitis media is an accumulation of fluid, called *effusion*, which occurs in the middle ear. When the fluid in the middle ear is clear and noninfected, it is called *serous otitis media*. When the fluid in the middle ear is infected, it is called *acute otitis media*. When the fluid becomes thickened or puss-like (with or without active bacteria), it is called *mucoid otitis media*, *purulent otitis media*, or *glue ear*. If fluid remains in the middle ear for an extended period of time, it is called *chronic otitis media*. Otitis media is a common cause of conductive hearing loss. Figure 9–3 summarizes the background and audiologic profile for a case with otitis media. The degree of conductive hearing loss with otitis media can range from mild to moderate depending on the amount and consistency of the fluid in the ear.

Otitis media can occur in all ages; however, young children have the highest prevalence of otitis media due to the anatomical and functional differences in the eustachian tube (see Chapter 1). The general sequence underlying the occurrence of otitis media begins with *eustachian tube dysfunction*, in which the eustachian tube is unable to equalize the air pressure in the middle ear, creating a negative pressure in the middle ear as the

remaining air becomes absorbed by the tissues of the middle ear. Eustachian tube dysfunction can be related to developmental differences or may be due to swelling of the nasopharynx that can occur with an upper respiratory infection, allergy, or enlarged adenoids.

Negative middle ear pressure may also result from a relatively sudden change in external air pressure, called *barotrauma*, as can occur during an airline flight or underwater diving. Prolonged negative middle ear pressure, in some cases, can lead to an effusion from the mucous lining of the middle ear, leading to serous otitis media. If the fluid becomes invaded with bacteria, which may occur when the person coughs or sneezes, the condition advances to acute otitis media. The acute otitis media stage can be painful and accompanied by fever or pulling at the ears.

For acute otitis media, the treatment options include prescribing oral antibiotics or simply allowing the ear to resolve the condition on its own over a few weeks. Persistent cases would generally require antibiotic treatment and possibly removal of the fluid with a needle-type syringe, a procedure called *myringotomy*, which is performed by a physician. For patients with chronic or reoccurring otitis media, a physician may recommend placement of a *pressure equalization* (PE) *tube*. A PE tube is a small grommet-like tube inserted into the tympanic membrane to allow the fluid to drain, and provides a mechanism to equalize air

OTITIS MEDIA (BILATERAL)

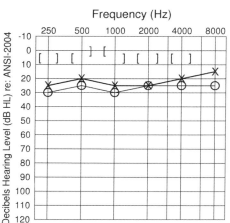

Location: Middle ear

Causes: Poor eustachian tube function and fluid build-up in middle ear; may become infected by way of the eustachian tube through coughing/sneezing. Common in young children.

Complaints: Difficulty hearing; lack of attention in school. Fever, tugging on ears, irritability.

Physical Signs: Tympanic membrane may be retracted, reddened, thickened, ruptured; may have visible discharge.

Audio: Mild to moderate conductive loss in both ears if bilateral. May also be unilateral.

Treatments: Medical observation; may need antibiotics for infection or PE tubes for chronic/reoccurring cases

Figure 9–3. Profile of a typical case with bilateral otitis media. **PE**, pressure equalization.

pressure in the middle ear. The PE tube remains in place for a few months and can be effective in reducing the chance of reoccurring ear infections. In most cases, as the tympanic membrane regrows over the incision, the PE tube is pushed out and the tympanic membrane is healed. Treatment decisions for otitis media are also guided by the extent and duration of hearing loss, as well as whether the age of the patient is an important learning period. In most cases, the conductive hearing loss will be resolved. It is important to realize that it is the fluid in the middle ear that causes the conductive hearing loss because it alters the transmission of vibrations across the ossicular chain. Antibiotics only kill the bacteria but do nothing about the fluid in the middle ear. A patient who does not have an active ear infection or who is being treated for an ear infection may continue to have the conductive hearing loss. The fluid in the middle ear is usually resolved naturally by the patient when the eustachian tube becomes functional over several weeks or through myringotomy and/or PE tubes.

Tympanic Membrane Perforation

A *perforation* is a hole that occurs in the tympanic membrane. Perforations can occur from trauma, such as a slap to the ear, explosion, or a patient-induced puncture from a cotton swab, paper clip, or hairpin. Your parents were right when they told you not to put anything other than your elbow in your ears. It is not uncommon for someone to be cleaning his or her ears with a cotton swab and another person bumps his or her arm when opening the medicine cabinet door. Trauma-induced perforations can be of different sizes and locations on the tympanic membrane. With relatively large perforations, there may be a mild conductive hearing loss; however, smaller perforations may not result in any appreciable conductive hearing loss. The hearing loss associated with trauma-induced perforations is usually unilateral, unless both ears were affected. A perforation can also occur from otitis media. In this case, there is considerable fluid buildup in the middle ear that erodes the tympanic membrane from the inside until it ruptures as a way to relieve the fluid pressure. Figure 9–4 summarizes the background and audiologic profile for a case with a mild perforation. Most tympanic membrane perforations spontaneously heal themselves but may cause scar tissue or an area in the tympanic membrane without the fibrous tissue layer, called a *monomere* (or monomeric tympanic membrane). The healed tympanic membrane does not usually have any associated hearing

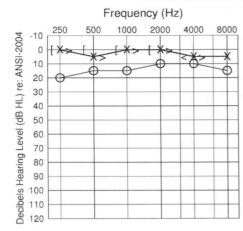

MILD PERFORATION (UNILATERAL)

Location: Tympanic membrane

Causes: Sharp object, slap to ear, otitis media, or PE tube.

Complaints: Usually not noticed. May have secondary problem if water gets in ear.

Physical Signs: Small hole in tympanic membrane; may have discharge if related to otitis media.

Audio: Normal hearing to slight conductive loss on affected side.

Treatments: None. Will usually heal itself. Swim plugs recommended when in water.

Figure 9–4. Profile of a typical case with unilateral tympanic membrane perforation. **PE,** pressure equalization.

loss. The presence of a *patent* (open) PE tube in the tympanic membrane acts like a very small perforation, and this usually does not cause any conductive hearing loss.

Cholesteatoma

A *cholesteatoma* is a benign mass that invades the middle ear space. It usually arises secondary to a perforation or otitis media. The mass consists of dead skin tissue and keratin that is normally sloughed off from healthy skin tissue but becomes trapped in a surrounding area of healthy skin, and the mass continually expands as more skin cells are sloughed off. This keratinizing, moist mass of tissue may lead to a foul-smelling otorrhea. The cellular makeup, growth pattern, and enzymes can destroy the middle ear structures and the bony shelf between the middle ear and the brain and/ or invade the mastoid; therefore, this disorder is considered a medical condition that requires immediate attention and surgical removal. The most common origin of an acquired cholesteatoma is from a *retraction pocket* (sucked in) in the pars flaccida region of the tympanic membrane, whereby the negative middle ear pressure pulls the pars flaccida into the middle ear space. The retraction

pocket is lined with the healthy skin cells, which continually slough off and are trapped in the retraction pocket. A cholesteatoma may also occur from the tympanic membrane tissue around a perforation or PE tube as the tissue is healing itself but migrates into the middle ear (Myerhoff, Marple, & Roland, 1997). Cholesteatomas are usually unilateral. The hearing loss associated with a cholesteatoma can vary. In the early stages, there may not be any symptoms or hearing loss; however, as the mass enlarges, and depending on the direction it grows, it may erode the ossicles or affect their vibration because of the increased mass. The cholesteatoma may cause a perforation in the tympanic membrane resulting in otorrhea, and in some cases the cholesteatoma may invade the round window and cause a sensorineural hearing loss or mixed hearing loss. Following surgery, the conductive or mixed hearing loss may persist depending on the damage caused by the cholesteatoma. Figure 9–5 summarizes the background and audiological profile for a case with cholesteatoma.

Otosclerosis

Otosclerosis is a disorder that is caused by an outgrowth of the bony wall around the stapes foot-

CHOLESTEATOMA (UNILATERAL)

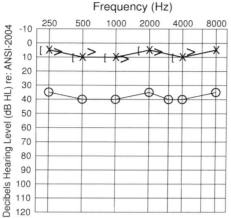

Location: Middle ear.

Causes: Skin flap grows into middle ear, e.g., from retraction pocket in pars flaccida. Sloughed-off skin becomes trapped causing pseudotumor to grow; becomes keratinized and infected.

Complaints: Hearing loss on affected side. May have otalgia and smelly drainage from ear.

Physical Signs: Whitish mass behind tympanic membrane. May have discharge in ear canal.

Audio: Normal to moderately severe conductive loss in affected ear depending on how it affects ossicles.

Treatments: Surgery is required to remove growth. Ossicular reconstruction may be option if needed. Hearing aids also option if conductive hearing loss due to removal of ossicles after surgery

Figure 9–5. Profile of a typical case with unilateral cholesteatoma.

plate. The otosclerosis begins as a spongy bony growth (*otospongiosis*) that eventually becomes hardened or sclerotic. Otosclerosis is more prevalent in females and begins to show up between the ages of 20 and 40 years (House, 1997). The cause of otosclerosis in not completely understood; however, a popular theory is that in many cases it appears to be due to a late-onset genetic disorder. This embryologic origin may be related to the incomplete developmental process of bone formation around the oval window, which is the last area that bone formation occurs (Myerhoff et al., 1997). In young adulthood, the otosclerosis begins to reveal itself, often exacerbated by hormonal changes, especially in women. When the bony growth encapsulates the footplate of the stapes (*stapes fixation*) and causes a conductive hearing loss, the otosclerosis becomes a clinical disorder.

Otosclerosis often shows up as a conductive hearing loss in one ear, but typically progresses to a bilateral conductive loss. There may be some asymmetry between the ears as well, but the conductive loss typically progresses from a mild to moderately severe degree in the low to mid frequencies. The audiometric pattern also shows a slightly poorer (notch) in the bone conduction threshold around 2000 Hz, known as *Carhart's notch*. This notch in the bone conduction is not a reflection of any sensorineural loss but is a result of a loss of middle ear resonance due to the conductive involvement of the ossicular chain. The bone conduction threshold at 2000 Hz usually returns to normal following surgical treatment of the otosclerosis. Immittance results often show a characteristic pattern for otosclerosis; they typically have a normal-shaped tympanogram (Type A) or reduced admittance (Type A$_s$), but also have absent acoustic reflexes. Figure 9–6 summarizes the background and audiometric profile for a case with bilateral middle ear otosclerosis. Surgical treatment is one option for otosclerosis and usually involves replacing part of the stapes with a prosthetic device that connects the incus to the oval window, called *stapedectomy*, or connecting the prosthesis through a hole drilled in the stapes footplate, called a *stapedotomy*. There are a variety of prostheses, including wires or pistons made out of metal or synthetic material. Surgery for otosclerosis is not required for medical reasons. Surgery for otosclerosis is quite successful in eliminating or significantly reducing the conductive hearing loss.

OTOSCLEROSIS (BILATERAL)

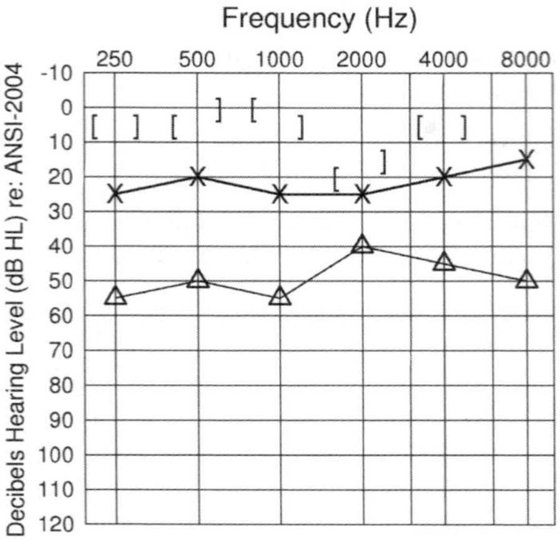

Location: Middle ear (footplate of stapes)

Causes: Bony growth of temporal bone around stapes footplate. Appears in second to third decade. May have a genetic link; exacerbated by pregnancy.

Complaints: Difficulty hearing. May hear better in noisy situations.

Physical Signs: May see a pinkish glow, otoscopically (called Schwartz's sign)

Audio: Progressive mild to moderate conductive loss as fixation increases. May begin unilateral and progress to bilateral. Characteristic bone conduction notch at 2000 Hz (Carhart's notch).

Treatments: Elective surgery to replace stapes with prosthesis (stapedectomy). Hearing aids/BAHA also options.

Figure 9–6. Profile of a typical case with bilateral otosclerosis with stapes fixation.

COCHLEAR OTOSCLEROSIS (BILATERAL)

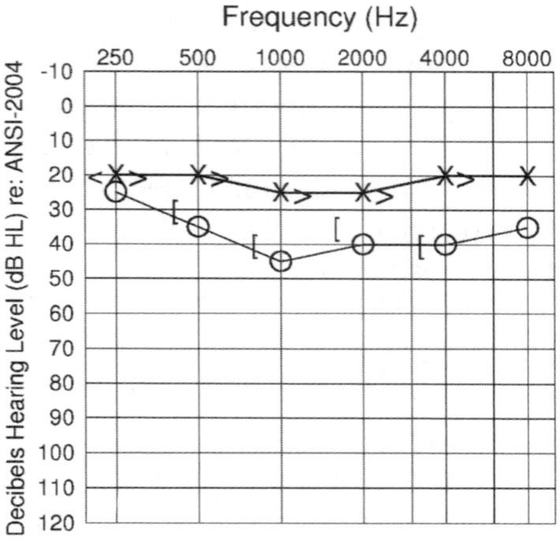

Location: Middle ear around oval window and cochlea.

Causes: Bony growth of temporal bone around oval window invades cochlea. Toxins destroy hair cells in the cochlea.

Complaints: Progressive difficulty hearing and understanding speech.

Physical Signs: None

Audio: Progressive mild to moderate bilateral sensorineural loss, usually worse in mid frequencies. May begin unilateral and progress to bilateral. No Carhart's notch. If combined with stapes fixation, there may be a mixed hearing loss and Carhart's notch.

Treatments: Sodium fluoride. Hearing aids when hearing loss affects communication.

Figure 9–7. Profile of a typical case with bilateral cochlear otosclerosis.

However, patients may also decide to be fit with a hearing aid or do nothing at all.

Otosclerosis can also invade the inner ear, which is called *cochlear otosclerosis*. In cochlear otosclerosis, the otospongiosis of the temporal bone around the oval window invades the inner ear and either produces toxins or alteration of the blood supply that destroys the hair cells (Myerhoff et al., 1997). Cochlear otosclerosis produces a slow, progressive, sensorineural hearing loss, usually stabilizing at a moderate degree of hearing loss. Figure 9-7 summarizes the background and audiometric profile for a case with bilateral cochlear otosclerosis. Treatment for cochlear otosclerosis may include sodium fluoride to slow or stabilize the process (Shambaugh, 1983) and/or hearing aids as needed for the sensorineural hearing loss.

Ossicular Disarticulation

A *disarticulation* refers to a separation of the ossicular chain or a break in one of the ossicles, typically dislocation of the long process of the incus from the stapes (Jordan & Roland, 2000). A disarticulation may occur as a result of damage from a variety of causes, including a slap on the side of the head, head injury, waterskiing accident, or necrosis (cell destruction) from otitis media or cholesteatoma. Ossicular disarticulations are usually unilateral and result in a moderate to moderately severe conductive hearing loss. The immittance results show a characteristic normal-shaped tympanogram with a high admittance (Type A_d) and acoustic reflexes are absent. Figure 9–8 summarizes the background and audiometric profile for a case with ossicular disarticulation. Disarticulations may be repaired or replaced with a prosthetic device, in a surgical procedure called *ossiculoplasty*. Surgery for disarticulation may not completely elim-

inate the conductive hearing loss in many cases (Jordan & Roland, 2000).

Glomus Tumors

Glomus tumor is a benign, slow-growing tumor of the middle ear. A glomus tumor is a highly vascularized tumor arising from the neural tissues (paraganglia cells) in the middle ear, usually associated with the jugular bulb that runs along the floor of the middle ear (called *glomus jugulare*) or other nerves running in the middle ear along the promontory (called *glomus tympanicum*). Glomus tumors are usually visible otoscopically as a reddish purple mass due to their vascularity. Glomus tumors occur more often in older female adults and may arise spontaneously or have a hereditary link (Lustig & Jackler, 1997). The effects of the glomus tumors vary depending on their size and location but may present with aural fullness, a pulsing sound related to the blood flow, and a conductive hearing loss in about half of the patients (Woods, Strasnick, & Jackson, 1993). Immittance results typically show a normal tympanogram (Type A) and acoustic reflex patterns depend on the extent of the conductive hearing loss. Treatment for glomus tumors is surgery to completely remove the mass.

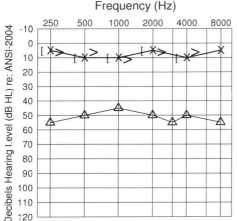

DISARTICULATION (UNILATERAL)

Location: Middle ear (ossicular chain).

Causes: Head injury, slap to ear, cholesteatoma

Complaints: Hearing loss on affected side.

Physical Signs: None. May notice hyperflaccid tympanic membrane, otoscopically.

Audio: Moderately severe conductive loss in affected ear.

Treatments: Ossicular reconstruction may be option if needed. CROS hearing aid or BAHA options if surgery not done or if hearing loss continues to exist after surgery.

Figure 9–8. Profile of a typical case with unilateral ossicular disarticulation.

Synopsis 9–2

- Hearing disorders of the middle ear typically result in a conductive hearing loss. Most middle ear pathologies occur unilaterally; however, some (e.g., otitis media and otosclerosis) occur or progress to involve both ears.

- Otitis media, an accumulation of fluid in the middle ear, is the most common cause of middle ear disorders. Otitis media begins with poor eustachian tube function leading to accumulation of fluid (effusion). If bacteria invade the middle ear, an acute infection may occur. Antibiotics treat the infection but do not eliminate the fluid. Otitis media often resolves on its own, but may require myringotomy or pressure equalization tubes.

- Trauma-induced middle ear disorders include tympanic membrane perforations and ossicular chain disarticulations. Tympanic membrane perforations usually heal spontaneously. Disarticulations can be managed with prosthetic reconstruction, called ossiculoplasty.

- Otosclerosis originates from a bony growth of the temporal bone around the oval window that may begin between 20 and 40 years of age. The bony growth may fixate the stapes leading to a conductive hearing loss, or may invade the cochlea where its toxins may damage the hair cells leading to a sensorineural hearing loss. The cause of otosclerosis is not known, but is thought to have a hereditary link (late onset). Surgical replacement of the stapes with a prosthesis is called stapedectomy.

- Tumors can also arise in the middle ear; the most common are cholesteatoma (pseudotumor) and glomus tumors.

- Table 9–2 summarizes disorders of the middle ear covered in this chapter.

Table 9–2. Summary of Middle Ear Disorders

Disorder	Description	Type of Hearing Problem
Otitis media	Inflammation of the middle ear, usually accompanied by fluid (effusion); acquired from poor eustachian tube function; common in children	Conductive hearing loss due to the fluid; hearing loss improves when otitis media is resolved, spontaneously or with surgery (PE tubes); antibiotics may be prescribed if accompanied by bacterial infection
Perforation	Puncture or rupture of the tympanic membrane; can vary in size; PE tube may act like a small perforation	Normal hearing to mild conductive hearing loss; membrane usually heals itself

Table 9–2. (*Continued*)

Disorder	Description	Type of Hearing Problem
Cholesteatoma	Skin flap growing in the middle ear, usually from retraction pocket; sloughed-off skin builds up and becomes infected; continues to grow in middle ear and may rupture tympanic membrane producing smelly discharge	Hearing loss depends on where cholesteatoma grows and structures that it damages; usually erodes the ossicles and results in moderate conductive loss; needs medical referral for surgery
Otosclerosis	Spongy growth of temporal bone around oval window; can encapsulate stapes or invade cochlear (cochlear otosclerosis); Begins in second to fourth decade; some hereditary link	Usually fixates stapes and causes moderate conductive hearing loss in affected ear; usually unilateral, but may progress to bilateral; cochlear otosclerosis causes sensorineural loss due to toxin damaging hair cells; stapedectomy to replace stapes with prosthesis
Disarticulation	Trauma-induced break in the ossicular chain or fracture in one of the ossicles	Moderate to moderately severe conductive hearing loss; elective surgical reconstruction (ossiculoplasty)
Glomus tumors	Benign vascularized tumors arising in the middle ear from paraganglia cells associated with jugular bulb or other nerves in middle ear; occur spontaneously	Hearing loss depends on location of tumor; about half present with a conductive loss; refer for surgical treatment

PE, pressure equalization.

Cochlear Disorders

Noise-Induced Hearing Loss

A *noise-induced hearing loss* (NIHL), also called *acoustic trauma*, is, as the name implies, a hearing loss that occurs from exposure to extremely loud impulsive-type sounds, like an explosion or gunshot, or more commonly from longer-term exposures to high-level industrial, military, and/or recreational noises, such as jackhammers, airplanes, machinery, or music. Noise-induced hearing loss is one of the most common causes of acquired sensorineural hearing loss. The hearing loss usually shows characteristic hearing thresh-old shifts in the 3 to 6 kHz region (called a *noise notch*). With prolonged exposure, the notch deepens and widens, and eventually the higher (and surrounding lower) frequencies will worsen. High pitched tinnitus (ringing in the ears) is a common complaint with NIHL. Figure 9–9 summarizes the background and audiological profile of a case with permanent NIHL.

The hearing loss associated with NIHL results from damage to the stereocilia, tectorial membrane, metabolic changes to the hair cell, rupture of Reissner's membrane, or complete destruction of the organ of Corti. The NIHL can be characterized by *permanent threshold shifts* (PTS) or *temporary threshold shifts* (TTS). The TTS may occur when exposed to loud noise levels for a few hours,

NOISE-INDUCED HEARING LOSS (PERMANENT)

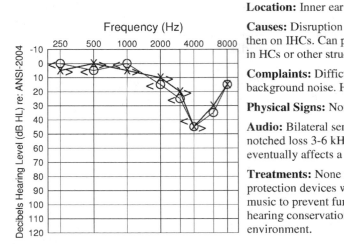

Location: Inner ear

Causes: Disruption of stereocilia, first on OHCs, then on IHCs. Can produce biochemical changes in HCs or other structural damage to cochlea.

Complaints: Difficulty hearing, especially in background noise. High-pitched tinnitus.

Physical Signs: None

Audio: Bilateral sensorineural loss. Begins as a notched loss 3-6 kHz region; progressive, and eventually affects a wider frequency range.

Treatments: None for existing damage. Ear protection devices when exposed to noise/loud music to prevent further damage. Should have hearing conservation program if in noisy work environment.

Figure 9–9. Profile of a typical case with permanent noise-induced hearing loss. **OHC**, outer hair cells; **IHC**, inner hair cells.

as might occur from a music concert or loud stereo; and one may notice that sounds seem muffled and there is a high pitched tinnitus. The TTS will, by definition, return to normal within a few hours. With continued exposure to loud sounds for several years, the hearing loss and tinnitus will become permanent and progressive, generally beginning with a loss of function in the outer hair cells, and then a loss in the inner hair cells with continued exposure. However, even a single occurrence to an impulsive, high-intensity sound can cause mechanical damage to the cochlea, or even to the tympanic membrane and ossicles. The sound pressure levels and durations of exposure that cause permanent hearing loss are complicated and may vary depending on the type of noise, one's susceptibility, other health factors, or exposure to chemicals or drugs that may damage the ear. In general, there are standards (National Institute for Occupational Safety and Health [NIOSH], 1998; Occupational Safety & Health Administration [OSHA], 1983) that set acceptable limits for industrial noise exposures within a 24-hr period, called *damage risk criteria*. The most conservative standard (NIOSH) begins with a maximum allowable exposure of 85 dBA for 8 hr (within a 24-hr period), and for every 3 dB increase in noise level, the maximum exposure time is cut in half; for example, 88 dBA = 4 hr, 91 dBA = 2 hr. The OSHA standards set 90 dBA as the minimum allowable exposure to which one can be exposed for a period of 8 hr (within a 24-hr period) to be considered relatively safe; and the duration of exposure decreases in half for each 5 dB increase in the noise level, for example, exposure to continuous noise level of 95 dBA would only be allowed for a maximum of 4 hr. Exposures less than the damage risk criteria are considered safe for most people. Continued exposure to levels exceeding the damage risk criteria can result in PTS.

It is not atypical for music venues to exceed 100 dBA; therefore, one would want to limit exposure to less than 2 hr. Of course, *hearing protection devices* (HPDs), such as noise reduction headsets or earplugs, can help reduce the level of noise (by about 15 to 20 dB) and are highly recommended (and required by industry) when in situations where the sounds are too loud. Workplaces with the potential for exposure to loud sounds should have in place a *hearing conservation pro-*

gram to educate the employees about effects of noise, monitor their hearing, provide HPDs, and make changes in the environment if possible. Other treatment options are to reduce exposure to excessive noise and consider hearing aids when the degree of hearing loss is more advanced.

Hearing Loss Due to Aging

Presbycusis is the term used for hearing loss related to aging. Presbycusis is the most common form of adult acquired sensorineural hearing loss. Close to half of persons 65 to 75 years of age have some degree of high frequency hearing loss, and the percentage increases with advancing age. Presbycusis is characterized by a bilateral sloping high frequency sensorineural hearing loss that can begin around the sixth decade of life and may slowly progress with age. Patients often complain of difficulty with understanding speech (Committee on Hearing, 1988; Humes, 1996). The sensorineural hearing loss associated with aging is typically a result of a loss of outer hair cell function and then inner hair cell function; however, involvement of the central auditory pathways or the stria vascularis has also been shown. Figure 9–10 summarizes the background and audiologic profile for a case

with presbycusis. Although there is high correlation between age and increasing sensorineural hearing loss, it is difficult to separate any concomitant effects of noise exposure, genetic predisposition, smoking, alcohol, diet, or other health factors (Roush, 1985). Treatment for presbycusis is primarily audiological with the fitting of hearing aids and aural rehabilitation programs as needed.

Ménière Disease

Ménière disease is a disorder that is characterized usually by four conditions: (a) episodes of vertigo, often severe with vomiting, (b) low frequency sensorineural hearing loss, which can fluctuate in early stages, (c) aural fullness, and (d) low pitched tinnitus ("ocean roar"). Ménière disease is related to a buildup of excessive endolymph in the scala media and vestibular labyrinths, called *endolymphatic hydrops*, the cause of which is not understood, and may occur spontaneously or with a viral attack or may have some genetic predisposition (Roland & Marple, 1997). Ménière disease occurs typically in the 30- to 60-year-old range. The hearing loss is sensorineural, which is usually unilateral, but may progress to bilateral in about 20% of patients (Jordan & Roland, 2000). Although the

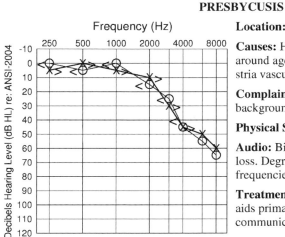

PRESBYCUSIS

Location: Inner ear

Causes: Hearing loss due to aging, beginning around age 50 years. Affects cochlear hair cells, stria vascularis, and/or neural auditory pathways.

Complaints: Difficulty hearing, especially in background noise. High-pitched tinnitus.

Physical Signs: None

Audio: Bilateral high frequency sensorineural loss. Degree of loss and range of affected frequencies increase slowly with age.

Treatments: None for existing damage. Hearing aids primary treatment when loss is affecting communication.

Figure 9–10. Profile of a typical case with presbycusis.

MÉNIÈRE DISEASE (UNILATERAL)

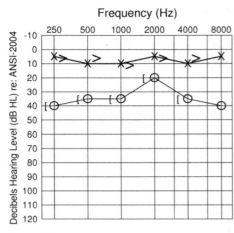

Location: Inner ear

Causes: Excessive build-up of endolymph in the scala media and vestibular labyrinths. May occur spontaneously, or from viral attack, or from late-onset genetic link.

Complaints: Vertigo, ocean roar tinnitus, aural fullness, and hearing loss in affected ear. Vertigo may be debilitating.

Physical Signs: None.

Audio: Fluctuating, low frequency, sensorineural hearing loss, initially. May end up with a permanent flat moderate sensorineural loss. Often see best thresholds at 2000 Hz.

Treatments: Eliminate salt and caffeine from diet. May benefit from a prescribed diuretic. Severe cases may require endolymphatic shunt operation or vestibular/cochlear nerve section.

Figure 9–11. Profile of a typical case with unilateral Ménière disease.

hearing loss may start out as a low frequency hearing loss, with time the hearing loss flattens out with a moderate hearing loss (often with the best hearing at 2000 Hz). Figure 9–11 summarizes the background and audiologic profile of a case with Ménière disease. The severity, duration, and repeatability of the vertigo attacks vary across patients. The fluctuating characteristic of the hearing loss has been shown to correspond to a buildup of endolymph (causing the hearing loss) and then a rupture of Reissner's membrane, causing a vertiginous attack, then improved hearing when the membrane repairs itself; then the process begins again. The patient may learn to predict the vertigo attacks by sensing the buildup of aural pressure, hearing loss, and tinnitus. Ménière disease requires medical evaluation, and most patients improve with treatment. Treatment may begin with elimination of caffeine, nicotine, and salt in the diet, followed by a prescribed diuretic. In severe cases without resolution from other treatments, an *endolymphatic shunt* operation may be performed to provide for drainage of the endolymph into tissues, or a more invasive approach may be used to destroy the vestibular organs by infusing vestibulotoxic drugs into the inner ear through the middle ear, or by surgery (*labyrinthectomy* or *vestibular nerve section*).

Ototoxicity

Ototoxicity (or *vestibulotoxicity*) is the hearing loss (or vestibular dysfunction) that occurs from therapeutic drugs. For the most part, the drugs are being used to treat some other disease and have known associated side effects that can cause hearing loss. Patients being treated with drugs that are ototoxic should have a baseline audiogram before treatment begins and regular audiograms during the treatment in order to monitor any changes in hearing. In some cases, if hearing loss begins to show up, the physician may alter the drug dose; however, most of the time the underlying illness is more important than the hearing. There may be the need for subsequent audiologic treatment with hearing aids and aural rehabilitation. It is important for the audiologist to be involved as early as possible with patients being treated with ototoxic medications.

There are five general categories of medications that are associated with hearing loss: (a) aminoglycosides, (b) chemotherapeutic agents, (c) loop diuretics, (d) salicylates (aspirin), and (e) antimalarial drugs (quinine). Aminoglycoside and chemotherapeutic agents can cause permanent bilateral sensorineural hearing loss, whereas the loop diuretics, salicylates, and antimalarial drugs usually cause temporary, bilateral sensorineural hearing loss that returns to normal soon after the drug therapy is stopped. *Aminoglycosides* (also referred to as the antibiotic "mycin" drugs) are the most damaging to the auditory and/or vestibular system. However, they are very important in treating infections and are commonly used. Some common aminoglycosides that are mostly cochleotoxic are amakicin, tobramycin, dihydrostreptomycin, and neomycin. Aminoglycosides that are more vestibulotoxic (and often used to preserve hearing) are streptomycin and gentamycin. Damage to the cochlea from aminoglycosides is dose and duration dependent, but occurs first in the outer hair cells and can progress to the inner hair cells over longer treatment periods. If a hearing loss occurs, it is bilateral and begins first in the ultra-high frequencies. Figure 9–12 summarizes the background and audiological profile of a case with aminoglycoside ototoxicity. Estimates of hearing loss caused by aminoglycosides range from 2 to 15% (Monsell, Teixido, Wilson, & Hughes, 1997). Evaluations of patients treated with aminoglycosides is one of the main clinical applications for performing ultra-high frequency audiometry. With time, the hearing loss may progress to the conventional frequency range. Although monitoring hearing during aminoglycoside treatment is a good idea, it may not always be possible because of the severity of the illness. In some cases, the hearing loss will continue to progress long after the treatment is terminated.

Chemotherapeutic (neoplastic) agents also pose a significant risk for cochlear damage. These drugs are used to treat some forms of cancer. The drugs most commonly associated with hearing loss are *cisplatin* and *carboplatin* (both also spelled *platinum*). Cisplatin is used to treat tumors of the head and neck as well as ovarian or testicular cancer. Hearing loss with cisplatin occurs in about 17% of patients (Martini & Prosser, 2003), and is typically a permanent, bilateral, high frequency

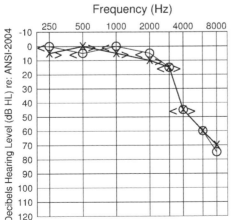

OTOTOXICITY (FROM AMINOGLYCOSIDES)

Location: Inner ear

Causes: Systemic biochemical damage to cochlear and/or vestibular hair cells from aminoglycoside antibiotic treatment.

Complaints: Slight hearing loss may be noticed. High frequency tinnitus. Often very sick from another medical disorder, which is why aminoglycosides were administered.

Physical Signs: None

Audio: Permanent bilateral high frequency sensorineural loss. Begins in ultra-high frequency range. Degree of loss and range of affected frequencies increase with dosage and time.

Treatments: None for existing damage. May alter drug therapy if appropriate. Hearing aids are the primary treatment when loss affects communication.

Figure 9–12. Profile of a typical case with ototoxicity from aminoglycoside antibiotics.

OTOTOXICITY (FROM LOOP DIURETICS OR ASPIRIN)

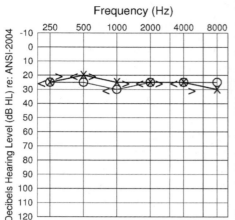

Location: Inner ear

Causes: Loop diuretics affect function of stria vascularis; aspirin affects biochemistry of cochlear hair cells.

Complaints: Noticeable hearing loss because of the involvement of speech frequencies. High frequency tinnitus is often prominent sign of beginning ototoxicity from aspirin.

Physical Signs: None.

Audio: Temporary mild to moderate relatively flat sensorineural hearing loss, bilaterally.

Treatments: Hearing should improve spontaneously when loop diuretic treatment is finished.

Figure 9–13. Profile of a typical case with ototoxicity from loop diuretics or aspirin.

sensorineural hearing loss, similar to that seen with aminoglycosides.

Loop diuretics are often used to treat patients with edema associated with congestive heart failure, edema of the lungs, or renal disease. These types of diuretics act upon the loop of Henley in the kidney and cause high levels of diuresis. The most common loop diuretics associated with hearing loss are furosemide, bumetanide, and ethacrynic acid. The hearing loss from loop diuretics is related to effects on the stria vascularis and is usually temporary and characterized by a bilateral, moderate sensorineural hearing loss (Gallagher & Jones, 1979). Figure 9–13 summarizes the background and audiological profile of a case of hearing loss from loop diuretics. The use of loop diuretics in conjunction with aminoglycosides or cisplatin may exacerbate their ototoxic effects and increase the risk for permanent sensorineural hearing loss (Brummett, Bendrick, & Himes, 1981).

Salicylates are anti-inflammatory drugs, the most common being aspirin. Aspirin in high doses, as sometimes used in the treatment of rheumatoid arthritis, can cause tinnitus and a bilateral, flat, mild to moderate, temporary sensorineural hearing loss. The audiometric pattern for aspirin-induced ototoxicity is similar to that for loop diuretics (see

Figure 9–13). The hearing loss and tinnitus disappear when the salicylate treatment is terminated. The amount of aspirin needed to produce tinnitus and hearing loss is about 6 to 8 g/day (Roland & Marple, 1997). *Antimalarial drugs*, like quinine and chloroquine, are also capable of producing hearing loss and tinnitus. These drugs are usually used to prevent malaria or severe leg cramps. The hearing loss is generally a bilateral, high frequency sensorineural loss. As with salicylates, the hearing loss is usually temporary.

Infections

Viral or bacterial infections that affect the inner ear are less common than those that affect the external and middle ear. Inner ear infections and hearing loss may be secondary to other infections like *meningitis*, gaining access through the cochlear aqueduct or internal auditory canal, or from otitis media and cholesteatoma, gaining access through the oval or round windows (Roland & Marple, 1997). Hearing loss from inner ear bacterial infections is usually severe and permanent. Treatment of bacterial infections is with antibiotics and corticosteroids. Hearing aids and aural rehabilitation

BACTERIAL INFECTION (MENINGITIS)

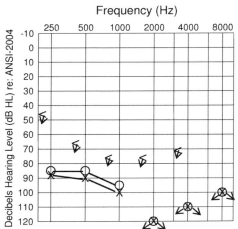

Location: Inner ear

Causes: System effects damage hair cell biochemistry and stria vascularis. Concomitant affects from any aminoglycosides antibiotics treatment.

Complaints: Sudden severe hearing and resulting communication problems.

Physical Signs: None.

Audio: Permanent bilateral severe to profound sensorineural loss. Some cases may be less severe; rare cases of unilateral loss.

Treatments: After recovery, treatment is with bilateral hearing aids and aural rehabilitation program.

Figure 9–14. Profile of a typical case with bacterial infection resulting in meningitis.

are required to treat and concomitant hearing loss. Figure 9–14 summarizes the background and audiological profile for a case with inner ear infection due to meningitis.

Viruses can also invade the inner ear and cause sudden sensorineural hearing loss of varying degrees and in some cases may even be temporary. Cytomegalovirus (CMV) is a common viral infection that generally does not cause hearing loss or much illness, other than a slight flu. However, if the mother contracts CMV during pregnancy, a small percentage of the time the baby will be born with a CMV infection that can lead to a progressive sensorineural hearing loss. CMV is a leading cause of sensorineural hearing loss in young children. Usually the hearing loss with CMV has a delayed onset and is progressive. Other childhood viruses, like rubella (German measles) or mumps, can also cause sensorineural hearing losses of varying degrees. Despite the systemic nature of the mumps virus, when there is a hearing loss it is almost always unilateral and profound. The unilateral hearing loss may go unnoticed until later in life and may be traceable to early childhood mumps. Syphilis and herpes zoster can also cause severe bilateral sensorineural hearing loss, especially if exposed in utero. These viral infections are relatively rare today in developed countries because of pediatric vaccinations.

Temporal Bone Fractures

A nonpenetrating trauma to the skull (also called *closed-head injury*) from car accidents, sports, physical abuse, or falls can cause fractures to the temporal bone and lead to hearing loss and vestibular symptoms. A *transverse fracture* of the temporal bone is one that is perpendicular to the petrous portion of the temporal bone and causes damage to the inner ear structures, leading to a sensorineural hearing loss (Bergemalm & Borg, 2001). If the fracture runs parallel along the edge of the petrous portion of the temporal bone it is called a *longitudinal fracture* and usually results only in middle ear involvement, including fluid/blood in the middle ear or a disarticulation of the ossicles. Transverse fractures are less common and can occur from a blow to the front or back of the head. A longitudinal fracture is most often caused by a blow to the side of the head. Temporal bone fractures are identified through computerized tomography. In some closed-head injuries, including concussions, there may be some stretching of nerves in the brainstem or temporal lobe lesion, causing some subtle hearing problems.

Sudden Sensorineural Hearing Loss

Sudden sensorineural hearing loss is not a disease per se, but a term used to describe a sensorineural hearing loss that comes on rapidly, typically in a few hours or when one wakes up at night. It is usually a unilateral hearing loss, but in some cases, depending on the causes, may affect the other ear at a later date. The hearing loss is usually accompanied by aural fullness and tinnitus. The degree of hearing loss varies and in some cases may spontaneously recover or can be restored with drug treatment if begun quickly; therefore, any sudden hearing loss should be treated as a medical emergency. There are many known causes of sudden sensorineural hearing loss, including viral attacks, vascular embolisms, autoimmune disorders, Ménière disease, acoustic neuroma, and closed-head trauma. A rupture in the oval or round window membrane, a *perilymph fistula*, may also result in a sudden sensorineural hearing loss and vestibular symptoms. In many cases, a cause cannot be identified, in which case it is referred to as an idiopathic sudden sensorineural hearing loss. When the cause is known, appropriate treatment can be administered. In many cases, like with autoimmune or idiopathic sudden sensorineural hearing loss, immediate treatment with corticosteroids may be prescribed in the hope of stabilizing or improving the hearing loss. Figure 9–15 summarizes the background and audiological profile for a case with sudden sensorineural hearing loss.

Neural Disorders

Hearing disorders of the 8th cranial nerve and the area around the nerve between the cochlea and the cochlear nucleus (cerebellar-pontine angle or CPA) are traditionally referred to as *retrocochlear* disorders. Although retrocochlear implies anything after the cochlea, disorders of the brainstem and cortical areas are usually considered central auditory disorders. The auditory nerve can be affected by a variety of factors, including presbycusis, vas-

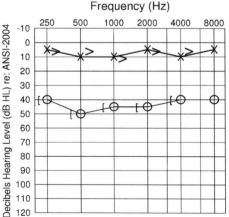

SUDDEN SENSORINEURAL HEARING LOSS

Location: Inner ear

Causes: Autoimmune disorder, viral attacks, or idiopathic disorders that produce damage to cochlear hair cells. Perilymph fistula can alter fluids and cause hearing loss and vertigo.

Complaints: Hearing loss in the affected ear that developed within a few hours or upon awakening. May have vertigo if from perilymph fistula.

Physical Signs: None.

Audio: Sudden unilateral relatively flat mild to moderate sensorineural loss. May progress and/or may spontaneously recover. May occur in other ear at a later date.

Treatments: Seek medical attention immediately to stabilize hearing and maximize potential for recovery. Typically treated with corticosteroids. Hearing aid should be considered after hearing loss has stabilized.

Figure 9–15. Profile of a typical case with unilateral sudden sensorineural hearing loss.

cular disorders, viral attacks, multiple sclerosis, diabetes, tumors, and a developmental condition that affects the firing of the neurons called auditory dyssynchrony (or auditory neuropathy). The latter two neural disorders are more commonly seen by audiologists and are described in more detail below.

Acoustic Neuroma

A benign tumor that involves the 8th cranial nerve and causes hearing loss and vestibular symptoms is called an *acoustic neuroma*. This tumor typically arises from the Schwann cells of the vestibular portion of the 8th cranial nerve, and is also called a *vestibular schwannoma* or an *acoustic schwannoma*. It is the most common type of tumor found in the CPA (Lustig & Jackler, 1997). As the tumor grows, it compresses or destroys the cochlear nerve; it can grow from the internal auditory canal into the CPA, where it can eventually involve the central auditory pathways. Although these tumors are benign and relatively slow growing, they need medical attention that generally involves surgical removal. The earlier the acoustic neuroma is identified and removed, the more likely that the hearing may be preserved. Many audiological tests (e.g., speech tests, acoustic reflexes, ABR) have been developed to differentially diagnose retrocochlear (acoustic neuroma) disorders from cochlear disorders. The hearing loss associated with an acoustic neuroma is a unilateral, high frequency, progressive, sensorineural loss that can range from mild to severe. The higher frequencies are affected first because of the early pressure exerted on the outside of the cochlear nerve that originates from the more basal area of the cochlea. In some cases, hearing may be normal but the patient has unilateral tinnitus or difficulty with understanding speech. Acoustic reflexes may be absent or elevated beyond those considered for the amount of hearing loss. The speech recognition scores may also be poorer than would be predicted from the amount of hearing loss. Sometimes there is dizziness or imbalance, but this is not always a presenting symptom. A common symptom of an acoustic neuroma is a unilateral high pitched tinnitus. Figure 9–16 summarizes the background and audiologic profile of a case with an acoustic

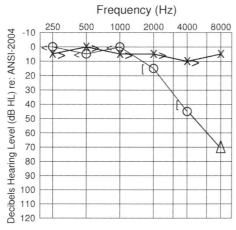

ACOUSTIC NEUROMA

Location: 8th Cranial Nerve. Usually arises from Schwann cells of vestibular branch of nerve.

Causes: Benign tumor of unknown origin. Compresses on cochlear nerve; first affects outermost layer of high frequency fibers. Damages cochlear blood supply with continued growth causing cochlear loss.

Complaints: Difficulty understanding speech, especially on the phone. Unilateral high frequency tinnitus. May have slight balance problem.

Physical Signs: None

Audio: Unilateral or asymmetrical high frequency sensorineural loss. Degree of loss and range of affected frequencies increase slowly as tumor grows.

Treatments: Surgical removal of tumor. With early detection and treatment, hearing may be preserved.

Figure 9–16. Profile of a typical case with acoustic neuroma.

neuroma. Referral to a physician is warranted, especially when an asymmetrical, high frequency, sensorineural hearing loss is present in an adult. Today, magnetic resonance imaging (MRI) and/or computerized tomography are quite sensitive in identifying acoustic neuromas, even when they are quite small.

Auditory Dyssynchrony (Neuropathy)

Auditory dyssynchrony or *auditory neuropathy* is a condition of the 8th nerve in which the neurons do not fire with the normal synchrony (at the same time) necessary to transmit the neural output from the cochlea to the brainstem (Berlin, Morlet, & Hood, 2003; Sinninger, 2002; Starr, Picton, Sinninger, Hood, & Berlin, 1996). Auditory dyssynchrony is not caused by any known disease. The cochlea is functioning fine, but the 8th nerve is somehow affected. Auditory dyssynchrony is often discovered in newborns or young infants who have had their hearing screened using auditory brainstem responses (ABR). The classic diagnostic picture of auditory dyssynchrony is that the ABR is absent or abnormal and the otoacoustic emissions are normal (as would be expected with normal outer hair cell function). The source of the auditory dyssynchrony could be at the level of the inner hair cell, its synapse, or in the nerve itself. Patients with auditory dyssynchrony have a wide range of hearing losses on the audiogram, from normal to profound. They also often have difficulty understanding speech and absent acoustic reflexes, beyond that predicted by the degree of hearing loss. The use of hearing aids as a treatment is not recommended; however, some success has been found with cochlear implants (Zeng & Sheng, 2006).

Central Auditory Disorders

Central auditory disorders are a general category that can include a variety of problems involving the central nervous system's auditory pathways and its related auditory processing, both at the brainstem and cortical levels. Disorders of the central auditory system can be localized to a discrete area of the brain, such as those that might be caused by tumors or vascular lesions/strokes, or more generalized, such as those that might be caused by developmental deficits, hereditary neuropathies, infections, presbycusis, chemicals, multiple sclerosis, or idiopathic causes. Depending on the source of the central disorder, there may be other more serious medical issues than hearing deficits. On the other hand, in some cases the disorder may only manifest as a subtle *auditory processing disorder* (APD), which may especially pose a problem with learning in school-age children. Disorders of the central auditory system do not typically affect hearing for pure tones or even basic speech measures because of the multiple neural pathways, including those that course through the brainstem along ipsilateral and contralateral routes (see Chapter 1). Even a stroke in the temporal lobe does not affect hearing per se but may affect receptive language abilities. Bilateral temporal lobe deficits are very rare but may result in deafness (Hood, Berlin, & Allen, 1994). Auditory deficits from central auditory disorders, if any, may show up on more complicated listening tasks, such as competing messages from the two ears, filtered speech, or time-compressed speech. Symptoms of central auditory disorders may include difficulty in noisy or reverberant environments, difficulty with complex directions, poor auditory memory, trouble localizing, distractibility, or inattentiveness. Tests for central auditory disorders are beyond the scope of this introductory text, and the interested reader is referred to other sources (Bellis, 2003; Musiek & Chermak, 2006; Stach, 2000).

Nonorganic (Functional) Hearing Loss

In audiologic practice, it is not uncommon to have patients who purposely feign or exaggerate their hearing loss, a situation which is labeled *nonorganic hearing loss, functional hearing loss, pseudohypacusis,* or *malingering.* In other words, these patients are "faking" their hearing loss. Most of these patients are fully aware of their actions; however, some may have underlying psychological problems for which the audiologist needs to make an appropriate referral to a psychiatrist or psychologist. The primary reason an adult patient might exaggerate a hearing difficulty is for financial gain, including employee or military compensation cases or accident liability. It is not unheard of for some military recruits to want to have a hearing test just for the distraction or to get out of an assignment. Children may try to feign a hearing loss for attention that they gain in their family or school environment. They may also believe that they can use a hearing loss as an excuse for poor school performance, or to get out of an assignment. Luckily, there are a variety of ways in which an audiologist can identify those with functional hearing losses, and they can usually end up getting the patient to provide fairly accurate test results. Testing these patients can often be challenging and interesting (or even entertaining). However, the audiologist should be careful about how the results are presented so that the patient is not actually labeled with any of the above terms. The audiologist's role is to end up with test results that are a reflection of the organic basis of the hearing loss and not be concerned about any underlying reason for the exaggeration (Martin, 2002).

Although it is beyond the scope of this text to present all of the test strategies used by audiologists when suspecting a functional hearing loss, a few of them will be mentioned. First of all, otoacoustic emissions can often indicate if the patient has normal peripheral hearing, and if this is not in agreement with the initial behavioral thresholds obtained during pure-tone testing, the audiologist should suspect a functional hearing loss and proceed accordingly. In these situations, pure-tone threshold searches should start at the lowest level of the audiometer, and the audiologists should spend some time presenting tones less than 20 dB HL, and, yes, even deviate from the down 10, up 5 rule. For example, if patients do not respond at 20 dB HL, you might even decrease the level of the signal for a few trials, and then come up to 15 dB HL (they might then respond). The intent is

to confuse them and wait them out; they may get nervous or they may even think you are testing at a higher level. Another strategy is to give them some instructions or make some comment through the earphones at a lower level and see what they do or if they respond. Of course, reinstructing patients as if they were not cooperating may also work well. You may also let them know that you are not getting consistent results and that you may need to do an auditory brainstem response test (where they do not have to do anything); often this will improve their cooperation.

There is also a very effective and easy test, the *Stenger test*, which can be used for patients who are feigning a hearing loss in only one ear. The Stenger test takes advantage of the Stenger phenomenon, where a tone (or word) presented simultaneously to both ears will only be heard in the ear where it is louder. In a clinical situation with a unilateral hearing loss, the level of the tone (or word) in the normal hearing hear is set at 10 dB above the reported threshold, and the level of the tone (or word) in the poorer hearing ear is set at a level 10 dB below their "threshold." The tones are then presented simultaneously to the two ears and the patient is asked to respond if he hears a tone (he is not told that he will be given a tone in each ear). The patient should respond because the tone is above threshold in the good ear; however, if he does not respond, that means that he only heard the tone in the poorer ear because it was louder than the tone in the good ear (he is not aware of the sound in the good ear). When the patient does not respond it is considered a positive Stenger and suggests that the patient's behavioral thresholds were being exaggerated. The Stenger should be used to verify any unilateral hearing loss. Of course, the ABR can be used as a more definitive test for objectively documenting thresholds in patients suspected of functional hearing loss, especially involving compensation cases.

Often, the audiologist, suspecting that a child may not be cooperating, will obtain some initial audiometric test results that indicate a hearing loss; however, after further testing, the child ends up with normal thresholds. In this case, it is usually sufficient to report to the parent that the child has normal hearing and leave it at that. When the audiologist is not confident that the hearing test results are an accurate reflection of a child's hearing abilities, this should be cautiously implied in the clinical report or in the discussion with the patient or family (e.g., "unable to get consistent responses"; "thresholds may be better than those obtained today"). Again, it is not useful to challenge the patient's behavior or motivation or label him as a functional hearing loss. In some cases, it may be suggested that further testing is needed, including the possibility of an auditory brainstem response test.

Tinnitus

. . . my ears whistle and buzz continuously day and night. I can say I am living a wretched life.
(Ludwig von Beethoven, 1801)

Tinnitus refers to auditory perceptions that are generated internally (within the head), without any externally applied stimulus. The word tinnitus (pronounced either "TIN-uh-tus" or "tin-EYE-tus," is derived from the Latin word *tinnire*, which means "tinkling" or "ringing." Tinnitus is not a disease but a symptom or consequence of many different types of disorders. It is estimated that about 17% of the world's population (50 million Americans) has tinnitus, with increasing percentages with age: In the United States, about 2 million of the 12 million people seeking medical attention for tinnitus are so affected by their tinnitus that they are unable to function on a daily basis (American Tinnitus Association, 2007).

Tinnitus is typically divided into two general types, subjective (nonvibratory) and objective (vibratory). *Subjective tinnitus* is typically described by the patient as "ringing, hissing, or roaring" and is the type of tinnitus commonly encountered by audiologists due to its association with many types of hearing loss. *Objective tinnitus* is most often described by the patient as "whooshing" or "pulsing" sounds, and is the type of tinnitus usually associated with a nonauditory condition, such as a vascular problem in the head or neck that is trans-mitted internally as an auditory stimulus. An audiologist should be knowledgeable about both types of tinnitus so she or he can properly counsel patients and make appropriate medical referrals.

Subjective Tinnitus

Subjective tinnitus is much more common than objective tinnitus. Most patients with hearing loss, when asked, say that they have some type of ringing in their ears. In many cases, the patient seeks medical or audiologic services because of the tinnitus. Subjective tinnitus is most commonly reported as a high pitched ringing or whistling in the head. Although the perceived level of the stimulus may be relatively loud, audiometrically it is usually matched to the loudness of a tone (in an area of good hearing) to about less than 25 dB (Goodwin & Johnson, 1980) and is usually comparable to the frequency range where there is the greatest amount of hearing loss. Subjective tinnitus can be constant or intermittent, unilateral or bilateral, tonal or noiselike, temporary or permanent.

Table 9-3 lists some disorders that are associated with subjective tinnitus. The most common cause of subjective tinnitus is noise exposure; up to 90% of tinnitus patients have some noise-induced hearing loss. High pitched tinnitus is most often associated with high frequency hearing loss; however, it can also occur without any measurable hearing loss. Unilateral high pitched tinnitus is often the first symptom of acoustic neuroma. In

Table 9–3. Disorders Associated with Subjective Tinnitus

Noise exposure	Otosclerosis
Presbycusis	Head injury
Ménière disease	Meningitis
Acoustic neuroma	Thyroid disorder
Ototoxic medications	Psychological
Sudden hearing loss	Depression
Central disorders	Anxiety

Ménière disease, tinnitus is a primary symptom; however, it is usually low pitched and characteristically described as an "ocean roar" or "buzzing" sound. In some cases, the cause of the tinnitus is idiopathic. In any case, underlying history and/or medical examination should be included in the evaluation of tinnitus patients to help determine the type and cause of their tinnitus. One must also be aware that some patients may feign tinnitus, especially in cases involving compensation. Documentation of these functional cases is difficult to disprove.

The physiological mechanisms of subjective tinnitus are not well understood; most likely there are a variety of sensory, neural, autonomic, and psychological mechanisms associated with tinnitus, and one or more of these may play a role in different disorders. A confounding factor is the inherent differences that individuals have in their ability to cope with their tinnitus or even cope with stresses in their lives that may be exacerbating the tinnitus. Patients with depression or anxiety may have tinnitus; however, it may not be clear which came first. The source of the tinnitus can be in the peripheral auditory system, brainstem, or cortical areas. Regardless of the tinnitus's origin, its conscious perception has a cortical component, perhaps located in the prefrontal–temporal area associated with attention, emotion, and memory (Pederen, Johannsen, Ovesen, Stodkilde-Jorgensen, & Gjedde, 1999).

Fortunately, most patients learn to cope with their tinnitus when they are given information about how tinnitus is related to their hearing loss and how tinnitus is quite common and not a sign of some medical emergency. For those patients with more severe tinnitus or psychological reactions to their tinnitus, treatment options are available; however, these may have different levels of success and may vary depending on the individual. For more severe cases of tinnitus, a medical, psychological, and audiologic management approach is warranted.

A popular and comprehensive approach to tinnitus and its management comes from the work of Pawel Jastreboff and colleagues (Jastreboff & Hazell, 1993), commonly referred to as the *neu-rophysiological basis of tinnitus*. The Jastreboff model proposes that, in the more severe cases of tinnitus, the limbic (emotional) and autonomic (unconscious control and alerting system) play important roles, especially in the annoyance factor associated with tinnitus. The Jastreboff neurophysiological model has a tinnitus treatment program, known as *Tinnitus Retraining Therapy* (TRT), that has become clinically popular. The TRT is a comprehensive approach to tinnitus assessment and management based on Jastreboff's neurophysiological model, and includes a structured counseling component and a prescribed masking therapy (Henry, Jastreboff, Jastreboff, Schechter, & Fausti, 2002; Jastreboff, Gray, & Gold, 1996). In the TRT masking therapy, the patient learns to habituate to the tinnitus over several weeks whereby the patient listens to a noise that is set at a level that almost masks out the tinnitus. The idea is to allow the tinnitus to be audible, but to reduce the annoyance and/or focus on the tinnitus by presenting an external noise. Over time, the level of the noise is reduced, which results in an additional reduction in the patient's perception of the tinnitus. In successful cases, the patient "learns" not to perceive the tinnitus even during periods of time when the noise is removed. To use TRT as a treatment option, the therapy provider must attend TRT training workshops.

Another tinnitus treatment that uses sound therapy is called *Neuromonics*. This is a patented sound therapy technique discovered and developed at Western Australia's Curtin University of Technology by Dr. Paul Davis (http://www.neuromonics.com). The Neuromonics approach uses a specially designed Neuromonics Processor (about the same size and weight of a cell phone) for the sound therapy part of its comprehensive tinnitus treatment, which presents customized sounds to the patient through earphones. The stimulus is based on the patient's audiometric profile up to 12.5 kHz and can be different for each ear. The Neuromonics approach is to embed the customized stimulus into a music-like stimulus rather than listening to a noise-like stimulus as in TRT or other tinnitus masking methods, thereby presenting a more pleasant stimulus to the patient. This type of sound activates the auditory pathways, as well as the limbic and autonomic systems, and with time reduces the perception and/or annoyance associated with the tinnitus through desensitization (Davis, 2005). With the Neuromonics approach, the musical, time-varying sound stimulus is set to be above the patient's audiometric thresholds in the areas where he or she has a hearing loss, in order to provide auditory stimulation. During the treatment stage, the stimulus is adjusted so that there are times when the tinnitus is heard within the Neuromonic's musical stimulus. The goal of the Neuromonics treatment, similar to TRT, is to have the patient habituate or become desensitized to the presence of the tinnitus. According to the manufacturer, after about 6 months of wearing the device (2 hr per day), successful patients are no longer bothered by their tinnitus and can stop wearing the device for a period of time.

A variety of other treatment options are also available and have been used as traditional methods of treating tinnitus, including the use of: (a) background noise/music as a distraction, (b) tinnitus masking instruments that are housed in a casing similar to that of hearing aids, (c) hearing aids (with their inherent noise), (d) biofeedback or other stress management techniques, and (e) counseling. A detailed comparison of the underlying theories and sound therapy treatment methods of TRT compared with traditional tinnitus masking techniques is detailed by Henry, Schechter, Nagler, and Fausti (2002). In addition, a variety of drugs and herbs have been investigated for the treatment of subjective tinnitus, but with little success. The most common medications currently used include corticosteroids or anticoagulants (Mora et al., 2003); however, their success still needs more validation.

A detailed audiometric description of the tinnitus is also helpful. In addition to a careful questionnaire, the audiologist: (a) determines the extent and type of hearing loss, (b) documents if there is a retrocochlear disorder, and (c) provides a detailed description of the tinnitus that can be of help in diagnosing the problem but also in providing information that may be useful for the sound therapy approaches to tinnitus management. The audiometric description usually includes *tinnitus matching*, which includes documenting the general frequency range of the tinnitus to a pure-tone frequency or narrowband noise, as well as documenting the perceived loudness of the tinnitus by matching the tinnitus to different stimulus levels (at the perceived frequency). An additional measure, *tinnitus maskability*, documents how much of a narrowband or white noise is needed to mask out the tinnitus (Mitchell, Vernon, & Creedon, 1993).

Objective Tinnitus

Objective tinnitus is much rarer than subjective tinnitus, especially in an audiological setting. Objective tinnitus is usually identified by a physician through a patient's medical visits, either because the patient is being treated for other related disorders or because the unusual sound in his head has caused some concern. However, audiologists should be familiar enough with objective tinnitus to be able to ask about it in the initial audiologic interview and to make the appropriate medical referral when encountered.

Objective tinnitus is caused by some vibration of tissues or structures within the head and neck

Table 9–4. Disorders Associated with Objective Tinnitus

Glomus tumors
Arterial bruits
Misplaced or thin jugular bulb
Arterial/venous malformations
Benign intracranial hypertension
Anemia
Palatomyoclonus
Stapedial muscle spasm
Patulous eustachian tube
Temporal–mandibular joint
Paget disease
Pregnancy

region that are audible to the patient, and in most cases, audible to the examiner through a stethoscope (some cases have been reported where these sounds are loud enough to be heard in the room without a stethoscope). Objective tinnitus is usually caused by vascular abnormalities around the temporal bone, usually heard as a pulsing or whooshing sound, and is commonly referred to as *pulsatile tinnitus*. The most common sources of pulsatile tinnitus are the carotid artery and the jugular bulb. Glomus tumors of the middle ear are usually accompanied by objective tinnitus. These vascular abnormalities can be caused by head injury, surgery, hypertension, or abnormal position of the jugular bulb (Crummer & Hassan, 2004).

Objective tinnitus can also originate from spasms in the middle ear muscles or palatal muscles brought on by neurological dysfunction (Fortune, Haynes, & Hall, 1999) and is typically described as a clicking or crackling sound. A patulous eustachian tube may also create objective tinnitus due to the patient hearing wind noise or breathing through the open tube. Table 9–4 provides a more complete list of causes of objective tinnitus. In some muscular spasm or eustachian tube related tinnitus, the breathing pattern can show up on the tympanogram. The audiologist usually becomes aware of objective tinnitus through the patient's history or complaints. Anytime objective tinnitus is apparent, the audiologist should make a medical referral. Treatment for objective tinnitus is dependent on the origin and is handled by the physician. Sound therapy methods (TRT, Neuromonics, and tinnitus maskers), which are useful treatments for subjective tinnitus, are not useful for treating objective tinnitus.

Synopsis 9–3

- Aural pathologies that affect the cochlea or the 8th nerve result in sensorineural hearing losses. Central pathologies do not produce any pure-tone hearing loss but are characterized by difficulty with other auditory processing tasks.

- Noise-induced hearing loss (NIHL) is a leading cause of acquired sensorineural hearing loss. Safe exposure limits allow for a maximum exposure of 85 dBA for 8 hr, and for each 3 dB increase in noise level, the maximum exposure time is cut in half. Temporary threshold shifts (TTS) and tinnitus can also occur from noise exposure, including loud music. NIHL occurs bilaterally.

- Presbycusis is a loss of hearing due to aging and is a leading cause of acquired adult hearing loss. Presbycusis can affect the hair cells, stria vascularis, or neural pathways. Susceptibility to aging hearing loss may also be related to noise exposure, diet, or genetics. Presbycusis occurs bilaterally.

- Ménière disease is related to an excessive buildup of endolymph (endolymphatic hydrops). It is characterized by a low pitched (ocean roar) tinnitus, vertigo, aural fullness, and fluctuating low frequency hearing loss in the early stages, followed by a permanent, moderate flat sensorineural loss. Ménière disease is usually unilateral but may occur later in the other ear.

- Ototoxic medications are divided into five general types: (a) aminoglycoside antibiotics, (b) anticancer drugs, (c) loop diuretics,

(d) aspirin in high doses, and (e) antimalarial drugs. The first two types result in permanent hearing loss; the hearing loss with the other types resolves when treatment ends. Ototoxic drugs affect the ultra-high frequencies first and are a primary population where high frequency audiometry is used. Ototoxicity occurs bilaterally.

- When a hearing loss comes on suddenly, medical treatment should be sought immediately in order to have the best chance of stabilizing or reversing the hearing loss with corticosteroid treatment by a physician. Sudden hearing loss may be caused by an autoimmune disorder, perilymph fistula, viral attack, or idiopathic causes. Sudden sensorineural hearing loss is usually unilateral but may occur later in the other ear.

- Bacterial infections (e.g., meningitis) or viral infections (e.g., mumps, measles, cytomegalovirus) often result in severe bilateral sensorineural hearing loss, especially in children.

- Temporal bone fractures from head injury can also result in hearing loss. A longitudinal fracture usually produces a conductive loss. A transverse fracture damages the cochlea and can cause a sensorineural hearing loss.

- The two most common 8th nerve disorders that produce hearing loss are acoustic neuroma and auditory dyssynchrony. The use of acoustic reflexes, OAE, and ABR are important for identifying these disorders. For example, auditory dyssynchrony is characterized by normal OAEs and abnormal ABRs. Acoustic neuroma occurs unilaterally; auditory dyssynchrony usually occurs bilaterally.

- Nonorganic (functional) hearing losses are those where the thresholds or hearing problems are exaggerated. Worker's compensation, military, or children seeking attention may present with functional hearing loss. With careful attention to hearing test techniques, the patient eventually volunteers accurate results.

- Tinnitus is a symptom commonly associated with a variety of hearing disorders, and not a disease per se.

- Subjective tinnitus (nonvibratory) is a perceived sound by the patient without any known source. It is often characterized as high pitched ringing in most disorders, or an ocean roar common with Ménière disease. Subjective tinnitus can be treated and/or alleviated with information or counseling, listening to background sounds, hearing aids, tinnitus maskers, or sound therapies, such as found with Tinnitus Retraining Therapy or Neuromonics tinnitus instruments.

- Objective tinnitus (vibratory) is caused by some abnormal structure or restricted blood flow that causes a vibrational stimulus that is heard by the ear. Treatment is usually medical and/or surgical depending on the source of the objective tinnitus.

References

American Tinnitus Association. (2007). *About tinnitus; frequently asked questions; how many people have tinnitus?* Retrieved January 10, 2008 from http://www.ata.org/abouttinnitus/patient_faq.php/.

Bellis, T. J. (2003). *Assessment and management of central auditory processing disorders in the educational setting: From science to practice* (2nd ed.). Clifton Park, NY: Thomson Delmar Learning.

Bergemalm, P.-O., & Borg, E. (2001). Long-term objective and subjective audiological consequences of closed head injury. *Acta Otolaryngologica, 121,* 724-734.

Berlin, C. I., Morlet, T., & Hood, L. J. (2003). Auditory neuropathy/dyssynchrony: Its diagnosis and management. *Pediatric Clinics of North America, 50,* 331-340.

Brummett, R. E., Bendrick, T., & Himes, D. (1981). Comparative ototoxicity of bumetanide and furosemide when used in conjunction with kanamycin. *Journal of Clinical Pharmacology, 21,* 629-636.

Crummer, R. W., & Hassan, G. A. (2004). Diagnostic approach to tinnitus. *American Family Physician, 69,* 120-126.

Davis, P. B. (2005). Music and the acoustic desensitisation protocol. In R. Tyler (Ed.), *Tinnitus treatments* (pp. 146-160). New York, NY: Thieme.

Fortune, D. S., Haynes, D. S., & Hall, J. W. I. (1999). Tinnitus. *Medical Clinics of North America, 83,* 153-162.

Gallagher, K. L., & Jones, J. K. (1979). Furosemide-induced ototoxicity. *Annals of Internal Medicine, 91,* 744-745.

Goodwin, P. E., & Johnson, R. M. (1980). The loudness of tinnitus. *Acta Otolaryngologica, 90,* 353-359.

Henry, J. A., Jastreboff, M. M., Jastreboff, P. J., Schechter, M. A., & Fausti, S. A. (2002). Assessment of patients for treatment with Tinnitus Retraining Therapy. *Journal of the American Academy of Audiology, 13,* 523-544.

Henry, J. A., Schechter, M. A., Nagler, S. M., & Fausti, S. A. (2002). Comparison of tinnitus masking and Tinnitus Retraining Therapy. *Journal of the American Academy of Audiology, 13,* 559-581.

Hood, L. J., Berlin, C. I., & Allen, P. (1994). Cortical deafness: A longitudinal study. *Journal of the American Academy of Audiology, 5,* 330-342.

House, J. W. (1997). Otosclerosis. In G. B. Hughes & M. L. Pensak (Eds.), *Clinical otology.* New York, NY: Thieme.

Humes, L. (1996). Speech understanding in the elderly. *Journal of the American Academy of Audiology, 7,* 161-167.

Jastreboff, P. J., Gray, W. C., & Gold, S. L. (1996). Neurophysiological approach to tinnitus patients. *American Journal of Otology, 17,* 236-240.

Jastreboff, P. J., & Hazell, J. W. P. (1993). A neurophysiological approach to tinnitus: Clinical implications. *British Journal of Audiology, 27,* 7-17.

Joint Committee on Infant Hearing. (2000). Year 2000 position statement: Principles and guidelines for early hearing detection and intervention program. *Audiology Today, 12,* 7-27.

Jordan, J. A., & Roland, P. S. (2000). Disorders of the auditory system. In R. J. Roeser, M. Valente, & H. Hosford-Dunn (Eds.), *Audiology diagnosis* (pp. 85-108). New York, NY: Thieme.

Kinney, W. C., Kinney, S. E., & Vidimos, A. T. (1997). Disorders of the auricle. In G. B. Hughes & M. L. Pensak (Eds.), *Clinical otology* (pp. 177-190). New York, NY: Thieme.

Lustig, L. R., & Jackler, R. K. (1997). Benign tumors of the temporal bone. In G. B. Hughes & M. L. Pensak (Eds.), *Clinical otology* (pp. 313-343). New York, NY: Thieme.

Martin, F. N. (2002). Pseudohypacusis. In J. Katz (Ed.), *Handbook of clinical audiology* (5th ed., pp. 584-596). Baltimore, MD: Lippincott Williams & Wilkins.

Martini, A., & Prosser, S. (2003). Disorders of the inner ear in adults. In L. Luxon (Ed.), *Textbook of audiological medicine* (pp. 452-475). London, UK: Martin Dunitz.

Mitchell, C. R., Vernon, J. A., & Creedon, T. A. (1993). Measuring tinnitus parameters: Loudness, pitch, and maskability. *Journal of the American Academy of Audiology, 4,* 139-151.

Monsell, E. M., Teixido, M. T., Wilson, M. D., & Hughes, G. B. (1997). Nonhereditary hearing loss. In G. B. Hughes & M. L. Pensak (Eds.), *Clinical otology* (pp. 289-312). New York, NY: Thieme.

Mora, R. M., Salami, A., Barbieri, M., Mora, F., Passali, G., Capobianco, S., Magnan, J. (2003). The use of sodium enoxaparin in the treatment of tinnitus. *International Tinnitus Journal, 9,* 109-111.

Musiek, F. E., & Chermak, G. D. (2006). *Handbook of (central) auditory processing disorders* (Vol. 1). *Auditory neuroscience.* San Diego, CA: Plural Publishing.

Myerhoff, W. L., Marple, B. F., & Roland, P. S. (1997). Tympanic membrane, middle ear, and mastoid. In P. S. Roland, B. F. Marple, & W. L. Myerhoff (Eds.), *Hearing loss* (pp. 155-194). New York, NY: Thieme.

Nance, W. E., & Dodson, K. (2007). 2007 Marion Downs lecture, Part 1: How can newborn hearing screening be improved? *Audiology Today, 19,* 14–19.

National Institute for Occupational Safety and Health (NIOSH). (1998). *Criteria for a recommended standard: Occupational noise exposure—Revised criteria.* NIOSH Pub. No. 98-126. Cincinnati, OH: NIOSH.

Occupational Safety & Health Administration (OSHA). (1983). Occupational noise exposure (29 CFR 1910.95, May 29, 1971, vol. 36). Amended (March 8, 1983, Vol. 48, pp. 9776–9785). Washington, DC: Federal Register.

Pederen, M. F., Johannsen, P., Ovesen, T., Stodkilde-Jorgensen, H., & Gjedde, A. (1999). Positron emission tomography of cortical centers of tinnitus. *Hearing Research, 134,* 133–144.

Roland, P. S., & Marple, B. F. (1997). Disorders of inner ear, eighth nerve, and CNS. In P. S. Roland, B. F. Marple, & W. L. Myerhoff (Eds.), *Hearing loss* (pp. 195–256). New York, NY: Thieme.

Roland, P. S., & Rohn, G. N. (1997). History and physical examination. In P. S. Roland, B. F. Marple, & W. L. Myerhoff (Eds.), *Hearing loss* (pp. 107–131). New York, NY: Thieme.

Roush, J. E. (1985). Aging and hearing impairment. *Seminars in Hearing, 6,* 99–219.

Shambaugh, G. E. J. (1983). Adult fluoride therapy for otosclerosis (otospongiosis). *Archives of Otolaryngology, 109,* 353.

Shprintzen, R. J. (2001). *Syndrome identification for audiology.* San Diego, CA: Singular Thomson Learning.

Sinninger, Y. S. (2002). Auditory neuropathy in infants and children: Implications for early hearing detection and intervention programs. *Audiology Today, Special Edition, Update on Infant Hearing;* 16–21.

Stach, B. A. (2000). Diagnosing central auditory processing disorders in adults. In R. J. Roeser, M. Valente, & H. Hosford-Dunn (Eds.), *Audiology diagnosis* (pp. 355–379). New York, NY: Thieme.

Starr, A., Picton, T. W., Sinninger, Y. S., Hood, L. J., & Berlin, C. I. (1996). Auditory neuropathy. *Brain, 119,* 741–753.

Toriello, H., Reardon, W., & Gorlin, R. (Eds.). (2004). *Hereditary hearing loss and its syndromes* (2nd ed.). New York, NY: Oxford University Press.

Woods, C. I., Strasnick, B., & Jackson, C. G. (1993). Surgery for glomus tumors: The Otology Group experience. *Laryngoscope, 103*(Suppl.), 65–72.

Zeng, F. G., & Sheng, L. (2006). Speech perception in individuals with auditory neuropathy. *Journal of Speech, Language, and Hearing Research, 49,* 367–380.

10

Screening for Hearing Loss

After reading this chapter, you should be able to:

1. List the principles and criteria established by the World Health Organization important for establishing early identification programs.
2. Understand the need for reliable and valid methods for screening.
3. Estimate/calculate the cost of doing hearing screening in the schools.
4. Discuss the history and use of a high risk register for hearing screening, and list some of the current high risk factors.
5. Describe the various methods used in screening newborns, school-aged children, and adults.
6. Discuss the pros and cons of OAE and AABR techniques for screening infants.
7. List the recommended fail and referral criteria for hearing screening of school-aged children.
8. List two hearing handicap inventories popular for hearing screening in adults
9. Understand screening outcome matrices and how a specified screening criterion can affect the sensitivity and specificity.
10. Appreciate how the prevalence of a disorder can influence a test's predictive values.

Hearing screening is a process of "testing" subpopulations of people with an efficient and cost-effective method in order to identify people with potential hearing disorders. Hearing screening programs are sometimes referred to as *identification programs* for hearing loss. Screening programs essentially involve a *pass* or *fail* measure to separate those who most likely do not have the disorder (the passes) from those who may possibly have the disorder (the fails). Those people who fail a screening are referred for a more complete evaluation to determine if they actually have the disorder. In general, hearing screening is conducted on groups of people who might not otherwise know they have a hearing problem or who are unable or reluctant to seek professional services. Deciding to do a screening for a targeted disorder must weigh a variety of factors before proactively taking it to the field to identify those who are not generally seeking any professional services. This is a different concept than developing diagnostic tests for those who come seeking professional services because of a perceived problem or symptom. For example, with regard to hearing disorders, newborns and young children will be unaware that they have anything wrong or may not be able to convey a complaint. Likewise, many elderly adults may discount or ignore hearing problems, or not realize that they are socially withdrawing due to unrecognizable changes in their hearing abilities. This chapter discusses some general components and issues common to any screening program, as well as some specific details and criteria used with different types of hearing screenings currently in use, including those for newborns, school-aged children, and adults.

Historical and Current Practice Guidelines

The modern day principles of screening have their foundations established by the World Health Organization (WHO) to address its commitment to early identification of several chronic diseases. Table 10–1 is a summary of the important WHO original criteria for developing a screening test and enhancements of those criteria that occurred over the following 40 years (Andermann, Blancquaert, Beauchamp, & Dery, 2008).

One of the main considerations of a screening program is that it should target a disorder that is recognized as an important health issue. Hearing disorders have recognizable consequences on a person's ability to learn speech and language, as well as on many other important auditory, listening functions per se, and the absence or decline of hearing may lead to other associated social, academic, and/or behavioral problems. Implicit in the idea of screening is that it should be applied at an early stage while the consequences are minimal or can benefit from early treatment.

A screening test should be reasonably safe, acceptable to society, and cost-effective. The positive benefits to the individuals and to society should outweigh any harm associated with the screening. It is also very important that there be adequate and appropriate follow-up diagnostic tests, available facilities, and personnel or resources to diagnose and treat those who fail a screening test. One can have the best screening test, but if there is a lack of adequate follow-up care, or if those who fail the screening are not motivated or monitored regarding their follow-up, the screening test may not be appropriate or sustainable. Finally, any successful screening program will have scientific evidence of its effectiveness and benefits.

Effective screening tests should have good *reliability*, such that similar results should occur when applied several times to an individual and that different testers obtain similar results from the same individual. A screening test must also be designed to have good *validity*, so you can be confident that the measure used is one that can provide the information sought. For example, if you want to identify central auditory processing disorders or middle ear disorders, you would not use a pure-tone screening measure; other more appropriate measures should be used.

Screening is generally applied to populations that do not show or act upon symptoms of some disorder, that there is a significant probability of finding those with the disorder, and/or that the

Table 10–1. World Health Organization Screening Criteria and Subsequent Enhancements

A. Classical screening criteria (Wilson & Jungner, 1968)

- The condition sought should be an important health problem.
- There should be an accepted treatment for patients with recognized disease.
- Facilities for diagnosis and treatment should be available.
- There should be a recognizable latent or early symptomatic stage.
- There should be a suitable test or examination.
- The test should be acceptable to the population.
- The natural history of the condition, including development from latent to declared disease, should be adequately understood.
- There should be an agreed policy on whom to treat as patients.
- The cost of case finding (including diagnosis and treatment of patients diagnosed) should be economically balanced in relation to possible expenditure on medical care as a whole.
- Case finding should be a continuing process and not a "once and for all" project.

B. Synthesis of emerging screening criteria proposed over the past 40 years (Andermann et al., 2008)

- The screening program should respond to a recognized need. The objectives of screening should be defined at the outset.
- There should be a defined target population.
- There should be scientific evidence of screening program effectiveness.
- The program should integrate education, testing, clinical services, and program management.
- There should be quality assurance, with mechanisms to minimize potential risks of screening.
- The program should ensure informed choice, confidentiality, and respect for autonomy.
- The program should promote equity and access to screening for the entire target population.
- Program evaluation should be planned from the outset.
- The overall benefits of screening should outweigh the harm.

disorder is considered to be important enough to identify in the larger population. A *universal screening test* is one that is applied to a relatively large population, such as all newborns. A universal screening must consider the disorder of high significance and have personnel and equipment costs that make it feasible and cost-effective. It may, however, be more cost-effective to do a *targeted (or selective) screening test*, in which case only a subgroup of the larger population is targeted for screening. A targeted screening will have a higher prevalence rate of the disorder of interests, as compared with universal screening of the larger population, and may be more cost-effective. Obviously, the cost of a screening program should not be prohibitive in light of the significance of the disorder that is to be identified. A generally accepted formula

to estimate the *cost per child* of hearing screening in the schools, as suggested by Cooper, Gates, Owen, and Dickson (1975), is:

$$cost\ per\ child = (S/R) + (C + [M \times L]/[N \times L]),$$

where S = hourly salary of screening personnel, R = rate of persons screened per hour, C = initial cost of equipment, M = annual cost of equipment maintenance, N = number persons screened per year, and L = labor costs/child screened.

We will now briefly discuss some details of hearing screening programs that are in current use, including screening for hearing loss in newborns, school-aged children, and adults. Following those sections, some issues regarding screening limitations, outcomes, and efficacy are presented.

Synopsis 10–1

- Hearing screenings are conducted on groups of people who might not know they have a hearing problem or who are unable or reluctant to seek professional services, and that there is a significant probability of finding those with the disorder, and/or that the disorder is considered to be important enough to identify in the larger population.

- Effective hearing screening programs (a.k.a. identification programs) should target subpopulations using efficient and cost-effective methods to identify people with potential hearing problems and have options for follow up measures. Criteria for effective screening programs evolved from work of the World Health Organization (WHO) over 40 years ago.

- Screening programs essentially involve a *pass* or *fail* measure to separate those who most likely do not have the disorder (the passes) from those who may possibly have the disorder (the fails).

- An effective screening test should have good reliability (similar results obtained each time) and validity (identifies what is intended).

- A *universal screening test* is one that is applied to a relatively large population. A more cost-effective approach to screening is to do a *targeted* (or *selective*) *screening*. A targeted screening will have a higher prevalence rate of the disorder as compared with universal screening of the larger population.

- An estimate of the cost of a school-based screening program uses the formula: *cost per child = (S/R) + (C + [M × L]/[N × L])*, where *S* = hourly salary of screening personnel, *R* = rate of persons screened per hour, *C* = initial cost of equipment, *M* = annual cost of equipment maintenance, *N* = number persons screened per year, and *L* = labor costs/child screened.

Screening the Hearing of Newborns

Hearing screening of newborns, also referred to *early hearing detection and intervention (EHDI)*, has evolved over the past 40 years from not being very applicable (using behavioral hearing measures), to targeted screening of high risk infants (using high risk registers and/or auditory brainstem response measures), to today's approach in which screenings are attempted on all newborns (using otoacoustic emissions and/or auditory brainstem response measures). Future developments in genetics may also play an important role in hearing screening of newborns, especially when an affordable DNA screening becomes available. The primary goal of an EHDI program is to identify permanent and significant hearing loss that can affect and/or delay development of audition and speech-language abilities, which if left untreated would impact educational and psychosocial factors. Keep in mind that newborn hearing screening is only the beginning of a more comprehensive program which requires follow-up confirmations (identification) of hearing loss and appropriate intervention, including the goal of fitting hearing aids or cochlear implants before 6 months of age (JCIH, 2007), and there must be close follow-up care, rehabilitation, and counseling. This text will not review the early history of newborn hearing screening using behavioral methods; however, the interested reader may want to review some of the early work and research in this area (Downs & Sterritt, 1967; Ling, Ling, & Doehring, 1970; Northern & Downs, 1974; Thompson & Thompson, 1972; Durieux-Smith, Picton, Edwards, Goodman, & MacMurray, 1985). The limitations inherent in behavioral screening of newborns was an impetus for the development of more objective, physiological measures that would be more useful for detecting hearing loss in the newborn period. As discussed in earlier chapters, auditory brainstem response (ABR) and otoacoustic emissions (OAEs) have been accepted as objective measures of auditory function that can be effectively applied to screening of newborns. As objective tests were being developed in the late 1970s to 1990s, others were developing a list of neonatal conditions that were associated with hearing loss, called

the *high risk register*. For a more comprehensive review of newborn hearing screening, the interested reader is referred to Driscoll and McPherson (2010).

Screening High-Risk Infants

Targeted hearing screening of newborns and young infants has been advocated since the early 1970s through the use of a high-risk register (HRR) developed through a Joint Commission on Infant Hearing (JCIH).[1] The use of the HRR is a useful way to focus screening and follow-up testing on a subpopulation, especially before more cost-effective methods of screening all newborns became available. However, in some circumstances the use of a HRR is extremely useful. For example, there are some congenital disorders that have later onset or progressive hearing loss that could be missed if one relied solely on newborn hearing screening measures. Also, in developing countries without adequate resources for screening newborns, the HRR allows more focused attention on those who are more likely to have a hearing problem. The risk factors that are on the HRR are periodically updated by the JCIH as new information becomes available. Table 10–2 lists the most current risk factors for congenital deafness as developed by

Table 10–2. Risk Factors for Congenital Deafness

Family history of deafness
Congenital perinatal TORCH infection
Malformation of the pinna, ear canal, face, or palate
Down syndrome or other syndrome known to include hearing loss
Birth weight < 1500 g
Hyperbilirubinemia
Bacterial meningitis
Perinatal asphyxia (5 min Apgar score < 7)
Use of ototoxic drugs (aminoglycosides)
Mechanical ventilation (>4 days)

Source: U.S. Preventive Services Task Force (2008).

---

[1]The JCIH was first formed in 1969 and includes members from the academies of Pediatrics, Ophthalmology and Otolaryngology, and the American Speech, Language, and Hearing Association.

the JCIH (2007) and the U.S. Preventive Services Task Force (2008). Many of those infants with factors on the HRR will be admitted to the Newborn Intensive Care Unit (NICU). For those in the NICU, and others on the HRR, hearing screening is generally performed using the ABR.

Even the most aggressive use of the HRR may fall short in identifying infants with hearing loss as shown by a study in New Zealand (HEID, 2004) in which only 40% of children with significant permanent hearing loss would be identified by using the risk factor screening approach (Leigh, Schmulian-Taljaard, & Poulakis, 2010). These shortcomings of the HRR and the development of cost-effective objective measures for screening for auditory impairment have led to the implementation and acceptance of programs to screen all newborns, as described more fully in the next section.

Universal Screening

Hearing screening of all newborns is now possible and widely implemented in most developed countries. The acceptance of universal newborn hearing screening was made possible by the development of more cost-effective and valid screening measures of otoacoustic emissions and automated auditory brainstem responses. Universal newborn hearing screening programs are very large scale operations that involve the collaboration of many professionals, including physicians, nurses, audiologists, and trained screeners. Of course, the reason we want to screen all newborns is to be able to identify early those with hearing loss who do not have or who are not known to have any of the factors on the HRR, and to identify, diagnose, and treat those with significant hearing loss at the earliest possible age. Again, keep in mind that a comprehensive program includes an initial screening (at birth), a follow-up screening (at birth or within 1 month), diagnostic testing of those who fail the screen (by 3 months of age), and initiation of treatment (by 6 months of age) of those confirmed to have a hearing loss. There has been a significant improvement in the average age of confirmation/initiation of treatment from about 20 months to

less than 6 months since universal newborn hearing programs have been implemented (Leigh et al., 2010). Also, those who pass the newborn hearing screenings should have follow-up screening or a diagnostic hearing test between 24 and 30 months (JCIH, 2007), and parents and pediatricians should monitor their child's hearing behavior and speech-language development, and follow-up with any concerns. Table 10–3 provides a list of principles for EHDI programs developed by the JCIH (2007).

The initial screening of newborns occurs in the hospital before the baby is discharged. Because we are talking about screening all newborns, there is a need for adequate personnel and coordination of activities during the 1 to 2 days that babies are in the well-baby nurseries. Parents should know when they leave the hospital the results of their baby's hearing screening and any follow-up recommendations needed. The hospital staff must also have a well-developed system for recording the information and a plan to actively follow-up on those who fail the hearing screenings to be sure they are seen for a diagnostic hearing test. Screening programs should also regularly evaluate the success of their procedures and outcomes, and make adjustments accordingly.

The two types of technologies used for hearing screening of newborns and young infants are otoacoustic emissions (TEOAEs and DPOAEs) and automated ABR (AABR). The basics of these physiological tests are described in Chapter 8 and can be successfully used within the well-baby nursery environment while the baby lies in their bassinet, as long as the baby is lying quietly (which requires personnel to be at the screen to judge and adjust the testing based on the baby's state). Although these physiological technologies are used for universal newborn hearing screening, they provide only limited information about auditory function and are not measures of hearing in the complete sense. With this caveat in mind, the use of either or both of these technologies have been recommended for newborn screening by ASHA (1997), and they meet the requirements of an adequate hearing screening program as outlined by the JCIH (2007). Each hospital needs to decide which one (or both) of the technologies they will incorporate into their newborn hearing screening

Table 10–3. Principles of the Joint Committee Infant Hearing for Effective Early Hearing Detection and Intervention (EHDI) Program

1. All infants should have access to hearing screening using a physiological measure before 1 month of age.
2. All infants who do not pass the initial hearing screening and the subsequent rescreening should have appropriate audiologic and medical evaluations to confirm the presence of hearing loss before 3 months of age.
3. All infants with confirmed permanent hearing loss should receive intervention services before 6 months of age. A simplified, single point of entry into an intervention system appropriate to children with hearing loss is optimal.
4. The EHDI system should be family centered with infant and family rights and privacy guaranteed through informed choice, shared decision making, and parental consent. Families should have access to information about all intervention and treatment options and counseling regarding hearing loss.
5. The child and family should have immediate access to high-quality technology, including hearing aids, cochlear implants, and other assistive devices when appropriate.
6. All infants and children should be monitored for hearing loss in the medical home. Continued assessment of communication development should be provided by appropriate providers to all children with or without risk indicators for hearing loss.
7. Appropriate interdisciplinary intervention programs for deaf and hard-of-hearing infants and their families should be provided by professionals knowledgeable about childhood hearing loss. Intervention programs should recognize and build on strengths, informed choices, traditions, and cultural beliefs of the families.
8. Information systems should be designed to interface with electronic health records and should be used to measure outcomes and report the effectiveness of EHDI services at the community, state, and federal levels.

Source: Joint Committee Infant Hearing (2007).

program after careful consideration of their costs, training, logistics, and outcomes.

The AABR screening technology has been available since the early 1980s, and has been used by many hospitals for universal newborn hearing screening. The AABR uses quick attaching disposable electrodes, a single pre-set click stimulus level (30 to 40 dB nHL), and incorporates an internal software algorithm to determine if specific criteria are met to consider the response a "pass." This automated decision eliminates the need for someone trained to make decisions based on a recorded waveform since the instrument does it. The AABR has been found to be quick (about 10 min), reliable, and has acceptable outcomes, including referral (fail) rates and false positive rates of about 2% (Hall, 2007; Spivak, 2007).

The OAE technology received wider acceptance during the 1990s as screening OAE units were developed specifically for use with newborn screening programs. Without the need for electrodes, and the discovery that infants had large robust OAEs, the OAE screener became a popular alternative to the AABR. Either TEOAEs or DPOAEs are used for OAE screening, and to date there are no known advantages of one over the other in determining if hearing is better or worse than about 25 to 35 dB HL. TEOAEs are thought to be more sensitive to the 500 to 1000 Hz region than are DPOAEs, whereas DPOAEs are more sensitive in the higher frequencies than TEOAEs. Like the AABR, the OAE screeners have built-in algorithms to determine if a baby meets the criteria for a "pass." Initially, the false positive rates for OAE screening were quite high (10 to 20%), but with experience and the introduction of a two stage screening procedure, the false positive outcomes have been improved to less than 4% (Spivak &

Sokol, 2004; Vohr, Carty, Moore, & Letourneau, 1998). One of the biggest disadvantages of OAE screening is that the response will be absent when there is the presence of any outer or middle ear involvement, including any middle ear fluid or vernix residue in the ear canal, but which resolves after a day or two. In the near future, the use of wideband power reflectometry (see Chapter 8) may become part of newborn hearing screening programs to rule out conductive problems that may compromise the recordings of OAEs. Another limitation of OAE screening is that it will miss infants with *auditory neuropathy spectrum disorder*, also called *auditory dyssynchrony disorder*, characterized by normal OAEs and abnormal ABRs, and which may account for up to 10% of children with hearing loss (Sininger, 2002). According to Sininger and Oba (2001), 80% of those infants with auditory dyssynchrony disorder will spend time in the NICU and have ABR testing; however, there may be 20% of them who would be missed in the well-baby nurseries who are not tested using AABR. For more information about deciding on which system to use for newborn hearing screenings see Leigh et al. (2010).

Screening the Hearing of School-Age Children

Hearing screening of children has been around for over 50 years and was one of the earliest health screening initiatives in the United States. Screening guidelines have been published by the American Academy of Audiology (AAA, 1997) and the American Speech-Language-Hearing Association (ASHA, 1997). Hearing screening is recommended for all preschool children, school-age children kindergarten through the 3rd grade, in the 7th and 11th grades, and at any time there is a concern about a child's hearing, speech, or learning. School screening programs require close cooperation between the school administrators, teachers, parents, and personnel who are doing the screenings. The screening personnel should also be sure to visit the site and room to be used for the hearing screenings in order to be sure the background noise levels are acceptable,[2] the environment is relatively free of visual or other distractions, there are appropriate electrical outlets, and has suitable table and chairs. Calibrated portable, screening audiometers and tympanometers are available for use in school-based hearing screening programs. Hearing screening programs should be coordinated and/or supervised by an audiologist in order to insure quality. The air conduction pure-tone hearing screenings per se can be performed with trained nurses, speech-language pathologists, supervised graduate students, or in some states persons holding an audiometrist certificate. For tympanometry and otoscopy components of a screening program, an audiologist should be directly involved during the screenings.

The screening guidelines recommend that pure-tone air conduction screening of preschool and school-age children be done using age-appropriate behavioral techniques (see Chapter 4) at frequencies of 1000, 2000, and 4000 Hz. The screening level should be set at 20 dB HL. Typically, two to three presentations are given at each frequency. A child fails the screening if he or she does not give an appropriate response at 20 dB HL for any of the three frequencies, for either ear. If a child fails the initial screening, it is recommended that he or she be rescreened again during the same day. A child who fails the pure-tone rescreening should be referred for a complete audiologic evaluation. In addition to the pure-tone air conduction screening, screening for outer and middle ear disorders is recommended through the use of a brief history questionnaire sent by the parents, otoscopic inspection, and tympanometry. A child should be referred for a medical examination if the screening finds drainage in the ear canal, structural abnormality, foreign object, impacted cerumen, infection, or tympanic membrane abnormality, perforation (e.g., flat tympanogram

[2]Allowable octave band acceptable noise levels based on ANSI (1991) and for screening at 20 dB HL are 39.5, 46.5, 48.0, and 54.5 dB SPL for 500, 1000, 2000, and 4000 Hz, respectively. *Source*: Bess and Humes (2008).

with large ear canal volume not due to pressure equalization tube). The AAA (1997) criteria for tympanogram failures are $Y_{tm} < 0.2$ mmho, and/or TW > 250 daPa. For patients who show a flat tympanogram with normal ear canal volume or for those with an abnormally wide tympanogram, a rescreening should be done in 4 to 6 weeks. If the tympanogram abnormalities are found on the rescreening, the child should be referred for a medical examination. Neither AAA (1997) nor ASHA (1997) include abnormal peak pressure (TPP) as a reason for medical or audiologic referral due to its transitory nature or unacceptable over-referral rates for middle ear involvement. If tympanometry is not included in a screening program, the addition of pure-tone screening at 500 Hz should be included if the testing environment has acceptable background noise levels.

Screening the Hearing of Adults

Hearing screenings for adults has not received as much attention as screening of children. However, given that hearing disorders can be acquired during the adult years, and often progresses during the senior years, hearing screenings of adults may be the first place where an adult might feel comfortable finding out if they might have a hearing problem. Health fairs or senior centers are places where adult hearing screening might be conducted. As with children, the ASHA (1997) guidelines recommend screening of adults using a case history questionnaire, otoscopic examination, and pure-tone air conduction audiometry. In addition, there are questionnaires available that allow for adults to do a self-assessment of their communication and hearing abilities. The case history questionnaire should include questions about any perceived hearing loss (one or both ears), its time course (sudden onset or gradual), ear drainage, ear pain, tinnitus, and/ or dizziness. If any of these problems are identified, further medical and audiologic evaluations should be recommended. Pure-tone air conduction behavioral screening is recommended every 10 years up to 50 years of age, and every three years above 50 years of age. Pure-tone screening should

be performed at 25 dB HL (ASHA, 1997) at 1000, 2000, and 4000 Hz. Self-assessment communication scales of hearing disabilities have been developed and are available for screening adults. Some examples of valid, reliable, and normed hearing screening scales include the *Hearing Handicap Inventory for the Elderly-Screening* (Ventry & Weinstein, 1983) and the *Self-Assessment for Communication* (Schow & Nerbonne, 1982).

Screening Outcomes and Efficacy

Screenings separate those who have a high probability of the targeted disorder from those who have a low probability of the targeted disorder. The pass or fail outcomes of a screening imply that there is a way to validate the results through some other follow-up indicator of those who fail the screening who have the disorder and those who pass the screening who do not have the disorder, referred to as the *gold standard* diagnostic test. Results from a gold standard test are generally accepted as proof that the disorder or disease exists or not. For example, an acceptable diagnostic test to determine the amount of a sensorineural hearing loss for adults is pure-tone audiometry. However, for infants and young children, this gold standard may not be applicable within a similar time frame. In the case of infants, diagnostic auditory brainstem responses might be a better gold standard in the early months. Ultimately, when the infant reaches 6 to 7 months of age, one may be able to use pure-tone audiometry to confirm the test results. In the case of infant screening, the gold standard comparison is delayed and one can never be absolutely sure that the outcome would have been the same at the time of the screening and the hearing problem resolved itself (in the case of middle ear problems) or developed between the time of the screening and the time of the gold standard audiometric test. However, until other diagnostic measures become available, the most valid solution is to have the behavioral pure-tone tests done at the earliest possible time.

The usefulness of any test, including screening tests, depend on its *validity*, which is an

Test Outcome	Disorder Present	Disorder Absent	TOTALS
FAIL (positive for disorder	True positives (TP) HIT	False positives (FP)	TP+TP
PASS (negative for disorder)	False negatives (FN) MISS	True negatives (TN)	FN+TN
TOTALS	Total Present = TP + FN	Total Absent = TN + FP	TP+FP+ FN+TN

$$\text{SENSITIVITY} = \frac{TP}{TP + FN}$$

$$\text{SPECIFICITY} = \frac{TN}{TN + FP}$$

$$\text{Positive Predictive Value} = \frac{TP}{TP + FP}$$

$$\text{Negative Predictive Value} = \frac{TN}{FN + TN}$$

Figure 10–1. Screening test matrix showing test outcomes (Fail or Pass) and actual patient condition (Disorder Present or Disorder Absent). Calculation components are shown from which one can derive sensitivity and specificity, as well as positive predictive value and negative predictive value.

indication of how well a test measures what it is supposed to measure. Figure 10–1 presents a commonly used matrix for a screening test.

There are typically four outcomes to any test:

1. *True positive (a hit)*. The test correctly identifies the targeted disorder.
2. *True negative*. The test correctly identifies the absence of the targeted disorder.
3. *False positive*. The test incorrectly identifies the targeted disorder (says the disorder is present, but the disorder turns out to be absent).
4. *False negative (a miss)*. The test incorrectly identifies the targeted disorder (says the disorder is absent, but the disorder turns out to be present.

With these four outcomes in mind, tests can be evaluated in terms of their:

1. *Sensitivity*. How well the test correctly identifies the targeted disorder (proportion of true positives).
2. *Specificity*. How well the test correctly identifies those without the targeted disorder (proportion of true negatives).
3. *Positive predictive value*. The percentage of true positives for the test (i.e., the level of confidence one has in the true positive outcome).
4. *Negative predictive value*. The percentage of true negatives for the test (i.e., the level of confidence one has in the true negative outcome.

Figure 10–2 shows an example of the screening matrix using numbers to show the calculations of the above four characteristics of a screening test. A screening test's sensitivity is the proportion of the true positive (TP) outcomes to the total who

Test Outcome	Disorder Present	Disorder Absent	Totals
FAIL (positive for disorder	4	30	34
PASS (negative for disorder)	2	180	182
TOTALS	6	210	216

SENSITIVITY = $\dfrac{4}{6}$ = 66.6%

SPECIFICITY = $\dfrac{180}{210}$ = 85.7%

Positive Predictive Value = $\dfrac{4}{34}$ = 11.7%

Negative Predictive Value = $\dfrac{180}{182}$ = 98.9%

Figure 10–2. Example of screening test matrix with hypothetical values to show how the various test parameters are calculated. See Figure 10–1 for help in understanding how the numbers are derived.

actually have the disease (TP + FN), whereas the specificity is the proportion of the true negative (TN) outcomes to those who actually do not have the disease (TN + FP). Although sensitivity and specificity are measures of how well a specific test is able to separate those with and without the targeted disorder, in a clinical setting the positive and negative predictive values may be more meaningful when trying to decide if a screening procedure is worth the effort, or if one is interested in knowing the probability for those patients who fail the screening to actually have the disease. The positive predictive value is the proportion of the true positive (TP) outcomes to those who failed the test (TP + FP). Predictive values are dependent on the *prevalence* of the targeted disorder, as can be seen in Table 10-4. A test could have an intrinsically good sensitivity, but may have a low positive predictive value if the targeted disorder is extremely rare (there is a very low prevalence within the population being screened). If most of the tested population is expected to pass (and very few expected to fail), then an important consideration of a test's predictive value would be related to its specificity (i.e., one might want a high negative predictive value). In other words, if one is screening for a low prevalence disorder within a population, it may be important to have a test with a high specificity so that there are not too many unnecessary referrals. Of course, if the rare disorder has significant health consequences, one may want to develop a screening test that would maximize sensitivity so that most of those with the disorder are identified; however, this may also result in a low specificity and high over-referral rate. Strategic targeting of the screening population and/or sequential screening programs will increase the prevalence as the "filter" is applied and will have a corresponding effect on the predictive values.

Of course, ideally one would want a test with 100% sensitivity (always detected the disorder when present) and 100% specificity (always identified

Table 10–4. Example of How Prevalence Can Affect Positive Predictive Value (*PPV*)

Prevalence	Test Outcome	Has Disorder	No Disorder	Totals	+ PPV
	Fail	95	1,485	1,580	
1%	Pass	5	8,415	8,420	95/1,580 = 6%
	Totals	100	9,900	10,000	
	Fail	475	1,425	1,900	
5%	Pass	25	8,075	8,100	475/1,900 = 25%
	Totals	500	9,500	10,000	

Note: For a test with 95% sensitivity and 85% specificity, based on testing 10,000 people.

those without the disorder). Unfortunately, this "super test" does not exist for hearing screening or any of the diagnostic hearing tests (nor is it ever likely to exist). Therefore, one must develop tests whereby the measurement criterion is set so that it can produce a balance between good sensitivity and good specificity. A measurement criterion (considered a lax criterion) can be set so that the screening is sensitive enough to get 100% of those with the disease; however, there will be a corresponding decrease in the specificity since it will have an increase in the false positive rate. On the other hand, if one is overly concerned about having a high false positive rate because of the resources needed for follow-up, a measurement criterion (considered a strict criterion) could be

---

Synopsis 10–2

- Screening for hearing loss in newborns is now in widespread use. With the advent of OAEs, universal screening of all newborns is an accepted standard of care in the United States and in many other countries.

- The JCIH (2007) states that infants should be screened for hearing loss at birth (with a physiological testing method), hearing loss identified by 3 months of age, and those with significant hearing loss be fit with hearing aids or cochlear implants before 6 months of age. A screening program is just the first step of a comprehensive program which must include close follow-up care, rehabilitation, counseling, and appropriate social and educational services.

- Newborn hearing screening programs use OAEs (TEOAEs or DPOAES) and/or AABR to screen all babies before they are discharged from the hospital. Upon failing the screen, and immediate rescreen is recommended to reduce the number of false positives. False positive rates are generally less than 5%.

- *Auditory neuropathy spectrum disorder*, also called *auditory dyssynchrony disorder*, which may account for up to 10% of children

- with hearing loss, may be missed by screening programs relying solely on OAEs (Sininger, 2002), that is, this disorder is characterized by normal OAE and abnormal ABR.

- Hearing screening is recommended for all preschool children and school-age children kindergarten through the 3rd grade, and those in 7th, and 11th grades.

- Screening of preschool and school-age children should include age-appropriate behavioral techniques at frequencies of 1000, 2000, and 4000 Hz at 20 dB HL. If a child fails the initial screening, it is recommended that he/she be rescreened again during the same day. A child who fails the rescreening should be referred for a complete audiological evaluation.

- Screening programs should also include a short history questionnaire, otoscopy, and tympanometry to identify middle ear disorders. A medical referral should be made if the screening finds drainage in the ear canal, structural abnormality, foreign object, impacted cerumen, infection, or tympanic membrane abnormality, perforation.

- The AAA (1997) criteria for tympanogram failures are $Y_{tm} < 0.2$ mmho, and/or TW > 250 daPa. Children who shows a flat tympanogram with normal ear canal volume or for those with an abnormally wide tympanogram should be rescreened in 4 to 6 weeks.

- Health fairs or senior centers are places where adult hearing screening might be conducted. In addition to otoscopy, audiometry, and tympanometry, adults are often screened through questionnaires designed for self-assessment of their communication and hearing abilities.

- Figure 10–1 presents a commonly used matrix of outcomes for a screening test resulting in true positives (a hit), true negatives, false positives, and false negatives (a miss).

- Sensitivity = how well the test correctly identifies the targeted disorder (proportion of true positives); specificity = how well the test correctly identifies those without the targeted disorder (proportion of true negatives)

applied in order to reduce the false positive rate and increase sensitivity, but there will be a corresponding decrease in the sensitivity and one will miss more of those who have the disorder. This concept of manipulating the measurement criterion to change sensitivity and specificity, referred to as receiver operating characteristics (ROC), is beyond the scope of this text; the interested reader is referred to Swets (1988) and Hyde (2011).

References

American Academy of Audiology (AAA). (1997). *Indentification of hearing loss and middle ear dysfunction in preschool and school-age children*. Reston, VA: Author.

American Speech-Language-Hearing Association (ASHA). (1997). Panel on audiologic assessment. *Guidelines for audiologic screening*. Rockville, MD: Author.

Andermann, A., Blancquaert, I., Beauchamp, S., & Dery, V. (2008). Revisiting Wilson and Jungner in the genomic age: A review of screening criteria over the past 40 years. *Bulletin of the World Health Organization, 86*(4), 241–320.

Bess, F. H., & Humes, L. E. (2008). *Audiology: the fundamentals* (4th ed.). Philadelphia, PA: Lippincott Williams & Wilkins.

Cooper, J. C. Jr., Gates, G. A., Owen, J. H., & Dickson, H. D. (1975). An abbreviated impedance bridge technique for school screening. *Journal of Speech and Hearing Disorders, 40,* 260–269.

Downs, M. P., & Sterritt, G. (1967). A guide to newborn and infant hearing screening programs. *Archives of Otolaryngology, 85,* 15–22.

Driscoll, C. J., & McPherson, B. (2010) *Newborn screening systems.* San Diego, CA: Plural Publishing.

Durieux-Smith, A., Picton, T., Edwards, C., Goodman, J. T., & MacMurray, B. (1985). The Crib-O-Gram in the NICU: An evaluation based on brain stem electric response audiometry. *Ear and Hearing, 6,* 20–24.

Hall, J. W. III. (2007). *New handbook of auditory evoked responses.* Boston, MA: Pearson, Allyn and Bacon.

Hyde, M. (2011). Principles and methods of population hearing screening in EHDI. In R. Seewald & A. M. Tharpe (Eds.), *Comprehensive handbook of pediatric audiology* (pp. 283–337). San Diego, CA: Plural Publishing.

Joint Committee Infant Hearing (JCIH). (2007). Year 2007 position statement: Principles and guidelines for early hearing detection and intervention programs. *Pediatrics, 120,* 898–921.

Leigh, G., Schmulian-Taljaard, D., & Poulakis, Z. (2010). Newborn hearing screening. In C. Driscoll & B. McPherson (Eds.), *Newborn screening systems* (pp. 95–115). San Diego, CA: Plural Publishing.

Ling, D. A., Ling, A. H., & Doehring, D. G. (1970). Stimulus response and observer variables in the auditory screening of newborn infants. *Journal of Speech and Hearing Research, 13,* 9–18.

Northern, J. L., & Downs, M. P. (1974). *Hearing in children.* Baltimore, MD: Williams & Wilkins.

Project HEID. (2004). *Improving outcomes for children with permanent congenital hearing impairment: The case for a national newborn hearing screening and early intervention programme for New Zealand.* Auckland, New Zealand: National Foundation for the Deaf.

Schow, R. L., & Nerbonne, M. A. (1982). Communication screening profile: Use with elderly clients. *Ear and Hearing, 3,* 135–147.

Sininger, Y. L. (2002). Identification of auditory neuropathy in infants and children. *Seminars in Hearing, 23,* 193–200.

Sininger, Y. S., & Oba, S. (2001). Patients with auditory neuropathy: Who are they and what can they hear? In Y. S. Sininger & A. Starr (Eds.), *Auditory neuropathy* (pp. 15–36). San Diego, CA: Singular Publishing.

Spivak, L. G. (2007). Neonatal hearing screening, follow-up and diagnosis. In R. J. Roeser, M. Valente, & H. Hosford-Dunn (Eds.), *Audiology diagnosis* (2nd ed., pp. 497–513). New York, NY: Thieme.

Spivak, L. G., & Sokol, H. (2004). *Factors affecting effectiveness of newborn hearing screening protocols.* Paper presented at NHS 2004 International Conference on Newborn Screening, Diagnosis and Intervention, Milan, Italy.

Swets, J. (1988). Measuring the accuracy of diagnostic systems. *Science, 240,* 1285–1293.

Thompson, M., & Thompson, G. (1972). Response of infants and young children as a function of auditory stimuli and test methods. *Journal of Speech and Hearing Research, 15,* 699–707.

U.S. Preventive Services Task Force. (2008). *Universal screening for hearing loss in newborns,* topic page. Agency for Health Care Research and Quality, Rockville, MD.

Ventry, I. M., & Weinstein, B. (1983). Identification of elderly people with hearing problems. *ASHA, 25,* 37–47.

Vohr, B., Carty, L. M., Moore, P. E., & Letourneau, K. (1998). The Rhode Island hearing assessment program: Experience with state-wide hearing screening. *Pediatrics, 139,* 353–357.

Wilson, J. M. G. & Junger, G. (1968). *Principles and practice of screening for disease* (Public Health Paper No. 34). Retrieved from World Health Organization: http://www.who.int/iris/handle/10665/37650

11

Hearing Aids

H. Gustav Mueller and Earl E. Johnson

After reading this chapter, you should be able to:

1. Describe the six major steps used in the hearing aid selection and fitting process.
2. Name three different factors that impact the hearing aid market in the United States today.
3. Explain the function of each of the basic components of hearing aids.
4. Provide a brief description of seven different special features of modern hearing aids.
5. Describe and differentiate the basic hearing aid styles.
6. Name the basic earmold styles, their function and acoustic effects.
7. List two different hearing aid fitting options for special cases.
8. Describe the design and function of a cochlear implant.
9. Name the key issues concerning hearing aid candidacy.
10. Identity four advantages of bilateral hearing aid fittings.
11. Recognize the equipment and software needed to program modern digital hearing aids.
12. Identify a commonly used hearing aid validation procedure.
13. Describe the basic 2-cc coupler measures conducted with hearing aids (Supplemental Topic).
14. Describe the different clinical procedures used for verification (Supplemental Topic).

Historical Perspective

The practice of audiology includes a wide range of areas and continues to expand. One area, however, which has been part of audiology practice from the beginning, is the selection and fitting of amplification devices called *hearing aids*. About the time that the word *audiology* was being coined in the mid-1940s, Dr. Raymond Carhart was involved with fitting returning World War II veterans with hearing aids at Deshon Army Hospital in Butler, Pennsylvania. This work prompted him to write an extensive hearing aid fitting protocol, and he carried this work experience on to his teachings at the first audiology program at Northwestern University. At the time, Northwestern University was a prominent training site for PhD audiologists, who subsequently went on to establish their own audiology training programs at Universities across the United States. Portions of the original Carhart fitting protocol are still used in some clinics today.

The fitting of hearing aids is a key component to the overall rehabilitative audiology program. While it is possible that simply obtaining some form of amplification is all that is needed in an auditory rehabilitation program (e.g., a consumer buys a pair of hearing aids on eBay), it is the role of the audiologist to conduct a comprehensive selection and fitting procedure, coupled with appropriate counseling at several stages before, during, and after the fitting of the hearing aids. Various types of auditory and acclimatization training may also be included for some patients. The general workflow for the treatment process involving hearing aids is shown in Table 11–1.

Table 11–1. Typical Workflow for the Selection and Fitting of Hearing Aids

- Step 1. Assessment: Determine the extent and cause of hearing loss. Determine candidacy for hearing aids based on pure-tone hearing loss, self-assessment inventories, and patient history.

- Step 2. Treatment Planning: Review the assessment results with the patient and/or family members. Identify areas of difficulty and explore different amplification options.

- Step 3. Selection: Determine the type of fitting (style, etc.). Decide on electroacoustic parameters and what special features are needed.

- Step 4. Verification (see Supplemental Topic): Determine that the hearing aids meet a set of standardized measures, including electroacoustic performance and patient's real-ear match to desired levels (presumably based on validated prescriptive targets). The hearing aids also should have good sound quality, be comfortable to wear, and have acceptable cosmetics.

- Step 5. Orientation: Counsel the patient on the use and care of the hearing aids. Discuss hearing aid adjustments and realistic expectations. Determine the need for a more comprehensive audiologic rehabilitation program.

- Step 6. Validation: Assess the effectiveness of the use of hearing aids in the patient's everyday environment, through the use of patient interview and/or formal self-assessment inventories of benefit and satisfaction. Readdress areas of need regarding the fitting.

Source: Mueller and Hall (1998).

As mentioned, audiologists always have been involved in the selection and fitting process for hearing aids. However, the actual business of "dispensing" hearing aids has changed over the years.

Until the mid-1970s, once the appropriate hearing aids had been selected, the patient was then referred by the audiologist to a licensed dispenser to purchase hearing aids. The patient usually returned to the audiologist for a reevaluation or "approval" of the fitting. As you might guess, this practice often led to controversy, with the patient in the middle, as two professionals easily could disagree on what was "best" for a given patient.

The reason for using an outside dispenser as a middleman was that the selling of hearing aids was considered unethical by the American Speech and Hearing Association (ASHA), although audiologists working in government facilities were allowed to dispense hearing aids free of charge. The ASHA ethical guidelines were changed around 1977, and audiologists quickly began selling hearing aids, and there was a sharp increase in the opening of audiology private practices. The enthusiasm of the time was reflected in the name of a new audiology organization formed the same year, the Academy of Dispensing Audiologists (now the Academy of Doctors of Audiology). Today, the majority of audiologists are involved with hearing aids, including selecting, fitting, testing, and dispensing/selling—hundreds of audiologists are employed by hearing aid manufacturers. In addition to audiologist-owned dispensing practices, there has been considerable progress with hearing aid design and selection over the years. But, before we get started with the actual technology part of this chapter, we thought it would be useful to provide a "market report" update.

Recent Hearing Aid Market Trends

In the past 3 decades, much effort has been devoted to tracking changes in the hearing aid industry, making estimates of current hearing aid adoption rates among hearing impaired listeners, and predicting future trends. One of the best resources for obtaining information on the hearing aid industry is the *Hearing Industry Association* (HIA). The HIA typically publishes a quarterly report of the trends in hearing aid sales, as well as special reports on dispenser practice trends. Another resource on the hearing aid industry, from a consumer/patient standpoint, is called *MarkeTrak*, which for the past 30 years has been organized by Sergei Kochkin, Ph.D. The results of his extensive surveys are typically published in trade journals, such as *The Hearing Journal* and *Hearing Review*, and are now available on the website of the Better Hearing Institute (http://www.betterhearing .org). Annual dispenser surveys from these same trade journals as well as *AudiologyOnline* also provide excellent viewpoints of dispensers regarding the hearing aid industry. We discuss some of the results of these annual dispenser surveys in a later section devoted to dispenser practice behavior. Right now, we thought you might be interested in recent data from the HIA and the MarkeTrak studies.

Table 11–2 highlights some interesting trends in the hearing aid market. According to recent HIA data, over 2.7 million hearing aids are sold each year in the United States. However, since about 80% of hearing aids are sold in pairs (for bilateral fittings), only about 1.62 million people actually purchase hearing aids each year, that is, about 1,080,000 people purchase two hearing aids and the remaining 540,000 purchase one hearing aid. The unit volume of hearing aid sales has been slow to increase over time, considering that 1 million hearing aids were sold for the first time back in 1983. In 2004, the unit volume of hearing aid sales reached 2 million, indicating only an average of 4.7% increase in sales per year over the 21-year period from 1983. These numbers become even more significant when the "aging of America" is considered.

One reason for the slow increase in hearing aid sales is that the hearing aid industry has been unable to convince a larger percent of the population who needs hearing aids to adopt their use. Since the HIA began tracking adoption rates in 1984, the percentage of those with an admitted hearing loss who actually own hearing aids has remained near 22%. Thus, the increase in number of unit sales is due to an increase in the use of bilateral hearing aids, an increase in the total United

Table 11–2. Interesting Data About the Hearing Aid Market

- More than 2.8 million hearing aids are sold annually in the United States.
- The largest single purchaser of hearing aids sold in the United States, purchasing approximately 20% of all hearing aids, is the Department of Veterans Affairs.
- About 80% of new hearing aid sales are bilateral fitting, compared with only 25% in 1984.
- About two-thirds of hearing aids in 2013 are BTE style (much like in the 1950s and early 1960s). The BTE style became popular again because digital feedback suppression systems, operating on phase cancellation technology, enabled more open ear canal fittings. Because of increased popularity, a number of variants on the traditional BTE style (to be elaborated on further) are now available to fill almost every conceivable market niche.
- Just over 70% of all hearing aid owners report satisfaction with their hearing aid(s).
- About 15% of hearing aid owners report never using their hearing aids (curiously, this percentage has not changed significantly as technology has improved over 20 years).
- Only 22% of individuals with an admitted hearing loss have a hearing aid.
- The average age of a first-time hearing aid owner is about 70 years.
- The average age of a hearing aid in use by all hearing aid owners is about 4 years.
- The average household annual income of a hearing aid owner is $56,000.
- In the United States, it is estimated that over a million dependents (children under the age of 21 years) have parents who admit their children have hearing difficulties but do not use amplification.
- In a survey conducted about 15 years ago, a large group of individuals who were hearing aid candidates but did not use hearing aids were asked if they would use hearing aids if they were "free and invisible." Only 35% said yes!

States population, and a general pattern of generations with the highest percentage of the population (e.g., baby boomers) coming of age to purchase hearing aids. Based on the unchanging adoption rates over the past 20 years, it is clear that the hearing aid industry has not been very effective in its attempt to market hearing aids to potential patients. One most recent technological advancement (binaural directional beam formers, also known as bilateral directional microphones, which we discuss in a following section) may begin to change this reality as these hearing aids are manufactured with the functionality to outperform even the normal hearing listeners in difficult listening situations; hence, instead of conceptualizing hearing aids as a means to offset a hearing disability, they will be a means to super hearing (outperforming the normal hearer) (Dillon, 2010). Unfortunately, regardless of the marketing, design, or technology, hearing aids continue to carry the stigma of a "device for when you get old."

Despite the slow increase in sales and flat market penetration, the hearing aid industry has substantial annual sales figures. Total sales for this industry in 2005 were approximately $2.8 billion in the United States alone and approximately $8.4 billion for the entire world (Edwards, 2006). Perhaps to the surprise of some readers, the biggest purchaser of hearing aids in the Unites States is the Department of Veterans Affairs, which purchases about 20% of the total hearing aids sold annually for the Veterans it serves.

The first MarkeTrak report by Sergei Kochkin was published in 1990, and since that time seven more MarkeTrak reports have been released. The latest report, MarkeTrak VIII, suggested that there are over 35 million people in the country who have a hearing impairment and could benefit from hearing aids. The potential benefits we speak of include not only increased improvements in speech understanding, but enhanced communicative competence and self-confidence that increase verbal exchanges, which have been shown to increase hearing aid wearers' overall quality of life. Yet, as stated above, only about 22% percent of people with hearing loss seek professional hearing services or hearing aid products. Accordingly, the maximum potential untapped market of hearing aid users may be around 30.8 million people!

Some industry leaders, however, believe the untapped market is not that large, due to an overestimation of the pool of potential hearing aid consumers. In other words, just because a person has an admitted hearing loss does not mean he believes that he needs hearing aids. Understandably, a person needs to perceive that his hearing loss is of sufficient magnitude to warrant the need for amplification. Data show that only 32% of the individuals with hearing loss who do not currently own hearing aids perceive themselves as having significant need for hearing aids (Edwards, 2006;

Kochkin, 1998). Thus, the real untapped potential market for hearing aids of people who perceive themselves as needing a hearing aid may be closer to 8 million (Edwards, 2006), which increases to about 11.2 million today (35 million × 0.32) considering the latest MarkeTrak VIII estimate of people in the country who have a hearing impairment.

MarkeTrak reports also have focused on a variety of other issues, such as correlates to consumer satisfaction and benefit with hearing aids in general as well as particular product features. These data have shown that consumer satisfaction rates with modern-day digital hearing aids are relatively high, around 81%. Referencing the American Consumer Satisfaction Index, the 81% satisfaction rating was similar to satisfaction with other consumer electronics. In comparison, food processing and automobiles had the highest rating of satisfaction at 89% and 86%, respectively, while some of the lowest satisfaction ratings were in the area of telecommunications and gas/electric at 56% and 58%, respectively. The high satisfaction ratings of hearing aids suggest that the real reason hearing aids are not highly regarded or at least not sought out by the typical person with hearing loss is not directly related to performance or consumer satisfaction.

As mentioned earlier, we know that a leading reason why consumers do not purchase hearing aids is the social stigma associated with their use. Currently, the average age of the first-time hearing aid user is 70 years. Although the prevalence of hearing loss is lower as age decreases, the adoption rate of hearing aids among those who do have a hearing loss also decreases, lending support to the idea that a social stigma of older age is attached to hearing aids (Kochkin, 2005a). One of the most surprising findings regarding hearing aid adoption rates from MarkeTrak VII was the incredibly low rate of 12.5% for children under the age of 18 whose parents acknowledged them as having hearing loss, that is, 87.5% of parents who reportedly knew or thought their child had a hearing loss, *had not* gotten a hearing aid for the child. Presumably, not all of these children need hearing aids as their hearing loss may have been transient in nature (e.g., due to middle ear effusion), but conservative estimates indicated that more than 1 million children may not be receiving needed hearing aids and are getting "left behind" as a result (Kochkin, Luxford, Northern, Mason, & Tharpe, 2007).

We close this section with a final thought regarding the need for increased market adoption. In a recent MarkeTrak report (Kochkin, 2005b), the financial impact on individuals with hearing loss who either used or did not use hearing aids showed, as might be expected, that as the severity of the individual's hearing loss increased, yearly income decreased. However, the data also revealed that the use of hearing aids could offset this decrease by approximately 50%. In other words, hearing aids—a common treatment option for hearing loss—closed the wage earning gap between those individuals with hearing loss and those with normal hearing by one half!

Basic Hearing Aid Components and Technology

Now that we have covered the general area of hearing aid use, let's get into details regarding how hearing aids work. Other than miniaturization, the basic technology of a hearing aid has remained the same over the years, that is, the system must detect an acoustic signal, amplify it (which means a power source is needed), and then deliver it to the ear. While earlier instruments were based on analog amplification technology, today essentially all hearing aids use digital amplification technology. The following list describes the basic components of a *digital hearing aid:*

- Microphone: An auditory transducer, which converts the acoustic signal from the sound field into an electrical signal that goes to the amplifier.
- Receiver: An auditory transducer, which converts the amplified signal from the hearing aid into an acoustic signal that is delivered to the patient's ear.
- Digital conversion: The electrical signal is converted into digital information to allow for computerized signal manipulation

and application of different processing algorithms. The digital signal is subsequently reconverted to an electrical signal that is sent to the receiver.
- Amplifier: The heart of the hearing aid circuitry where the input signal is increased in level and filtered in frequency, and then sent to the digital converter.
- Battery: Provides the power source for the hearing aid. Batteries come in different sizes to match the size and power requirements of the hearing aid. Some models have rechargeable batteries.
- Volume control: Many hearing aids have a volume control that can be a wheel or button on the aid itself or could be a function part of a remote control device that also can be used to change the programmed settings.
- Telecoil: An alternative input source that converts the electromagnetic signal from a telephone or from an assistive listening device and delivers it to the amplifier; available on all but the smallest hearing aids.

Other Hearing Aid Features and Signal Processing

The basic technologies listed above are essential to provide basic amplification. Today's hearing aids, however, have many other features and algorithms designed to improve the amplified signal and to provide added audibility in different environments, more listening comfort, and easier operation for the patient. We first review a few of the features typically found on many digital hearing aids.

Multiple Memory Programs

Using a push-button selector or a remote control, several stored settings can be retrieved that modify the programmed amplification provided to the wearer and/or activate or modify some of the features listed below. For example, a patient could have a memory program dedicated to listening to music, which might be programmed quite differently from a memory dedicated to listening to speech-in-noise. Often, four or more memories are available, although not all patients are ready to work with several memory choices. Most hearing aids have a signal classification system, which can be used to automatically switch programs—that is, if the hearing aid detects that the user is in background noise, the "noise program" is implemented.

Multiple Channels

Digital hearing aids have many frequency channels (frequency processing regions), which means that adjustments in gain and output can be made to individual frequency regions, usually based on the hearing loss. Other special features can operate independently in different channels. Channels may be as few as two or four, or as many as 48 or more. Although one might think that "more is better," and this is generally true, the differences are not as striking as may seem.

Automatic Gain Control for Output (AGCo)

AGCo is one type of compression used in hearing aids. *Compression* simply means that the signal is no longer amplified in a linear (1:1) manner. These systems have what is referred to as a kneepoint (point where compression begins), and a ratio (amount of "squash effect"). For example, when a low kneepoint (around 40 dB SPL) is used, the compression ratio may be relatively small (e.g., 2:1, meaning that for every 10 dB increase in input, output increases by 5 dB). When high kneepoints are used (around 100 dB SPL), then quite large ratios are used (e.g., 10:1). Most hearing aids have the ability to amplify sounds to the extent that they could become uncomfortable to the listener. It is necessary, therefore, to use some compression after the amplifier, referred to as output compression (AGCo) to limit the maximum output of

the signal. The audiologist adjusts this compression based on the measured loudness discomfort level of each individual. The maximum power output (MPO) can be set independently for different frequency regions based on the patient's loudness discomfort ratings. This setting is critical, as "loud sounds are too loud" is one of the leading reasons that individuals stop using their hearing aids.

Automatic Gain Control for Input (AGCi)

AGCi is a second type of compression employed in hearing aids. As the name suggests, it compresses the signal at the input stage of the amplifier. Usually AGCi utilizes low kneepoints and small compression ratios. It is used in conjunction with AGCo, as it provides a different patient benefit. Many individuals with sensorineural hearing loss have *recruitment*, which is a loudness growth pattern that is more rapid than normal (see Chapter 8). For example, even when the hearing loss is 40 to 50 dB HL, the loudness judgments for loud sounds often are the same as those of normal hearing listeners. This means that the hearing aid may have to provide 30 dB of gain for soft speech, but little or no gain for loud speech. This is accomplished using AGCi, or input compression, often referred to as wide dynamic range compression (WDRC). The degree of compression employed using WDRC is adjusted based on the gain needed for soft speech compared with the gain needed for loud speech, which usually varies for different frequencies. To review, AGCi is used to repackage the input signal into the patient's residual dynamic range. AGCo is used to assure that the "ceiling" of that dynamic range is not exceeded.

Expansion

Expansion operates more or less the opposite of WDRC. Expansion reduces gain *below* the kneepoint rather than *above*. It is designed to reduce the gain for sounds softer than soft speech. For example, a patient may need 30 dB of gain to hear soft speech, but amplifying low-level ambient room noise by 30 dB would be annoying.

Signal Classification System

Modern hearing aids classify the incoming signal into as many as five or six categories (e.g., quiet, speech in quiet, speech in noise, noise, music, etc.). This classification process then can be used to control gain and output, and to trigger noise reduction or the directional microphone technology. To some extent, the classification system reduces the need for multiple memories, as the function of the processing can change according to the classification within a single memory.

Automatic Digital Noise Reduction

As mentioned above, the signal classification system analyzes the incoming signal in several different channels, and if the signal is determined to be noise, an automatic gain reduction occurs in that channel. Typically the speech versus noise decision is based on the modulations of the signal. Other types of noise reduction use a filtering approach. Noise reduction has not been shown to improve the signal-to-noise ratio significantly, and hence, there is little or no intelligibility improvement. It does, however, seem to improve listening comfort and reduce listener fatigue, which indirectly could improve intelligibility because of reduced cognitive load (see Mueller & Ricketts, 2005, for a review). Noise reduction usually is activated by default in the fitting software.

Adaptive Feedback Reduction

Historically, *acoustic feedback* or "whistling" has been a common problem with hearing aids. In fact, this has added to the negative stigma surrounding hearing aids, and contributes significantly to nonuse. Automatic feedback reduction can detect the feedback frequency and reduce or eliminate the problem. This usually is accomplished by using implementations of phase cancellation. In most products this allows the user an additional 5 to 15 dB of gain without feedback. This extra gain leads to audibility of soft speech inputs, which leads to hearing aid benefit, making feedback reduction algorithms one of the most beneficial features introduced in hearing aids in recent years.

Directional Microphone Technology

The goal of directional microphone technology, sometimes referred to as array microphones due to the use of multiple omnidirectional microphones and internal time delays to create directivity, is to reduce the output of the hearing aids for sounds coming from the sides and back, without changing the output for sounds from the front (Ricketts, 2001). Hearing aids can have a dedicated directional microphone, but usually two omnidirectional microphones are used to accomplish the directional effect electronically by creating phase delays. If we assume that the desired talker is from the front, and noise is from the sides and back, then this technology will indeed improve the signal-to-noise ratio and improve the patient's speech intelligibility in noise. Most modern directional hearing aids are both automatic and/or adaptive. Automatic means that the hearing aid will automatically switch back and forth between omnidirectional and directional depending on the listening situation (information from the signal classification system discussed earlier). Adaptive means that while in the directional mode, the hearing aid will automatically change the strength and pattern of the directional amplification based on the intensity, spectrum, and location of the noise source. In recent years, algorithms have been developed so that the pattern will even reverse, to enhance speech from the back when necessary (e.g., when listening to someone in the back seat while driving a car).

Binaural Beamformers (Bilateral Directional Microphone Technology)

Made possible by the capability of linked hearing aids (introduced in the next few pages), hearing aids can now share the audio signal with the best signal-to-noise ratio (SNR) between hearing aid devices. In other words, should the left hearing aid have a SNR advantage over the right hearing aid, the audio signal from the left hearing aid can be "streamed" over the right hearing aid, and vice versa. Not coincidentally, the streaming can change between ears in a matter of milliseconds such that the listener is almost always getting the best audio signal; for example, when the listener turns his or her head from side to side. While the best SNR ensures the best speech understanding performance, listening to the same signal in both the left and right ears (a diotic signal more or less) degrades other abilities, such as localization, as all interaural timing and level differences are no longer present. Advanced binaural beamformers have nonetheless addressed this issue in decidedly clever ways. One implementation of a binaural beamformer (Mejia & Dillon, 2010; Mejia, Keidser, Dillon, Cong-Van Nguyen, & Johnson, 2011) first routes (by a matter of 3 to 4 ms) the independent left and right hearing aid signals to each ear separately to allow localization via the precedence effect (Wallach, Newman, & Rosenzweig, 1949; Litovsky, Colburn, Yost, & Guzman, 1999), before routing the hearing aid signal with the best SNR to both ears immediately afterward.

Frequency Lowering

Currently, there are several implementations of frequency lowering in use by manufacturers; the primary goal of all implementations is to lower frequencies in a manner that makes the spectral energy at higher frequencies audible again and hopefully usable for speech understanding, albeit at a lower frequency. The target population for this algorithm is the patient with mild to moderate hearing loss in the low to mid frequencies, and a severe to profound loss in the highs—a loss so severe that audibility is not possible and/or audibility is not usable for speech recognition with traditional amplification. Presently, the implementation and recommended use of frequency lowering varies substantially between manufacturers. The best frequency lowering parameters have

not been clearly defined. Some manufacturer-independent research has proposed the face-valid approach of ensuring audibility of the /s/ sound while making sure that that /s/ and /sh/ sound are perceptually dissimilar (e.g., Glista & Scollie, 2009). Although this feature has been introduced by most of the major manufacturers, the true patient benefit has yet to be determined.

Data Logging

The hearing aid automatically keeps a record of various listening situations experienced by the patient, such as input level and signal-to-noise ratio, as well as the attributes of the hearing aid function, such as volume control position and the listening program/memory setting. After the patient has used the hearing aid for a period of time, the audiologist can read out (in the fitting software) the amount of time the hearing aid (presumably on the patient's ear) was in different environments. For example, the software will inform the audiologist of how much time was spent listening to speech in quiet, speech in noise, music, etc., and what setting (e.g., gain) the patient preferred to use in those different settings. Some hearing aids, termed "trainable," even make automatic adjustments based on this logged information (see related section below).

Linked Hearing Aids

Hearing aids are now available that "talk to each other." Through a type of near field magnetic induction transmission, the hearing aids (a bilateral fitting) share information. This has some direct patient benefit in that the patient only has to change gain on one hearing aid, and the gain of the other hearing aid will automatically change the same amount. The same result occurs when changing different programmed settings (memories) for different listening situations. The feature is advancing to the point of allowing even the audio signal (with the best SNR) between hearing aids to be shared across both hearing aids (recall the earlier bilateral beam-formers section).

Trainable Hearing Aids

For brevity, trainable hearing aids can be simplified into two types: (a) training that occurs as a result of control over the hearing aid which has been given to the user—direct patient-controlled training, and (b) training as a result of pre-programmed adjustments to the hearing aid that automatically occurs over time—hearing aid self-training.

For the first type, the ability to control or train the assigned gain and output as well as even the frequency response in some devices as a function of input level is transferred to the patient. In other words, in lieu of or after a prescriptive fitting of the gain and output parameters of the hearing aid, the patient can adjust much more than just the overall volume. Moreover, the hearing aid will be "trained" for all different types of listening situations (e.g., speech, noise, music, etc). Direct control of AGC-I processing occurs via interaction with a volume control on either the hearing aid itself, a remote control for adjusting the hearing aid, or both. The hearing aid simultaneously logs the input level of the listening environment, the classification of the environment, and the volume control adjustment. In advanced systems, the frequency response also can be altered with a simple graphic equalizer such as a three-band manipulator of bass, mid, and treble frequencies, although commercial hearing aids have only made treble adjustments available thus far. Reasons for using trainable hearing aids are many: allowing the patient to fine-tune their loudness perceptions, individualizing gain and output for different settings (noise, music, etc), and allowing the patient to become more vested in his/her hearing rehabilitation—getting the "best" fitting then becomes a shared task between the patient and the audiologist.

The second type of training exists because some evidence indicates that new users cannot accept the loudness provided by common gain prescriptions at the initial fitting visit. As a result, some hearing aids have been built with the option to "auto-acclimatize" to prescriptive settings over the time course of the first several months of hearing aid usage. That is, a hearing aid could be programmed 8 dB below prescriptive target, and then set to increase gain by 1 dB/week over an eight-week period. One alternative to using auto-acclimatization, though, is to select more recent hearing aid prescriptions that have different amplification recommendations, less for the new average user and more for the experienced user.

Wireless Connectivity

The most significant advancements in the past decade of hearing aids has not been in advancements to digital technology but rather in wireless electromagnetic induction. In fact, Dillon (2012) has labeled "wireless" as the new era in hearing aid development, while concomitantly labeling only five other eras in all of hearing aid history: acoustic (for the type of horned-shape amplifiers), carbon (for the type of microphones), vacuum tube (for the type of amplifier), transistor (for the type of amplifier), and digital (for the type of amplifier and processing capabilities).

In addition to creating the possibility of the already mentioned features of binaural beamformers and linked hearing aids, wireless connectivity allows for remote reception (the ability to receive signals from a microphone and transmitter worn by a talker from a far distance away), as well as connectivity to communication devices (such as audio signals from devices like mobile phones, computers, personal audio players, navigations systems, and the like). Not only does this provide a huge convenience for the patient, but in most cases, the signal-to-noise ratio also is improved.

Basic Hearing Aid Styles

There are five fundamental hearing aid styles. They are commonly referred to as: (a) body aid, (b) behind-the-ear (BTE or mini-BTE), (c) in-the-ear (ITE), (d) in-the-canal (ITC), and (e) completely-in-the-canal (CIC). These styles differ in size, in application, and also somewhat in features and components. It is important not to confuse the hearing

Synopsis 11–1

- Hearing aid selection and fitting has always been part of audiology practice; however, the actual selling of hearing aids by audiologists was not sanctioned by the profession until the late 1970s.

- A comprehensive selection and fitting procedure should consist of the following steps (see Table 11–1 for details):
  - Assessment of hearing loss and candidacy for hearing aids
  - Treatment planning to review results and options with patient
  - Selection of hearing aid style, electroacoustic parameters, and any special features
  - Verification that hearing aids meet expected performance standards and/or targets, both electroacoustically and with real-ear measures
  - Orientation on the use and care of the hearing aids, providing realistic expectations, and determining need for other rehabilitation
  - Validation measures to assess the patient's subjective satisfaction and benefit to determine any changes that might be needed

- There appears to be a large and growing untapped population who may benefit from hearing aids; however, the ability of the hearing aid industry to increase the penetration rate has remained relatively constant over the years.

- Hearing aid satisfaction with today's digital technology is fairly high (81%) and is not a primary reason for the relatively low penetration rate. Instead, people are primarily reluctant to use or purchase hearing aids because of the social stigma that is attached to their use.

- The basic operation of a hearing aid involves components that detect an acoustic signal, amplify it, and then deliver it to the ear. Today, almost all hearing aids use some digital (computer chip) technology. The basic components of a hearing aid include: (a) microphone, (b) amplifier, (c) battery, (d) digital converter, (e) volume control, and (f) receiver. Some instruments include a telecoil for use with a telephone.

- Additional features and options available in hearing aids include: (a) multiple memory programs for different listening situations, (b) multiple frequency channels, which can be individually adjusted to fit the hearing loss, (c) automatic gain control (AGC) on the output and input sides that limit the maximum levels to the patient and to adjust (compression) the gain depending on the level of sound, (d) directional microphone technology, (e) digital noise reduction circuits, (f) adaptive feedback reduction, (g) data logging of patient's real-world listening environment that can be used to train the hearing aid, and (h) linked hearing aids and wireless features.

aid style with the technology contained within the hearing aid. Manufacturers have different models of hearing aids (with more features added for the more expensive models). However, a given product model will have the same digital processing chip across the various styles offered by a manufacturer, and, therefore, different styles of the same product model will tend to sound similar to the patient.

Body Hearing Aid

The *body aid* is seldom used in the United States today, but it is still commonly used in developing countries, as it is inexpensive to produce and does not require custom fitting. Simply described, it is a square or rectangular hearing aid worn on the body. The amplified signals are delivered to the ears by wires that connect to external receivers mounted in custom earmolds, headphones, or earbuds. From a design standpoint, these may look similar to a large iPod or other digital music player. The main difference is that the hearing aid unit has a microphone to pick up environmental sounds, which are then amplified and sent to the earphones. Body aids typically do not have the digital signal processing that is present in the other more common hearing aid styles. However, because the body aid is the largest of the hearing aids, it may have some additional features, like Bluetooth or a powerful telecoil, that are not available with the smaller custom instruments.

Behind-the-Ear Hearing Aid (BTE)

The *behind-the-ear hearing aid*, called a BTE, is a hearing aid that is worn behind the ear (or one on each ear). The traditional BTE is a curve-shaped unit that has a hard tube coming off the receiver end of the hearing aid, called the earhook, which rests on the helix of the auricle and helps keep the hearing aid unit in place behind the ear. The amplified sound from the hearing aid's receiver is delivered through the earhook and through a flexible tube attached from the earhook to a custom-made earmold that fits into the auricle. Today, the earhook and

tubing sometimes is replaced with a one-piece thin tubing. There are two general categories of BTE, the traditional BTE and the mini-BTE.

Traditional BTE

The traditional BTE style (Figure 11–1) continues to be used for fitting some individuals with severe to profound hearing losses, individuals with visual or dexterity issues, and young infants and children with hearing loss. For severe to profound hearing losses, the BTE offers the benefit of increased gain and output compared with smaller hearing aid styles. In addition, the increased receiver-to-microphone distance separation is useful in reducing feedback (whistling) that often occurs when high amounts of gain are required. The traditional BTE style may often be selected for those with visual and dexterity issues because the hearing aid components (e.g., volume control and battery) are larger and more accessible than on smaller custom styles, and the hearing aid is easier to remove. The BTE

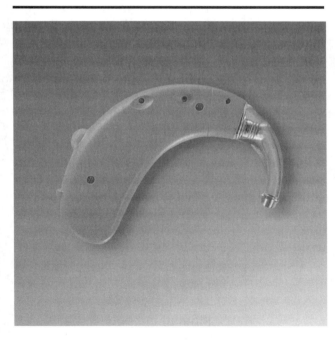

Figure 11–1. Traditional full-sized behind-the-ear hearing aid (BTE) without an earmold. Courtesy of Siemens Hearing Instruments, Piscataway, New Jersey.

style is also appropriate for an infant or young child because the outer ear will continue to grow for a number of years. In this situation, the earmold will need to be replaced every 6 months to 1 year due to the developmental changes. Purchasing a new earmold for a BTE is much easier and less expensive than the replacing required for some of the other models, where all of the hearing aid components are housed within the custom shell casing. In addition, the child would not have to be without the hearing aid while the new earmold is being made, unlike the other styles where the entire hearing aid must be sent to the manufacturer for recasing.

Mini-BTE

Soon after small custom in-the-ear instruments were introduced, the traditional BTE style began losing market share to these smaller in-the-ear styles. This was, in part, due to the BTE's bulkiness, requirement for a separate earmold, and its overall cosmetic visibility. However, this trend began to turn around, beginning around 2003, with the advent of *mini-BTE hearing aids*.

One type of mini-BTE hearing aid has all of the hearing aid components (microphone, amplifier, receiver, and battery) housed within the hearing aid casing, the same as for a traditional BTE, but the casing is typically smaller. In addition, the sound from the receiver is sent to the ear through a much thinner and smaller diameter tube (nearly invisible) than that used with traditional BTEs. A second type of mini-BTE does not house the receiver in the casing, but instead places the receiver in the earmold (often simply a soft plastic sleeve), which is connected to the casing via an electrical wire encased in thin tubing (Figure 11–2). Although a standard labeling of this style has not yet been established, it is usually called a receiver-in-canal (RIC) type of mini-BTE.

The mini-BTE has become popular because of its small case and thin tube, and also because it

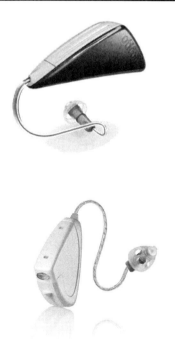
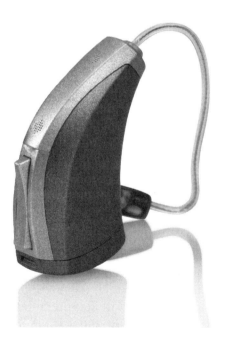

Figure 11–2. Mini-BTE hearing aids employing open fitting with receiver-in-canal technology. Courtesy of Oticon, Somerset, New Jersey, Unitron Hearing, Plymouth, Minnesota, and Starkey Hearing Technologies, Eden Prairie, Minnesota.

often is used with an open ear canal fitting. The open ear canal fitting is one in which the end of the tubing is loosely inserted into the ear canal or held in place by an open earmold or tip made of a flexible, thin material that comes pre-made in a variety of sizes, thus allowing for more natural sound quality, a more comfortable feel, and no need for a custom earmold (Figure 11–3). Often the mini-BTE has the added abbreviation of OC to imply an *open canal*. The OC fitting is only suitable for high frequency hearing losses. However, high frequency hearing losses are typical of those who are in the untapped market of potential hearing aid users that was discussed earlier. Recent marketing efforts of hearing aid manufacturers have redirected professionals and patients to products specifically promoted as mini-BTE OC fittings. Also, to fill the market niche of those dispensers preferring receiver-in-the canal placements, mini-BTEs have also been produced and sold as closed canal fittings now from nearly all brands (Figure 11–4).

To reinforce the hope that these smaller mini-BTEs will be attractive to baby boomers, one manufacturer offers these hearing aids in a choice of colors with the catchy names of Crème Brulee, Pinot Noir, Pure Passion, and Flower Power. Almost any color seemingly conceivable has now been made available. With the renewed interest brought about by mini-BTEs, the BTEs comprise about 66% of hearing aid sales as compared with 10 years ago when they represented only 20 to 25% of all sales. However, the increased popularity of the mini-BTE OC hearing fittings mostly has resulted in reduced sales of other hearing aid styles (e.g., the ITE, ITC, and CIC) instead of bringing more new consumers into the hearing aid market.

All BTE products require some type of *earmold*. For traditional BTEs, the earmold is custom made to fit into each patient's ear. The earmold is made by taking an ear impression made of special materials, which when mixed together form a solid impression after 2 to 3 min. To make the impression, a cotton ball or foam plug, with an attached string that remains outside the ear, is inserted partway into the ear canal to prevent the material from going too far into the ear canal. Then the *earmold impression* material is mixed and inserted

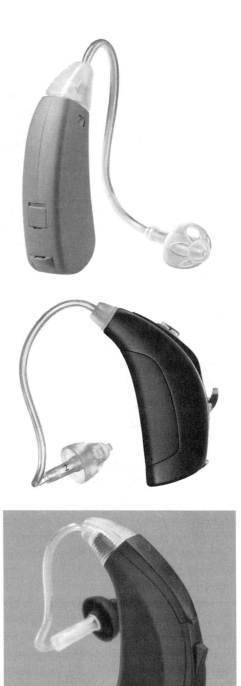

Figure 11–3. Mini-BTE hearing aid employing thin tubing and open ear canal fitting. Courtesy of Siemens Hearing Instruments, Piscataway, New Jersey, Unitron Hearing, Plymouth, Minnesota, and Starkey Hearing Technologies, Eden Prairie, Minnesota.

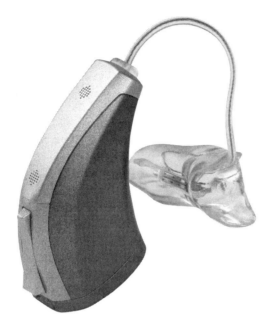

Figure 11–4. Mini-BTE hearing aid employing a closed fitting with receiver-in-canal technology inside an earmold. Courtesy of Starkey Hearing Technologies, Eden Prairie, Minnesota.

moved from the ear. The ear impression is sent to the selected hearing aid company, which uses it to make the custom hard-shell or custom soft material earmold and tubing that will be used to attach to the BTE. Some audiologists box-up and mail the impression itself, whereas others use an especially designed scanner and e-mail a scanned version of the impression to the manufacturer.

Earmolds come in various styles, ranging from large ones that fill the entire concha of the outer ear, to others that fit into the ear canal, or even some which are only a small piece of tubing or flexible tip that extends into the ear canal. The earmold's size, material, and other features (e.g., a small air vent) are determined by the audiologist when the earmold is ordered. Regardless of style, earmolds attach to the *earhook* of a traditional BTE via tubing and serve to route sound into the ear canal. With mini-BTEs the thin tubing or the wire connector of the RIC attaches directly to the hearing aid. In general, the greater the hearing loss, the larger and tighter fit the earmold needs to be in order to reduce the likelihood of feedback (whistling) that is related to the high-gain requirements. Figure 11–5 shows samples of some of the many earmold styles that are available.

relatively quickly into the ear canal, the concha, and part of the auricle. Taking good impressions of the ear is an art that must be learned by the audiologist. Bad impressions result in bad earmolds, which result in bad fittings and unhappy patients. After the impression material solidifies, it is re-

Custom In-the-Ear Hearing Aid

Hearing aids that have the components inside the earmold casing are generally referred to as *custom*

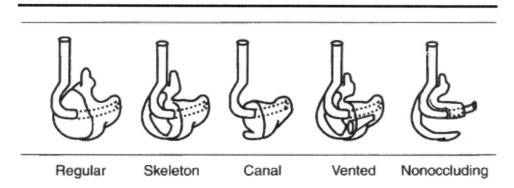

Regular   Skeleton   Canal   Vented   Nonoccluding

Figure 11–5. Examples of five different earmold styles. Courtesy of Westone.

hearing aids. The largest custom style hearing aid is the in-the-ear (ITE), which uses a full casing that fills a portion of the ear canal as well as most or all of the concha. The ITE hearing aid was first produced in the late 1950s when transistors replaced vacuum tubes for the hearing aid amplifier components (Dillon, 2001). Today, the digital integrated circuit has replaced transistors, and this has allowed hearing aid sizes to be reduced to the point where all of the hearing aid components can be fit into a customized case that fits into the ear canal. Discussed more fully below, the smallest of the custom styles is referred to as completely-in-the-canal, or CIC. For all of the custom style hearing aids, the audiologist makes the ear impression in the same way that was discussed above for the BTE. The manufacturer uses the ear impression (either the impression itself or a scanned version), sent to it by the audiologist, to customize the casing used for the custom hearing aid to be fit into the patient's ear.

As an expansion to the options with custom in-the-ear style hearing aids, some companies have introduced hearing aids that separate the microphone from the main hearing aid casing (a remote microphone design); or more simply and with less hype applying the same concept as RIC technology (separating the receiver from the casing) to the separation of the microphone from the casing. In general, the casing of the hearing aid is made smaller and placed deeper into the ear, like the CIC style, but the microphone is placed in the concha symba portion of the pinna.

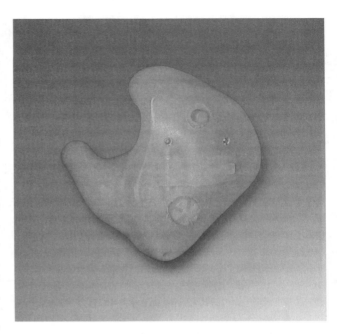

Figure 11–6. Example of full-concha ITE style hearing aid. Observable on the faceplate (*top to bottom*): button for changing program memories, port to each one of the two microphones, battery door, and volume control. Courtesy of Siemens Hearing Instruments, Piscataway, New Jersey.

the outer ear. The low-profile ITE fills the inner half of the concha, but does not protrude outward as much as the full-shell ITE. The half-shell ITE only fills the lower half of the concha.

In-the-Ear (ITE) Hearing Aid

The *in-the-ear* (ITE) hearing aid has all of the hearing aid components built inside of the customized casing (made from the ear impression), and the hearing aid is placed in the concha portion of the auricle with the receiver portion extending a little way into the ear canal (Figure 11–6). There are three general variants of the ITE style, the *full shell*, the *low profile*, and the *half shell*. The full-shell ITE fills the entire concha portion of

In-the-Canal (ITC) Hearing Aid

Like the ITE, the *in-the-canal* (ITC) hearing aid has all of the hearing aid components built inside of the customized casing (Figure 11–7). The ITC hearing aid only partially fills the lower approximate one quarter of the concha; thus, the ITC is even smaller than the half-shell ITE. With the smaller size of the ITC there is a tradeoff of less amplifier gain. For this reason, the selection of an ITC may be most appropriate for those with some cosmetic

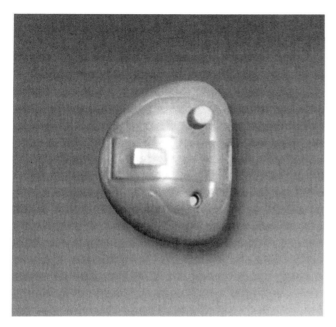

Figure 11–7. Example of ITC style hearing aid. Observable on the faceplate (*top to bottom*): button for changing program memories, battery door, port to microphone. Courtesy of Siemens Hearing Instruments, Piscataway, New Jersey.

concerns regarding hearing aids, and who have less severe hearing loss and relatively good manual dexterity. The ITC is also the smallest hearing aid style that can accommodate the space needed for directional microphone technology. Also, for patients who want to have controls for volume, or changing programs, and do not want to use a remote, the ITC often is the smallest custom hearing aid that can accommodate this.

Completely-in-the-Canal (CIC) Hearing Aid

The *completely-in-the-canal* (CIC) hearing aid is the smallest of the custom style hearing aids, and resides completely in the ear canal of the patient (Figure 11–8). The CIC is often selected by the pa-

tient who is looking for the "invisible" hearing aid. If the patient has a large enough ear canal, and the hearing aid can be fitted fairly deeply in the ear canal, the CIC is, indeed, barely noticeable. In case you are wondering, there is a small, clear filament that sticks out from the hearing aid that the patient can grasp in order to remove the aid (see Figure 11–8).

Traditionally, the CIC has not offered enough amplification for patients with moderate to more severe hearing losses. However, there are some new high powered CICs with advanced electronic feedback reduction systems; these newer models have been challenging the long-standing belief that CICs cannot be fit to individuals with severe hearing losses. One disadvantage of the CIC style is that the repair rate is higher than for other hearing aid styles; thus, the patient will be without his

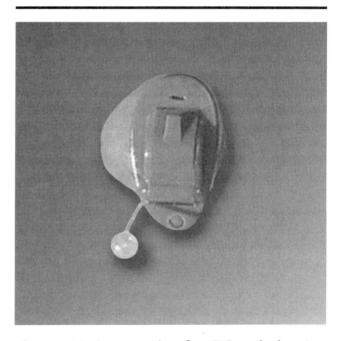

Figure 11–8. Example of a CIC style hearing aid. Observable on the faceplate (*top to bottom*): port to microphone, battery door, acoustic vent, and removal string. Courtesy of Siemens Hearing Instruments, Piscataway, New Jersey.

or her hearing aid more often during times when the hearing aid is returned to the manufacturer for a repair. Repairs are more frequent with CICs because components contained within the casing are more susceptible to perspiration and cerumen due to their deeper placement in the ear canal.

A variant of the CIC is what is sometimes called mini-CIC. This product fits even deeper into the ear than the standard CIC. Moreover, at least one model of this type needs to be inserted and removed by the audiologist, and is designed for extended wear (several months). These products indeed are invisible when placed in the ear canal.

Specialized Hearing Aids and Cochlear Implants

Sometimes other hearing aid styles are recommended as treatment options, depending upon individual patient characteristics. In these cases, the audiologist would generally work with an otologist or otolaryngologist when managing the patient's case. Two such specialized hearing aid styles that are used for conductive hearing loss are the bone-anchored hearing aid (BAHA) and the middle ear implanted hearing aid (MEI). Specialized hearing aid fittings may also be considered for patients with unilateral hearing loss, including the BAHA and the CROS (contralateral routing of signals). In addition, cochlear implants are a different type of hearing aid, in which the acoustic signals are delivered to electrodes that are implanted into a cochlea. Each of these types of hearing aids is discussed in the following sections.

Bone-Anchored Hearing Aid (BAHA)

A *bone-anchored hearing aid* goes by the acronym BAHA. At present, this product is available from two different manufacturers. The BAHA is a hearing aid that is surgically implanted by an otologist into the mastoid area behind the ear (Figure 11–9). The BAHA is most often advocated for listeners with bilateral conductive or mixed hearing losses, but can also be used in cases with unilateral hearing losses—that is, a type of CROS fitting (see following section). With the BAHA the

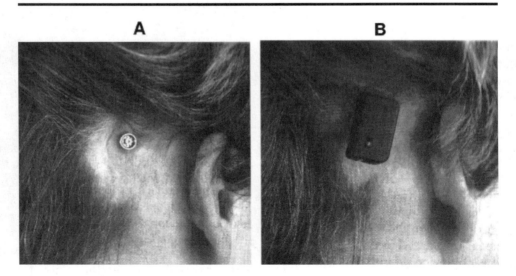

Figure 11–9. The Baha® percutaneous abutment is shown (**A**) with the Baha® device attached to the abutment (**B**). Courtesy of Cochlear Corporation, Sydney, New South Wales.

sound is transduced to the cochlea in a way similar to other bone conduction transducers, such as the ones used for bone conduction audiometry. Acoustic signals are picked up by the BAHA's microphone and transduced into vibrations that stimulate the skull, thus creating the normal vibratory energy in the normal hearing cochlea.

Middle Ear Implant (MEI)

A *middle ear implant* is typically abbreviated MEI. This specialized hearing aid has had some success in Europe but is rarely used in the United States. The MEI is most often used to treat sensorineural hearing losses. The MEI is surgically placed in the middle ear. Piezoelectric and electromagnetic transduction mechanisms are two common methods used in MEIs. The piezoelectric implementation uses an external microphone placed by the ear to detect sounds around the listener. From this, an electrically encoded signal is sent to an implanted middle ear crystal placed on the ossicular chain. The crystal moves in response to stimulation from the sound transduction and propagates this electrical activity onto the cochlea, where it is processed by the remaining hair cells and 8th nerve fibers. The electromagnetic implementation is larger than the piezoelectric version; therefore, it is only partially implantable. Most of the electromagnetic implants have an external coil that is connected to a microphone and an amplifier. An implanted magnet located at or near the incus–stapedial joint of the ossicular chain oscillates as electromagnetic waves move past the magnet; thus, the electromagnetic energy is converted to mechanical energy (ossicular movement).

Cochlear Implant (CI)

A *cochlear implant* (CI) is a biomedical device that bypasses the middle ear, the traveling wave, and the sensory cells on the basilar membrane, and electrically stimulates neurons of the cochleovestibular nerve. The purpose of a cochlear implant is to provide people with substantial hearing losses hearing improvement beyond that which can be offered by conventional hearing aids. Even individuals with severe to profound hearing losses have some functional auditory nerve fibers that can be stimulated electrically through a cochlear implant. Much like a hearing aid, a cochlear implant can provide reasonably good detection and correct identification of environmental and speech sounds. A simulation showing how cochlear implants work can be found on the Internet at http://utdallas.edu/~loizou/cimplants/.

Cochlear implants are regulated by the Food and Drug Administration (FDA), which requires data on safety and efficacy in clinical trials. Examples of safety data include prevalence of facial nerve paralysis, infection, device migration, and implant failure necessitating another implant. Efficacy data include studies on the benefits of the implant related to speech understanding as well as promoting the development of language and speech production. Approval from the FDA is directly related to coverage of cochlear implants by health insurance programs.

Often, the actual success and the functional level obtained with a cochlear implant depend on many factors. Some of these factors include time of onset of hearing loss, length of deafness prior to implantation, residual function of auditory neurons, appropriate programming of the implant, and consistent use of the implant. Some limitations to cochlear implants include surgical risk (complications less than 1%), implanted electrode array destroys most of the remaining functional hair cells, expense (~$40,000), the need to travel to and from a CI center for remapping and/or programming and checks, limited hearing of speech and environmental sounds, and unpredictable benefits and outcomes before surgery. Fortunately, the cost associated with cochlear implants, including the surgery, device, and programming visits, are covered by most medical insurances. Multichannel, multielectrode cochlear implants available in the United States may be found at the following cochlear implant manufacturers' Web sites: http://www.advancedbionics.com, http://www.cochlear-americas.com, or http://www.medel.com/.

A cochlear implant may be conceptualized as a device divided into external and internal components (Figure 11–10). The external components consist of a microphone, speech processor, and external transmitter. As with all amplification devices, the microphone changes the acoustic energy into electrical energy. The speech processor then converts the electrical signal into a speech strategy-specific electrical code. Cochlear implants have several different ways to process speech, called speech coding strategies. These strategies are the way in which the cochlear implant changes the sounds into patterns of electrical signals delivered to the cochlea needed to convey frequency, intensity, and duration information. Three common processing strategies used in cochlear implants are the Simultaneous Analog Stimulation (SAS), Continuous Interleaved Sampler (CIS), and Spectral PEAK extraction (SPEAK). Some more recent developments have incorporated parts of these strategies to form hybrid speech strategies; these include Advanced Combination Encoders (ACE) and Multiple Pulse Sample (MPS). Thirdly, the external transmitter coil of a cochlear implant sends the coded electrical signal to internal components. Information processed by the speech processor is transmitted to the internal receiver by a radio frequency carrier signal.

The internal receiver coil picks up the carrier signal from the transmitter and sends an electrical code along to the electrode array (e.g., 22 channels of electrodes). Electrodes along the array are placed along the scala tympani of the cochlea and the nerve fibers are activated in accordance with the electrical code arising from the output of speech strategy processing.

Two important criteria for cochlear implant referral are: (a) the patient must have a severe to profound bilateral sensorineural hearing loss (some corner audiograms are now also considered even when hearing thresholds at 250 and 500 Hz are less severe), and (b) more importantly, little or no benefit from hearing aids. An evaluation by a team of medical professionals is required for consideration of a cochlear implant. The cochlear implant team at minimum consists of the surgeon and audiologist. When a child is considered for implantation, a speech-language pathologist, psychologist, social worker, and educator may also be involved. The entire cochlear implant team usually participates in the evaluation and final decision on whether a patient is appropriate to receive a cochlear implant.

A medical evaluation includes a CT scan to determine the presence of a cochlea and auditory nerve, as well as an assessment of the patient's ability to cope physically with surgery. The audiology evaluation includes air conduction and bone conduction thresholds (or ABR thresholds for children too young to be tested behaviorally), tympanometry, acoustic reflex thresholds, speech reception thresholds, word recognition ability under insert earphones, and, last, aided word recognition in the sound field. A speech-language pathology evaluation will include a determination of current speech and language development.

As mentioned before, cochlear implants are approved for both children and adults. Typically, the earlier the age of implantation and/or the sooner the implantation after the onset of hearing loss, the better the prognosis for outcomes will be for the patient. Since the cochlea is adult size at birth and infant temporal bone growth can be compensated for by lengthening the electrode array, cochlear implant surgeries may be completed as early as 1 year of age.

Once a patient is determined to be eligible for a cochlear implant, surgery is scheduled. In general, cochlear implant surgery is a relatively uncomplicated surgery, at least for well-trained surgeons. The surgery can be completed in less than 3 hours under general anesthesia. The cochlear implant is programmed by an audiologist 3 to 6 weeks after the surgery (after ample time to heal). The programming visit is often referred to as *cochlear implant mapping*. The cochlear implant is programmed utilizing a computer, a device-specific software program developed by the manufacturer of the implant, and an interface box. The electrical thresholds for soft inputs and the upper limit of comfort thresholds are established at the initial visit, as well as the speech processing strategy to be used. It is often common to turn off the electrodes in which stimulation causes pain, facial twitches, and/or no improvement in hearing sensitivity. The patient may return multiple times

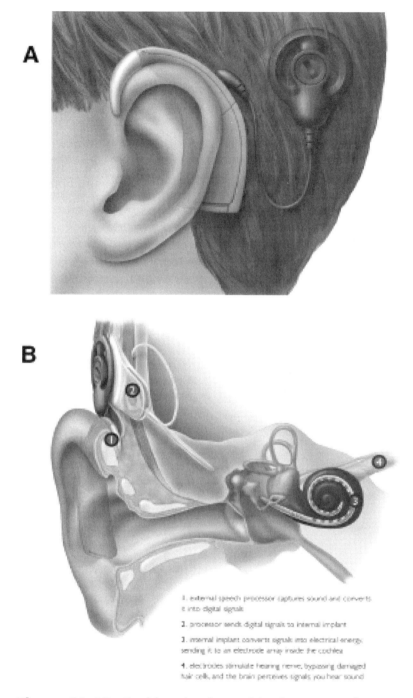

Figure 11–10. Cochlear implant with placement of external and internal CI components. Courtesy of Cochlear Corporation, Sydney, New South Wales.

within the first 6 months to 1 year for additional cochlear implant mapping sessions in order to fine-tune the cochlear implant.

Most adults with post-lingually acquired hearing loss show significant improvements in speech recognition abilities after implantation. The speech recognition abilities appear to improve and plateau for most individuals within the first 3 months and may continue to improve up to 1 year post-implant.

Outcome performance is negatively correlated with the duration of deafness and age. Following a cochlear implant, pre-lingually deafened children vary substantially with respect to their final communication mode. Some children may use spoken language only, whereas others show some use of spoken language with continued used of sign language, or rely heavily on sign language as their primary means of communication. After implantation, the road to rehabilitation is still a long and arduous process. Individuals may need counseling regarding realistic expectations, additional training with communication strategies, speech-

---

Synopsis 11–2

- There are five basic styles of hearing aids: (a) body aid, (b) behind-the-ear (BTE), (c) in-the-ear (ITE), (d) in-the-canal (ITC), and (e) completely-in-the-canal (CIC).

- The major manufacturers typically provide all of the different styles of hearing aids. A manufacturer may have different models of hearing aids (e.g., entry level, mid-level, premier) that have different features or options; however, for a given model the same processing chip usually is used in each style.

- Body aids are not used much today in the United States but may be used in developing countries.

- Body aids and BTEs have an earmold that is separate from the hearing instrument. The dispenser makes an earmold impression for a patient's ear that is sent to the manufacturer along with the request for the hearing aid. Generally, more output power can be obtained with larger instruments like a body aid or BTE; however, a good fitting earmold is essential to avoid feedback. BTEs are appropriate for young children, so that only the earmold needs to be replaced as children grow and they would not have to be without a hearing aid when the earmold is being remade.

- Mini-BTEs have become popular recently and have some of the advantages of the traditional BTE, with additional advantages of being smaller and having a very thin tube connecting to the ear canal. The mini-BTE often is used for high frequency hearing losses with an open ear fitting for more natural sound quality.

- ITEs have all of the components built into the custom-made hearing aid casing. There is no need for an earmold, since the earmold impression is used to create the custom hearing ITE aid. The ITEs were a product of technological miniaturation and became very popular for cosmetic reasons.

- ITCs and CICs are smaller versions of the ITE and have a less visible case. While these may be cosmetically appealing, they have limitations in their output levels and special features. Newer technology is being developed to reduce the feedback issue of CICs allowing an increase in the output levels and increasing the fitting range.

- BAHA (bone-anchored hearing aid) is a special hearing aid that is surgically implanted into the mastoid bone and can provide good bone conduction hearing in cases with conductive or mixed hearing losses.

- MEI (middle ear implant) is a special hearing aid (more popular in Europe than the United States) that is surgically placed into the middle ear, where the normal middle ear transduces mechanical activity into electrical stimulation of remaining hair cells and nerve fibers in the inner ear.

- Cochlear implants are composed of an array of electrodes that are implanted into a nonfunctioning cochlea and a processor on the side of the skull. The processor transduces acoustic signals into electrical signals along the electrode array to stimulate auditory nerve fibers. A candidate for a cochlear implant must have a severe/profound hearing loss and only marginal benefit from traditional amplification.

language therapy, academic support, continued instruction, and additional fine-tuning of the cochlear implant.

Hearing Aid Candidacy

As shown earlier in the workflow of the overall hearing aid fitting process, one of the steps is to determine if the patient is an appropriate candidate for hearing aids. There are several audiometric, personal, and psychological factors that impact on determining *hearing aid candidacy*. In many respects, the most straightforward factor is the hearing loss. In general, to be considered a candidate, the person should have a hearing loss (e.g., hearing thresholds of 25 dB or worse) in the frequency range of the key speech sounds (e.g., 500 to 4000 Hz). Because most hearing losses are downward sloping, a typical marginal candidate would be someone with normal hearing through 2000 Hz and a hearing loss at 3000 Hz and above, or even more marginal if he has normal hearing through 3000 Hz. It is very unlikely that someone with normal hearing through 4000 Hz would be considered a candidate for a hearing aid. Results for speech-in-noise tests also are sometimes considered in candidacy determination, that is, a person may be having considerably more speech communication difficulties than suggested by the audiogram alone.

When is a hearing loss too severe for conventional hearing aid amplification? Today, the question is whether or not to recommend a hearing aid or a cochlear implant. There are guidelines available to help make these distinctions, and often the decision is based on a combination of factors, including degree of impairment and the benefit that can be obtained using conventional hearing aids, coupled with the desires of the patient.

The patient's opinions about the use of hearing aids, of course, are critical to determining candidacy. First, the patient must believe that the hearing loss is causing a problem. A mild high frequency hearing loss could be a problem for a school teacher but perhaps not a problem at all for a retired person living alone. Secondly, the patient must have a desire to obtain treatment (the wearing of hearing aids). Along with this comes the "ownership" of the hearing problem and the desire to make things better. It is common for family members to coax or even push a loved one into the audiologist's office for the fitting of hearing aids. To satisfy their family, these individuals often purchase hearing aids, but the chances are poor that they will become satisfied hearing aid users. The prudent audiologist needs to pull together all the audiometric data and then carefully examine the thoughts and feelings of the patient when hearing aid candidacy is being decided. There are several self-assessment inventories that can be used to help determine the patients readiness for hearing aid use. These inventories measure such things as motivation, expectations, and perceived handicap and disability.

Fitting Strategies

The audiologist must work with the patient to come to some decision regarding the best hearing aid fitting arrangement. The two main fitting decisions that need to be made are:

1. When a bilateral hearing loss is present, are bilateral hearing aids the best option or would the person be better served using only one hearing aid?
2. When a unilateral hearing loss is present (i.e, one ear is unaidable) is some type of a CROS (contralateral routing of signals) hearing aid arrangement the best option?

Bilateral Hearing Aid Fittings

If we think of fitting hearing aids like we do fitting eyeglasses, then it would seem logical that two impaired ears would be fitted with two hearing aids. Unfortunately, it is not that simple. Dispensers report that approximately 80% of patients are fitted bilaterally (Johnson, 2007a). Assuming that about 90% of these individuals are candidates for two hearing aids, bilateral fittings certainly are the predominant fitting strategy. We know, however, that many of the people who purchase two hearing aids eventually become unilateral users. Although the monetary concerns of purchasing two versus one hearing aid are well understood (which partially accounts for the 20% who originally purchase one hearing aid), the decision to return or not use one of the hearing aids is not fully understood. It is difficult to identify the reason why these people do not obtain significant benefit with two hearing aids, but it may be related to the symmetry of the patient's hearing loss, the patient's central auditory processing capabilities, his ability to handle two instruments, as well as other unknown factors.

In theory, two hearing aids should provide more benefit than one, and some of the common reasons cited for this are listed in Table 11–3. Given that most patients with relatively symmetrical hearing will benefit from a bilateral fitting, and the fact that it is difficult to identify those who will not benefit, it is generally recommended to start with a bilateral fitting arrangement; then, through follow-up visits, determine if the expected benefit is present.

CROS Hearing Aid Fittings

When the hearing loss in one ear is so severe that it is unaidable, and the other ear has near normal hearing, the *contralateral routing of signals* (CROS) *hearing aid* fitting may be considered. The CROS arrangement transmits sounds that originate from the side of the head with the poor hearing ear over to the normal hearing ear. This involves placing a hearing aid on the poor hearing ear so that the microphone can pick up the sounds on that side and transmit the electrical signals to the hearing aid receiver in the good ear. This gives the patient "two-sided" hearing, although not two-eared hearing. In other words, the sounds from the poor hearing side sound different than the sounds on

Table 11–3. Some Potential Benefits of a Bilateral Versus Unilateral Hearing Aid Fitting

- Sound localization: Interaural cues for time, phase, intensity, and spectrum are required for localization in the horizontal plane.
- Speech understanding in noise: When inputs from both ears are compared in the central auditory system, there often is a "release" of noise, resulting in an improvement in the signal-to-noise ratio of 2 to 3 dB. Moreover, listening with two ears adds redundancy to the auditory system.
- Reduction of head shadow: When a hearing aid is worn on each ear, it is not necessary to position the head so the aided ear is near the talker.
- Loudness summation: At threshold, the summation effects for input from both ears are 2 to 3 dB. This effect can be as large as 5 to 8 dB at suprathreshold levels (less gain needed equals less feedback problems).
- Sound quality: When the input from two ears is balanced, and the perceived sound is "across the head," sound quality is rated higher than when the input is at an individual ear.

the good hearing side because they are going through an electronic circuit. On the good hearing side, the sounds are more natural. If the good hearing ear also has a hearing loss, then a fitting called a *bilateral CROS* (BiCROS) may be used, in which a microphone is placed on both sides, and all sounds are amplified and channeled into the good ear. There are several methods that can be used to implement a CROS fitting (see Valente, 2007, for review):

- Traditional CROS: Using a pair of BTEs, or possibly eyeglasses, the signal is transferred from the poor hearing side to the good hearing side using a wire (either behind the neck, or through the frame of the eyeglasses).
- FM CROS: Using a pair of BTEs, or a BTE and an ITE, the signal is transferred from the poor hearing ear to the good hearing ear using an FM signal.
- Transcranial CROS: Using a power custom instrument in the poor hearing ear, the signal is transferred to the good ear (actual transfer occurs via bone conduction).

- Transcranial bone conduction CROS: Using a power BTE and a bone conduction receiver in the ear, the signal is transferred to the cochlea of the good hearing ear.
- Implantable bone conduction CROS: Using an implantable BAHA device (discussed earlier), the signal is transferred from the poor hearing ear to the cochlea of the good hearing ear.

Electroacoustic Analysis

All hearing aids must meet certain performance requirements based on an *electroacoustic analysis*. There are standards from the American National Standards Institute (ANSI) that describe how hearing performance is measured. In general, this involves attaching the hearing aid to a 2-cc metal coupler, and using sweep tones and noise signals to test the aid in an isolated sound enclosure (normally referred to as a test box). When new products are developed, detailed specifications are established. These specifications (e.g., the gain and output results from the test box evaluation) are used for quality control when each product is manufactured. In other words, the product is not shipped to the audiologist unless it meets the specifications.

In general, audiologists use 2-cc coupler measures for three reasons:

- To assess the performance of the hearing aid when it arrives from the manufacturer to assure that it is performing according to specifications.
- To assist with the fitting and verification process, that is, corrections are made to the 2-cc coupler findings to predict performance in the patient's ear. This approach is commonly used with infants and young children.
- To troubleshoot a patient complaint of a faulty hearing aid, or to simply conduct an annual check of the hearing aid's performance.

Additional information regarding the electroacoustic evaluation of hearing aids can be found in the supplemental section of this chapter.

Hearing Aid Programming

The title of this section prior to the 1990s would have most likely been something like "hearing aid adjustment." At that time, adjusting the frequency characteristics of a hearing aid (with analog circuits) was accomplished using different adjustment potentiometers, which were changed with a small screwdriver. The most common adjustment was to change the frequency response, although some hearing aids also had a potentiometer for compression and maximum output. In general, even when going from max to min, the range of change was small, often imperceptible to the patient. It is likely that as students reading this book, you may never fit or even see a hearing aid with screwdriver-controlled adjustment. Instead, the audiologist does *hearing aid programming*.

Today, the audiologist clicks on handles or buttons in the computer software to change the hearing aid settings. The hearing aid settings are programmed digitally between the computer and the digital hearing aid circuit. The programmed settings can be saved to the hearing aid's memory and to a patient database in the software and stored on either a local hard drive or network server. With digital hearing aids, it is now possible to make changes on 20 or more different parameters for a single hearing aid. Moreover, the changes are significant, for example, changes in gain of up to 70 dB are achievable.

This brings up two important points: First, because there are so many parameters that can be changed, it is now possible for the trained audiologist to tailor a hearing aid fitting to achieve an optimum setting for a given patient (of course it is also possible for the untrained to really mess it up). Second, because large changes can be made in gain and output, a single model hearing aid can be used for a wide range of patients.

Computer software for hearing aids is nearly always manufacturer specific, that is, each manufacturer develops and maintains ongoing versions of a software application for fitting its hearing aid products. These software applications may either be stand-alone or may be programming modules within a larger, more universal computer software platform called *NOAH*. Stand-alone software programs are installed and assessed much like other software programs on a computer. NOAH, on the other hand, is a software system that has programming modules from different manufacturers (Figure 11–11), and a dispenser may see a wide variety of patients fit with different brands of hearing aids; thus, nearly all software programming modules need to be available to such a dispenser. The downside to multiple stand-alone software applications is the difficulty it imposes on maintaining one central patient database, as each stand-alone application has its respective patient database. In contrast, NOAH allows for execution of many different manufacturer software modules, and uses only one central patient database. NOAH even has other capabilities, such as storing real-ear probe microphone verification results, and can provide office management necessities such as scheduling, accounting, and marketing. Table 11–4 describes some of the current terminology associated with

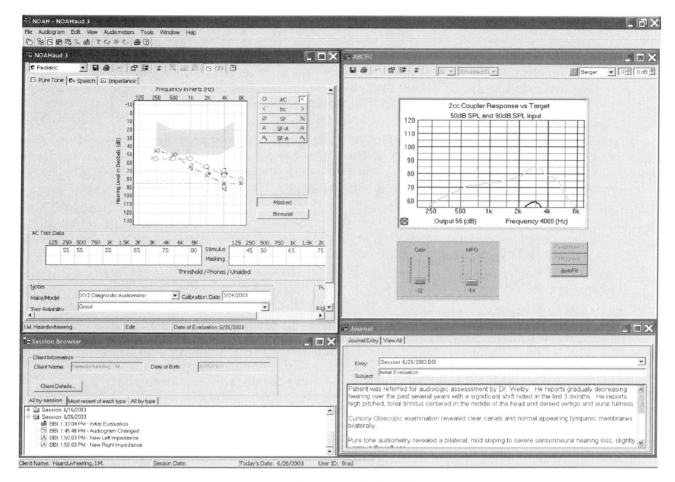

Figure 11–11. Screenshot of NOAH 3.0 software with data for sample patient entered. Courtesy of HIMSA, Eagan, Minnesota.

Table 11–4. Hearing Aid Programming Terminology

- HIMSA: Founded in 1993, HIMSA is an abbreviation for the Hearing Instrument Manufacturer Software Association. Its goal was and continues to be creating standards for integrating hearing care software. Now over 100 companies support the development and maintenance of HIMSA's primary software application, NOAH.

- NOAH: Instead of an abbreviation, NOAH is the actual name of the software application that manages modules from different hearing care companies, that is, the software is a program interface (office systems, audiometric and probe mic equipment, and hearing aids) designed to assist with managing the entire database of modules; thus, without these modules NOAH, in and of itself, is not capable of programming hearing aids. NOAH is reportedly used by approximately 70% of all hearing aid dispensers.

343

Table 11–4. (*Continued*)

- Stand-alone applications: These software applications are designed to function using general operating systems, such as Microsoft Windows, without the use of NOAH; thus, in essence, these applications are again hearing aid manufacturer specific and much akin to modules used within NOAH to program hearing aids.

- HI-PRO: HI-PRO is an acronym for a hearing instrument programmer, which is an interface between the software applications and the hardware (i.e., the hearing aid). It connects to a computer via a serial port and connects to hearing aids via programming cables. At this time, the cables are not standard across manufacturers and remain the bane of hearing instrument programming.

- NOAHlink: A wireless hearing instrument programmer that was popular just a few years ago and still is somewhat popular. It communicates with the computer via Bluetooth technology and is much faster than the HI-PRO with its serial port connection. However, the NOAHlink still connects with the hearing aids via a wired connection.

- Manufacturer-specific wireless interface between hearing aid and computer: Finally, there are no cables connecting the hearing aids back to the computer. A number of manufacturer-specific wireless interfaces are in current use. Many such interfaces attach to the computer via a universal serial bus (USB) connection and operate with Bluetooth and other wireless technology. Some interfaces still require close proximity to the hearing aid and have an intermediary device while programming that is placed over the neck and on the chest of the patient. The wireless connection has freed up a lot of real estate, particularly on small pinnae for use of real-ear verification measures, which is in essence all about making sure the hearing aids are programmed as the professional and/or patient desires and that the hearing aid settings are documented.

hearing aid programming. Although the software from different companies is similar, it is different enough that each has a significant learning curve. Most audiologists fit the majority of their hearing aids from two or three companies, and therefore become familiar with this specific software.

The interface device that connects the hearing aid that is to be programmed and the software application needs further discussion. Traditionally, the most commonly used device has been the *Hearing Instrument Programmer* (HI-PRO) (Figure 11–12). The HI-PRO uses a serial port and specially designed cables, again manufacturer specific, to link the hearing aids to the HI-PRO box. More recently, the HI-PRO is being replaced with wireless transmission systems. The most common device is called the NOAHlink (Figure 11–13). This system, even though it is wireless, is much faster than serial ports, with maximum transmission speeds of 115,000 bits per second and connection rates of 3 megabytes per second (Mbps) in a Bluetooth 2.0 implementation. The Hearing Instrument Manufacturers' Software Association (HIMSA) recently reported that programming that used to take 30 seconds with the HI-PRO is completed in only 3 to 6 seconds with a NOAHlink.

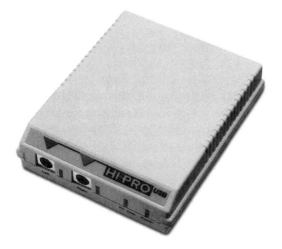

Figure 11–12. HI-PRO hearing aid interface unit that is used to program hearing aids. Courtesy of GN Otometrics, Schaumburg, Illinois.

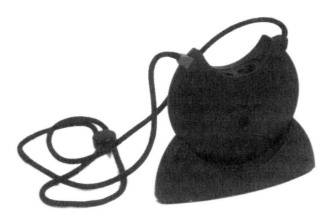

Figure 11–13. NOAHlink interface unit, used to program hearing aids. Courtesy of GN Otometrics Schaumburg, Illinois.

Today, almost all manufactures have begun introducing their own wireless programming interfaces in part because of new product model introductions with wireless capabilities but also to further speed up the connection between the hearing aid and the programming software.

Prescriptive Fitting Methods

In the preceding section we discussed "programming" the instruments. A reasonable question might be: "What do we program them to?" Desired hearing aid gain and output for the patient is first selected using a validated *prescriptive fitting method* (for review, see Mueller, 2005), that is, a mathematic model of selecting gain and output, based on the patient's hearing loss that has been shown to provide the best outcome, should be used when programming the hearing aids. Ear canal gain and output target levels are used as the prescription. Although the exact prescriptive targets may not be the ideal fitting for all patients, it has been shown that they will optimize the fitting for the *average* patient. Given the large variety of hearing aid settings, it is important to have a good starting point. Two fitting methods that are currently used are:

■ National Acoustic Laboratories' (NAL) Non-Linear method v.2 (*NAL-NL2*). See http://www.nal.gov.au
■ Desired Sensation Level method v.5 (*DSLm[i/o]*). See http://www.dslio.com

In general, most audiologists use the NAL method with adults and the DSL method with children. However, in Australia, where the NAL-NL2 method was developed, it is also used with children, whereas in Canada, where the DSLv5 was developed, it remains popular for adult hearing aid fittings. In essence, the methods are appropriate for both populations and ongoing comparison work between the two methods continues. In addition to the desired targets for gain and output, these software programs also provide guidance for the selection of compression parameters. Some hearing aid manufacturers have developed their own prescriptive approaches, which are implemented in their fitting software. However, these methods do not have the supporting research of the NAL-NL2 or the DSL *m*[i/o]. Screenshots of NAL-NL2 and the DSL *m*[i/o] are shown in Figure 11–14 and Figure 11–15, respectively.

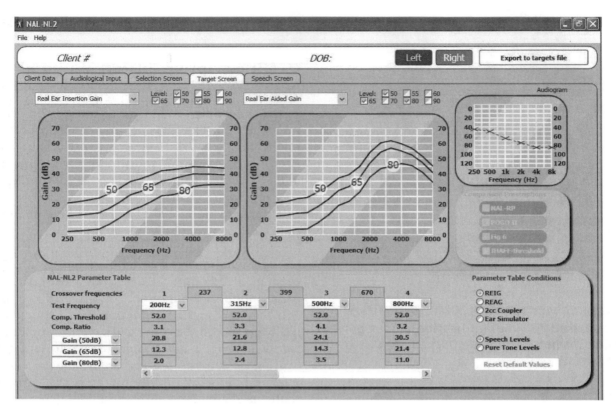

Figure 11–14. NAL-NL2 software screenshot. Courtesy of the Australian National Acoustics Laboratory, Sydney, New South Wales.

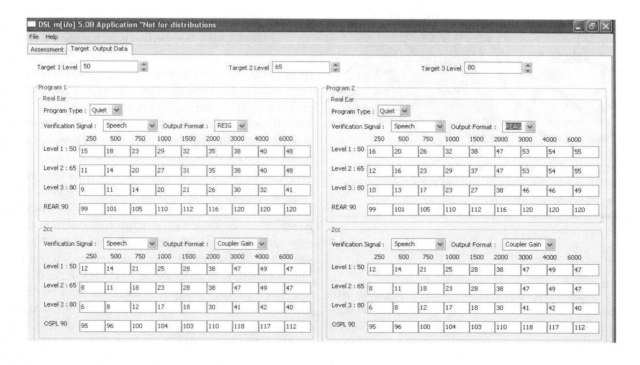

Figure 11–15. DSL Multiple input/output software screenshot. Courtesy of University of Western Ontario, London, Ontario.

Hearing Aid Verification

As mentioned in the preceding section, hearing aids typically are programmed according to a prescriptive fitting method that is appropriate for the patient's hearing loss. It is important to verify that the prescriptive fitting method produces the appropriate ear canal output when the hearing aids are actually being worn by the patient. In other words, just because prescriptive targets are met on the simulated version shown on the fitting screen, this does not assure that the SPL values are correct in the individual's ear. This measurement is accomplished using probe-microphone *real-ear measures* in which a thin silicone tube is placed in the ear canal and is attached to a measurement microphone, which measures the aided ear canal levels for externally produced signals such as speech. The preferred method is to deliver calibrated real speech at input levels ranging from soft to loud. This procedure is often referred to as "speech mapping." In addition to probe-mic measures, *verification* can take many other forms, but in general the audiologist is looking for a fitting that maximizes audibility and speech understanding, has good sound quality, restores loudness perceptions, and is acceptable to the patient (see Mueller, 2007, for review). The verification process, therefore, could address any or all of these factors, and ideally would include aided speech testing and aided loudness measures. More information regarding probe-microphone measurements and the verification process is included in the Supplemental Topic section of this chapter.

Hearing Aid Orientation

Following the verification of hearing aid performance, the patient then receives a *hearing aid orientation* involving extensive counseling and hands-on instruction on the use and care of the new hearing aids. This portion of the fitting process cannot be slighted, as the first few weeks of ownership are critical regarding hearing aid use and acceptance (recall the earlier statistic that about 15% of people who own hearing aids do not use them).

Many times the hearing aids are not used simply because the patient becomes frustrated with the basic operation and handling of the instruments during those first few days. The best circuitry is the world doesn't help much if the patient is unable to properly fit the hearing aid in the ear. Frequent follow-up phone calls and clinic visits are essential. Some clinics offer group classes for new hearing aid users that are very helpful.

Validation of Hearing Aid Benefit

The next step in the fitting process is to conduct some measure of *validation*. By validation we mean one or more measures to determine if the fitting was successful during real-world use. Typically, this involves using a self-assessment inventory, which is completed by the patient. There are many of these types of questionnaires available; some are rather informal and others have been researched extensively. One reason there are so many different questionnaires is that there are many different ways to measure success with hearing aids. Normally, we are interested in both benefit and satisfaction, although you could have one without the other. Hearing aid use is highly correlated with satisfaction, so this is an important area of interest, too. We also, of course, would like to know if the hearing aids improved the patient's social and emotional well-being; and maybe most importantly, did the intervention improve his or her quality of life?

One easy to use and well-researched questionnaire which incorporates many of the factors related to success is the *International Outcome Inventory for Hearing Aids* (IOI-HA). It is displayed in Table 11–5. This inventory is relatively easy to administer and score and is available in several languages. An advantage of this scale is that it addresses many of the different areas of "hearing aid success" that we have mentioned. Again, the purpose of the validation process is to assure that the fitting is beneficial and that the patient is satisfied. If low scores are observed, the patient should be targeted for more counseling, and in some cases, adjustments to the fitting should be considered.

Table 11–5. INTERNATIONAL OUTCOME INVENTORY—HEARING AIDS (IOI-HA)

- Think about how much you used your present hearing aid(s) over the past two weeks. On an average day, how many hours did you use the hearing aid(s)?

none	less than 1 hours a day	1 to 4 hours a day	4 to 8 hours a day	more than 8 hours a day
❏	❏	❏	❏	❏

- Think about the situation where you most wanted to hear better, before you got your present hearing aid(s). Over the past two weeks, how much has the hearing aid helped in that situation?

helped not at all	helped slightly	helped moderately	helped quite a lot	helped very much
❏	❏	❏	❏	❏

- Think again about the situation where you most wanted to hear better. When you use your present hearing aid(s), how much difficulty do you STILL have in that situation?

very much difficulty	quite a lot of difficulty	moderate difficulty	slight difficulty	no difficulty
❏	❏	❏	❏	❏

- Considering everything, do you think your present hearing aid(s) is worth the trouble?

not at all worth it	slightly worth it	moderately worth it	quite a lot worth it	very much worth it
❏	❏	❏	❏	❏

- Over the past two weeks, with your present hearing aid(s), how much have your hearing difficulties affected the things you can do?

affected very much	affected quite a lot	affected moderately	affected slightly	affected not at all
❏	❏	❏	❏	❏

- Over the past two weeks, with your present hearing aid(s), how much do you think other people were bothered by your hearing difficulties?

bothered very much	bothered quite a lot	bothered moderately	bothered slightly	bothered not at all
❏	❏	❏	❏	❏

- Considering everything, how much has your present hearing aid(s) changed your enjoyment of life?

worse	no change	slightly better	quite a lot better	very much better
❏	❏	❏	❏	❏

English Version

Translations of the International Outcome Inventory for Hearing Aids (IOI-HA)   Cox/Stephens/Kramer   9

Dispenser Practice Characteristics

Now that we have provided a brief review of hearing aid technology, selection, strategies, fitting procedures, and validation measures, we end with a general discussion about hearing aid dispensing.

Who Can Dispense Hearing Aids?

The term *dispenser* may refer to either a hearing instrument specialist or an audiologist, both of whom may legally dispense hearing aids if they have a professional license to do so in their state of practice. Hearing instrument specialists (non-audiologists) must have a hearing aid dispenser's license. Audiologists in many states can dispense hearing aids as part of their audiology license; however, in some states, they must also hold the dispensing license. In addition to a state dispensing license, dispensers may also have special certifications as well. The most popular certification for hearing instrument specialists is the BC-HIS, which stands for Board Certified in Hearing Instrument Services. In addition, audiologists are typically certified by professional organizations, such as the American Speech-Language-Hearing Association (ASHA) or the American Board of Audiology (ABA). Board certification is not required for dispensing hearing aids; however, a state license is always required. It is estimated that outside of the Veterans Affairs (where essentially all hearing aids are dispensed by audiologists), approximately 60% of hearing aids are dispensed by audiologists.

Where Do Dispensers Work and How Much Do They Earn?

The most common work locations for hearing instrument specialists are personally owned private practices, manufacturer owned practices, retail chain practices (e.g., Costco), and physicians' offices. Dispensing audiologists usually work in similar environments, but may also be employed in schools, hospitals, government agencies, and universities or colleges. On the whole, the salaries of audiologists and hearing instrument specialists are pretty similar. Typically, dispensers and audiologists working for themselves in private practice have the highest earned salaries (in the $100,000 range), while dispensers working as full-time employees of an agency report earnings in the $50,000 to $70,000 range (Kirkwood, 2006a). While many factors certainly affect salary, the top correlates are work experience, gender, educational degree, and work location (e.g., school versus private practice) (Kirkwood, 2006a).

How Many and What Kind of Hearing Aids Are Sold?

Dispensing audiologists and hearing instrument specialists generally report selling between 15 and 25 hearing aids a month. While 25 hearing aids per month may sound daunting, given that the percentage rates of bilateral fitting (a hearing aid for each ear) is approximately 80%, it translates to about 15 new patients per month. A general rule of thumb for successful practice is to sell, on average, one hearing aid per workday.

The average patient price per hearing aid is around $1,800 to $2,000 for a mid-level hearing aid product (Johnson, 2007a; Kirkwood, 2006b). The price range can extend from approximately $800 to $1000 for low-end products to $2700 to $3300 for high-end products. In general, smaller, custom products, such as CICs, are more expensive. The BTE aid does, however, require an earmold that costs around $50. These data have not changed significantly since the 2006 survey.

Perhaps surprisingly to some readers, the dispenser's cost of the hearing aid is usually about 25 to 45% of the patient's price, depending on the negotiated sales contract with each manufacturer. The dispenser's markup helps ensure that he can cover all practice-related expenses, as well as ensure a salary for his hired employees and himself. Moreover, it is common among dispensing audiologists to provide all hearing aid follow-up service free-of-charge, so to some extent the patient is pre-paying for their care for the life of the hearing aid. One of the biggest factors that can decrease the unit cost per hearing aid to the dispenser is by dispensing more hearing aids from a particular manufacturer; this is sometimes referred to as a volume discount. Some ethical concerns exist on this topic, as some audiologists believe that this incentive biases dispensers toward choosing a particular manufacturer, rather than selecting a hearing aid to address the unique needs of a patient. Other audiologists, however, contend that as long as the manufacturer offers enough unique products and product features in its hearing aid product line, a suitable hearing aid for almost any patient can be chosen from that manufacturer's product line; thus, the use of a particular manufacturer to obtain a volume discount is not an ethical concern (Hawkins, Hamill, & Kukula, 2006).

Although the specific manufacturer and product model can vary from dispenser to dispenser, the available choices are now decreasing due to consolidation of hearing aid companies. There are a number of smaller companies (20 to 25) that manufacture hearing aids or purchase and rebrand products from bigger manufacturers; however, may of these smaller companies are owned by the larger ones. Strom (2006) identified the six largest companies referring to them simply as the "Big 6": these included GNReSound, Oticon, Phonak, Starkey, Siemens, and Widex. Generally, each of these companies carries four to six distinct product models, covering a low- to high-end product range, in several different hearing aid styles (e.g., BTE, mini-BTE, ITE, and CIC).

The naming of product models is a complex coordination of marketing and advertising efforts by the manufacturer. These efforts may not be directed as much toward selling hearing aids to patients as they are for selling hearing aids to audiologists. Often, the audiologist makes the decision regarding the specific hearing aid, although most audiologists usually ask their patients several questions about their individual hearing needs and likes/dislikes. Kochkin (2002) reported that only 4 out of 10 patients were even aware of the name of the manufacturer of their hearing aids prior to purchase, and fewer were knowledgeable about the names of the different models. While most dispensing practices use two to four manufacturers (Strom, 2006), 95% of dispensers have a preference for one manufacturer and approximately 75% of an individual dispenser's hearing aid products are sold from that manufacturer (Johnson, 2007b; Johnson, Mueller, & Ricketts, 2009).

Summary

As the discipline of audiology has evolved and progressed over the years, the evaluation and fitting of hearing aids has been a constant companion. As we have outlined in this chapter, there are several important steps in the overall fitting process. The digital technology of today's hearing aids has improved to the extent that it is not so much *what* the hearing aid can do, but rather, does the audiologist have the skills to program this technology to make the hearing aid perform at its maximum for a given patient? The theoretical fitting algorithms and real-ear verification techniques allow a tailoring of the hearing aid fitting that was not possible only a few years ago. Of course, it is critical to involve the patient in the decision making along the way, and to provide the post-fitting counseling that is necessary for optimum benefit and satisfaction. Properly fitted hearing aids can change a person's life, and the audiologist is the person to make this happen.

Synopsis 11–3

- The hearing aid evaluation begins by determining candidacy for a hearing aid. Generally, there should be some degree of hearing loss that involves frequencies 3000 Hz and lower. The decision should also include the needs, motivation, and abilities of the patient.

- Bilateral fittings are generally recommended when there is a bilateral hearing loss, and about 80% of fittings are bilateral; however, there are some patients who do not seem to get the expected benefit from two hearing aids, possibly due to asymmetric hearing loss, central auditory problems, difficulty handling the instruments, or other unknown reasons.

- CROS fittings are options for unilateral hearing loss. CROS hearing aids pick up sounds on the poorer hearing ear and transmit them to the better hearing ear. A BiCROS hearing aid arrangement can also include some amplification in the better hearing ear if needed.

- Electroacoustic analyses are obtained in a hearing aid test box with the hearing aid attached to a small (2-cc) coupler, in order to see if it meets certain standards (ANSI) (see Supplemental Topic for more details of the electroacoustic analysis as part of the verification steps).

- The frequency and output settings, as well as other special features, are programmed by a computer (to which the hearing aid is attached). NOAH is a computer platform that has many of the manufacturers' software packages installed for easy access.

- The dispenser programs a digital hearing aid using accepted prescriptive algorithms, which have been validated by research to provide the best gain across the frequencies for a particular hearing loss. These prescriptive algorithms provide targets that the programmer tries to meet in order to optimize the hearing aid fitting for a particular patient. The two most popular prescriptive fitting methods are the NAL-NL2 (National Acoustics Laboratory Nonlinear method used mostly for adults) and the DSL-5 (Desired Sensation Level v.5) used mostly for children.

- In the verification step, the dispenser determines if the prescriptive fittings are actually achieved and are acceptable to the patient. The verification is done using real-ear probe microphone measures obtained from the patient's ear canal while he is wearing the hearing aid (see Supplemental Topic for more details).

- In the validation step, the dispenser is interested in the patient's opinion on the benefits he is getting from his hearing aids, and how satisfied he is with their use. These opinions are usually obtained using various self-assessment inventories, such as the International Outcome Inventory for Hearing Aids (IOI-HA).

- Hearing aids can only be dispensed by licensed practitioners. Audiologists can dispense hearing aids if they have a state license to do so. Most audiologists have extensive academic graduate education as well as professional certification. Hearing aids may also be dispensed by hearing instrument specialists (nonaudiologists) who typically do not have an advanced degree and who are primarily operating a business practice.

Supplemental Topic: Electroacoustic and Real-Ear Verification

Electroacoustic Characteristics of Hearing Aids

The standard for electroacoustic performance characteristics of hearing aids is the American National Standards Institute (ANSI) S3.22. Revisions to the original standard written in 1977 have occurred in 1987, 1996, and 2003. An electroacoustic analysis takes only a few minutes and is an important quantifiable method of documenting hearing aid performance. Electroacoustic analysis can be performed before a hearing aid fitting to be sure that the instrument is performing according to specifications and can be performed after a hearing aid fitting to ensure that the desired electroacoustic performance is maintained.

Electroacoustic measurements are performed inside a hearing aid test box using a reference microphone to monitor the level of the input signal and another microphone to measure the hearing aid output in a 2-cc coupler (a hard cavity that estimates the volume of an ear canal with the hearing aid in place). This standard 2-cc coupler may either be an HA-1 or HA-2 style. With an HA-1 coupler, the receiver of the hearing aid is placed into a large opening, and puttylike material is placed around the case of the hearing aid to seal off the opening. An HA-2 coupler can be used for attaching to a body aid button type receiver or a BTE aid, by using an additional snap-on earmold tubing attachment. Table 11–6 defines the main electroacoustic measures obtained on most hearing aids.

Table 11–6. Simplified Definitions of Electroacoustic Measurements

- Output Sound Pressure Level (OSPL90): Represents the maximum output level in dB SPL the hearing aid is able to produce with an input of 90 dB.
- High Frequency Average (HFA) OSPL90: The average output for a 90 dB input at 1000, 1600, and 2500 Hz, or at three special-purpose average frequencies.
- High Frequency Average Full-On Gain (HFA FOG): Average difference between the output SPL in a 2-cc coupler and the input SPL set to the hearing aid's full-on position at 1000, 1600, and 2500 Hz, or at three special-purpose average frequencies.
- High Frequency Average Reference-Test Gain (HFA RTG): Average difference between the output SPL in a 2-cc coupler and the input SPL in a 2-cc coupler at 1000, 1600, and 2500 Hz, or at three special-purpose average frequencies with the hearing aid set to its RTG position. The RTG position is described as HFA-OSPL90: 77 dB.
- Frequency Range: The useful range of frequencies that fall within a lower and upper designated frequency. The useful range is defined as the frequencies that have greater output SPL values than the HFA output response level: 20 dB at the hearing aid's RTG position.
- Total Harmonic Distortion (THD): Unwanted signals created by the hearing aid that occur at integer multiples of an input sine wave. It is most often reported at test frequencies of 500, 800, and 1600 Hz. For each test frequency, the power of all distortion products is summed and expressed relative to the power of the wanted output signal in a percentage value.
- Equivalent Input Noise (EIN): The internal noise generated by microphones and amplifiers in the hearing aid.

Clinical Verification Procedures for Hearing Aid Fittings

Verification can take many forms, but in general the audiologist develops a "gold standard" of what is an acceptable fitting, and then conducts testing to determine if that standard has been met. Typically, verification procedures fall into one of these following four categories, and often is a combination of these categories.

Probe Microphone (Real-Ear) Measurements

The most reliable method to verify the performance of a hearing aid and its relation to the preferred validated fitting method (following published protocols and best practice guidelines) is to measure the output of the hearing aid at the tympanic membrane of the hearing aid user. This is referred to as *probe microphone verification* or *real-ear verification*. The verification is accomplished by placing a small silicone tube in the ear canal that is attached to a measurement microphone. A loudspeaker is used to present the input to the hearing aid while being worn by the patient, and the output near the tympanic membrane is analyzed using computerized equipment (Figure 11–16 and Figure 11–17). It is usually desirable to use calibrated real speech as the input signal, although other signals (e.g., speech-shaped noise) also are satisfactory. As mentioned before, when speech is used as the input signal, the verification process often is referred to as "speech mapping."

As the term "verification" suggests, the purpose of these measurements is to assure that the hearing aid output meets a pre-determined standard—the most basic is simply that soft speech has been made audible. The prudent audiologist will deliver the speech signal at different input levels and make changes in the hearing aid programming and verify these changes on the patient until the programming meets the recommended standard. In addition to verification of gain and frequency response, the equipment has a variety of other uses in the evaluation of hearing aids and

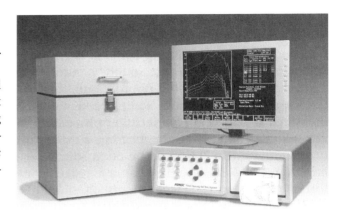

Figure 11–16. Test equipment used to assess 2-cc coupler and real-ear performance of hearing aids. Courtesy of Frye Electronics, Tigard, Oregon.

assistive listening devices: It can be used to assess the real-ear function of compression characteristics, directional microphones, digital noise reduction, frequency lowering, feedback suppression, telecoil sensitivity, and many other features.

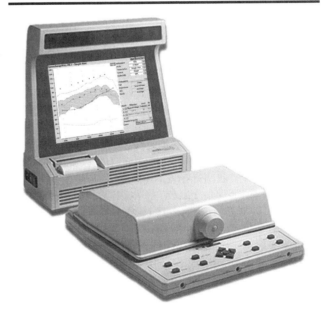

Figure 11–17. Test equipment used to assess 2-cc coupler and real-ear performance of hearing aids. Courtesy of Audioscan Dorchester, Ontario.

Ratings of Loudness

A general goal of the fitting process is to make soft sounds audible, average sounds comfortable, and loud sounds loud—but not too loud. It is useful, therefore, to conduct some aided loudness measures as part of the verification procedure. In general, when wearing the hearing aids, inputs of around 45 dB SPL should be rated soft, inputs around 65 dB SPL should be rated average (comfortable), and inputs around 85 dB SPL should be rated loud, but not uncomfortably loud (see Mueller, 1999). Gain and compression can be adjusted to assure that these ratings are appropriate. The fitting software from different manufacturers also has several different types of speech and real-world environmental sounds that can be used for this testing. An important measure, using environmental sounds, is to ensure that high level inputs do not exceed the patient's loudness discomfort level. Protocols for this testing are available (Mueller & Hall, 1998).

Clinical Speech Measures

Because the patient usually enters the hearing aid fitting process because of difficulty understanding speech, it seems logical that the verification procedure should measure his ability to understand aided speech. Although this seems logical, because of the poor sensitivity of most speech material, it is difficult in clinical practice to use outcomes of speech testing for selecting the best hearing aid frequency response or signal processing strategy—the probe-mic measures are used for this. However, in some cases, speech testing can provide useful information as to the suitability of the hearing aids. In other words, is wearing the hearing aids better than not wearing the hearing aids, as determined by scores on unaided versus aided clinical speech measures? This unaided testing can be conducted for speech in quiet, or in background noise. Although this is not useful for selecting the *best* hearing aid setting or arrangement, it may be useful in demonstrating to the patient the benefits of amplification. The aided speech re-

sults, especially if background noise is included, adds useful information for counseling.

References

Dillon, H. (2001). *Hearing aids*. Turramurra, Australia: Boomerang Press.

Dillon, H. (2010, August). *Mild hearing loss is serious business*. Keynote address presented at the International Hearing Research Conference, Lake Tahoe, CA.

Dillon, H. (2012) *Hearing aids* (2nd Edition) New York: Thieme Medical Publishers.

Edwards, B. (2006). What outsiders tell us about the hearing industry. *Hearing Review, 13*, 88–93.

Glista, D., & Scollie, S. (2009). Modified verification approaches for frequency lowering devices. Retrieved November 20, 2009 from http://www.audiology online.com/articles/modified-verification-approaches -for-frequency-871/.

Hawkins, D., Hamill, T. A., & Kukula, J. (2006). Ethics in hearing. *Audiology Today, 18*, 22–29.

Johnson, E. E. (2006). Segmenting dispensers: Factors in the selection of open-canal fittings. *Hearing Journal, 59*(11), 58–64.

Johnson, E. E. (2007a). Survey finds higher sales and prices, plus more open fittings and directional mics. *Hearing Journal, 60*(4), 52–58.

Johnson, E. E. (2007b). Survey explores how dispensers use and choose their preferred hearing aid brands. *Hearing Journal, 60*(3), 23–36.

Johnson, E. E., Mueller, H. G., & Ricketts, T. A. (2009). Statistically-derived factors of varied importance to audiologists when making a hearing aid brand preference decision. *Journal of the Academy of Audiology, 20*(1), 40–48.

Kirkwood, D. (2006a). Survey probes the economic realities of the dispensing business. *Hearing Journal, 59*(3), 19–32.

Kirkwood, D. (2006b). Survey: Dispensers fitted more hearing aids in 2005 at higher prices. *Hearing Journal, 59*(4), 40–50.

Kochkin, S. (1998). MarkeTrak IV: Correlates of hearing aid purchase intent. *Hearing Journal, 51*(1), 30–41.

Kochkin, S. (2002). Factors impacting consumer choice of dispenser and hearing aid brand: Use of ALDs and computers. *Hearing Review, 9*(12), 14–23.

Kochkin, S. (2005a). MarkeTrak VII: Hearing loss population continues to increase along with satisfaction ratings for hearing instruments. *Hearing Review, 12*(7), 16, 18, 19, 22-29.

Kochkin, S. (2005b). *Hearing loss and its impact on household income: A special report on new data generated by the Better Hearing Institute. Hearing Review, 12*(10), 16-24.

Kochkin, S., Luxford, W., Northern, J., Mason, P., & Tharpe, A. M. (2007). Hearing loss in America being left behind? *Hearing Review, 14*(10), 10-34.

Litovsky, R. Y., Colburn, H. S., Yost, W. A., & Guzman, S. J. (1999). The precedence effect. Review and tutorial paper, *Journal of the Acoustical Society of America, 106,* 1633-1654.

Mejia, J., & Dillon, H. (2010). A system and method for producing a directional output signal. *WIPO Patent Application* WO/2010/051606.

Meija, J., Keidser, G., Dillon, H., Cong-Van N., & Johnson, E. (2011). *The effect of linked bilateral noise reduction processing on speech in noise performance.* International Symposium on Auditory and Audiological Research, Nyborg, Denmark (August).

Mueller, H. G. (1999). Just make it audible, comfortable and loud but okay. *Hearing Journal, 52*(1), 10-17.

Mueller, H. G. (2005). Fitting hearing aids to adults using prescriptive methods: An evidence-based review of effectiveness. *Journal of the American Academy of Audiology, 16*(7), 448-460.

Mueller, H. G. (2007). Hearing aid verification: Old concepts and new considerations. In C. Palmer & R. Seewald (Eds.), *Hearing care for adults 2006* (pp. 155-165). Staefa, Switzerland: Phonak AG.

Mueller, H. G., & Hall, J. W. (1998). *Audiologists' desk reference.* San Diego, CA: Singular.

Mueller, H. G., & Ricketts, T. A. (2005). Digital noise reduction. *Hearing Journal, 56*(1), 10-17.

Ricketts, T. (2001). Directional hearing aids. *Trends in Amplification, 5*(4), 139-176.

Strom, K. (2006). The HR 2006 dispenser survey. *Hearing Review, 13*(6), 16-39.

Valente, M. (2007). Fitting options for adults with unilateral hearing loss. *Hearing Journal, 60*(8), 10-17.

Wallach, H., Newman, E. B., & Rosenzweig, M. R. (1949). The precedence effect in sound localization. *American Journal of Psychology, 62,* 315-336.

PART III

PERSPECTIVES ON THE PROFESSION OF AUDIOLOGY

Now that you have a good foundation in hearing sciences, basic audiological tests, and hearing aids, you might find yourself intrigued by the possibility of joining the audiology profession. Yes, even if you have been thinking about speech-language pathology, nursing, optometry, rehabilitation counseling, or some other field, it is OK to change directions and pursue a career in audiology. According to the U.S. Bureau of Labor Statistics (2012) there is a 37% (much faster than average) projected job growth in audiology over the next decade.

In this final part of the textbook, we provide you with some basic information about the profession of audiology. I hope this section provides you with an appreciation for the rewarding aspects of being involved in a professional career and interactions with other professionals. In Chapter 12, you will learn what is required to become an audiologist. You will also learn what kinds of settings audiologists practice in, and what kinds of activities might fill their week. You will become familiar with the varied paths you might take within audiology, and the extensive scope of practice that defines the skills of audiologists. Chapter 12 also presents some current demographic trends in audiology, as summarized from regular surveys conducted by our professional organizations. Finally, in Chapter 13, Dr. James Jerger, a pioneer and continuing contributor to clinical research that has defined our field, concludes this textbook with a chapter, co-authored with Dr. DeConde Johnson, on the history of the profession of audiology and how the field has changed over the past half century. I trust that you will gain an appreciation of audiology as a career, either for yourself or in your interactions with audiologists.

12

Audiology as a Career

Audiology is a discipline that focuses on the study of normal hearing and hearing disorders. More precisely, audiology is a health care profession devoted to hearing identification, assessment, treatment/rehabilitation, prevention, and the effects of hearing loss on related communication disorders. An *audiologist* is a professional who has the appropriate degree and license (in their state) to practice audiology, and who is, typically, certified by a professional board. The expanded definition of an audiologist would also include their involvement with the assessment and treatment of vestibular disorders. The main professional organization for audiologists is the *American Academy of Audiology (AAA)* (http://www.audiology.org). In addition, many audiologists are associated with the *American Speech-Language-Hearing Association (ASHA)* (http://www.asha.org), *Academy of Doctors of Audiology (ADA)* (http://www.audiologist.org), *American Auditory Society (AAS)* (http://www.amauditorysoc.org), *Educational Audiology Association (EAA)* (http://www.edaud.org), and/or *Academy of Rehabilitative Audiology (ARA)* (http://www.audrehab.org). A wealth of information about the field of audiology and career as an audiologist can be found on these and other websites.

Audiologists are educated and clinically trained as generalists in the areas of diagnostic assessment of patients with hearing or balance disorders, as well as performing hearing aid evaluations. Although many employment settings involve a wide range of activities and populations, there are different disciplines on which an audiologist may choose to concentrate, and many audiologists choose to be involved in more than one of these disciplines. Some examples of different disciplines (not necessarily mutually exclusive) include:

■ **Pediatric audiologist:** interested and skilled in special audiological techniques of assessment and treatment of infants and children; good at counseling and working with families and referral agencies. Often works in a facility primarily serving children, such as a children's hospital.

■ **Geriatric audiologist:** interested and skilled in assessment and treatment of elderly patients; experienced with the Medicare system; typically works in a Veteran's Hospital or university clinic.

■ **Hearing aid dispensing audiologist:** engages in the fitting and selling of hearing aids as part of their audiologic practice; typically works in a private practice, but may also work in a medical or university setting.

■ **Educational audiologist:** provides hearing assessment and hearing aid management of children in schools; part of a team that provides input to the child's educational plan and needs as they relate to their hearing abilities; may also engage in evaluation of auditory processing disorders; works in a school district, often as an itinerant that services several schools.

■ **Military audiologist:** an enlisted audiologist who performs assessment and treatment of armed services personnel, recruits, and their families; works in a community-based military hospital.

■ **Industrial audiologist:** specializes in consulting with industrial companies with potentially excessive noise levels, to establish appropriate hearing conservation programs to monitor noise levels, assess hearing, and educate employees and employers about protecting their hearing; contracts with companies.

■ **Academic audiologist:** a clinically educated and credentialed faculty member who is part of a university audiology program; may teach, conduct research, and supervise students in a university-based clinic.

■ **Research audiologist:** engages in hearing research, usually of an applied nature; funded by a grant; works in private research institutes or in companies that provide test equipment or hearing aids.

■ **Forensic audiologist:** specializes in legal cases related to hearing loss cases, and issues related to environmental or industrial noise; gives occasional depositions or testimony on trial cases; usually done outside of a regular job as an audiologist.

■ **Intraoperative monitoring specialist:** skilled in evoked potentials in a variety of modalities; high level of knowledge in neurology and anatomy; assists surgeons in the operating room; often contracts with hospitals.

Audiologists work with many other professionals. The medical expert in hearing disorders is the physician. The medical specialty related to the ears is called *otology*, which is practiced by appropriately trained and certified *otologists*, also called neuro-otologists, otolaryngologists, or ear, nose, and throat (ENT) specialists. The *American Academy of Otolaryngology-Head and Neck Surgery (AAO-HNS)* is one of the professional organizations for otologists. Another professional organization, called the *American Auditory Society (AAS)*, is a multidisciplinary professional organization that includes otolaryngologists, audiologists, and hearing scientists. Audiologists also work closely with *speech-language pathologists*, who are ASHA certified and/or licensed professionals who engage in prevention, assessment, and treatment of speech and language disorders, including those who have hearing loss.

Education and Professional Requirements

Today, the entry-level degree to practice clinical audiology is a professional doctorate, most commonly the *Doctor of Audiology (AuD)*. The AuD is a 4-year graduate degree composed of a comprehensive curriculum with about 2,000 to 3,000 hr of clinical experiences under the supervision and precepting of licensed audiology preceptors. The AuD is different from the research doctorate (PhD), which has been available in audiology and hearing sciences since its inception for those interested in research and/or an academic position. The move from a clinical master's degree to a professional doctoral degree began in the late 1980s and was a mantra of the AAA from its inception. In 1993, ASHA endorsed the plan to transition to the doctoral degree, with a final implementation by 2007. The first AuD program became available in 1993 at Baylor College of Medicine in Houston (which subsequently closed). As of 2012, there

are 74 audiology doctoral programs in the country (http://www.audiology.org).

Students entering audiology clinical doctoral programs come from a variety of disciplines, such as speech and hearing, psychology, engineering, music, physics, computer science, neuroscience, medicine, nursing, and business to name a few. Most doctoral programs expect entering students to have had some prerequisites in physical, life, social, and behavioral sciences, as well as some statistics or advanced level math. Audiology is a scientific discipline and requires a relatively strong science foundation and an ability to meet the challenges of a rigorous curriculum.

The curricula for AuD programs are quite similar across programs, and are partially driven by the professional accreditation standards, as well as specific requirements for professional certification. A list and links to doctoral programs can be found on the AAA and ASHA websites. There are, however, differences across programs in the number of faculty, the breadth of academic courses, the variety and amount of clinical experiences, and the amount of research available to students. While programs share a similar general core of courses, a program may have strengths in one or more areas, or may provide more advanced preparation in core areas, such as hearing aids, electrophysiology, vestibular assessment, cochlear implants, business practice, and/or otology. As part of the program, students typically obtain supervised clinical experiences. Some programs have on-campus clinics where students begin their clinical experiences, and then obtain additional clinical experiences in community hospitals, clinics, or other agencies. Other programs may rely solely on the community resources for the clinical experiences. Students should explore several programs prior to making a decision on where to apply and/or attend—after all, you will be there for 4 years.

Typically, the fourth year of the doctoral program is called an *externship*, which is usually the equivalent to full-time clinical experience (for 12 months) at an approved clinical site, which has agreed to provide a preceptor to supervise, educate, and mentor the extern during that final year of their program, prior to entering the profession as an audiologist. Externships are often located throughout the country and in many cases where one does the externship may be in a different location than where the program resides. Externships are established with agencies through specific affiliation agreements developed between the externship site and the doctoral program's institution. Most externship placements require the student apply for an available position, interview, and wait to see if offered the position. In the best case scenario, the student may be in a position to choose among more than one offer. Keep in mind, however, that the externship is part of the doctoral program, and the extern's progress is monitored by a designee of the doctoral program, and the externship preceptor is in regular contact with the doctoral program regarding the extern's performance and professionalism. Upon completion of the AuD degree, including all of the clinical rotations and externship requirements relevant for the state in which one chooses to practice, and upon passing a national examination in audiology, the student is eligible to apply for a license to practice audiology through his or her state's licensing board.

In addition to the legal requirement of having a state license, most audiologists choose to obtain professional certification through AAA and/or ASHA. But do not think that the education and training is over after obtaining a license and certification; there are mandatory continuing education hours that must be fulfilled to maintain license and certification throughout your professional career. For those who wish to continue their education and obtain a research doctorate (PhD), the AuD can be an excellent foundation and a valuable asset in an academic position.

Development of the Profession

Audiology is a relatively new profession that took on its own identity shortly after World War II, mostly as a result of returning service men who were in need of hearing assessment and care resulting from unprotected exposures to high-level noises. These returning servicemen were handled, initially, by otologists and speech-language pathologists, but soon evolved into a specialty practice in the United States that developed into the field of audiology (Martin & Clark, 2003). After the war, audiology-specific educational programs were developed in universities to prepare professionals for clinical work, as well as becoming the stage for research efforts that would define the practice of audiology. In the early years, audiology was focused on rehabilitation, including lipreading, auditory training, and hearing aids (Katz, 2002).

The late 1960s and early 1970s saw the development of immittance (known then as impedance) testing. The mid to late 1970s brought our attention to the clinical use of auditory brainstem responses (ABRs). Otoacoustic emissions were discovered in the late 1970s and become an accepted part of clinical practice by the late 1980s and was the primary impetus for most states to adopt universal newborn hearing screening programs. Also during this period, there was considerable research in the technological aspects of hearing aid design, and by the 1990s digital hearing aids were becoming the standard. Prior to 1977 it was considered unethical by ASHA for audiologists to dispense hearing aids, except in the Veteran's Hospitals. However, through the continuing interests and activities of audiologists in the dispensing of hearing aids throughout the 1970s, ASHA changed its perspective in 1979, and hearing aid dispensing soon became a large part of audiology practices. Cochlear implants were another milestone is audiology, beginning with the first implants in the 1960s, followed by a 30-year slow but steady convincing of the profession that cochlear implants were able to produce remarkable results in adults and children that are now well accepted in the audiology community. See Chapter 13 for a detailed and interesting look at some of the historical highlights that have occurred in audiology over the past 70 years.

The American Speech-Language-Hearing Association (ASHA) was the original (and only) main professional organization for audiologists and speech-language pathologists since the beginnings of audiology. In 1988, the American Academy of Audiology (AAA) was founded in order to establish an organization devoted entirely to the needs of audiologists and the interests of the audiology profession (see AAA at http://www.audiology .org). Originally, the AAA was focused on transitioning audiology to a doctoral level profession, which became a reality by 2007. Membership in AAA quickly skyrocketed during the first 10 years, and today AAA has a membership of over 12,000 audiologists.

The AAA and ASHA are both strong advocates for the hearing impaired and related services by audiologists, both at the state and national levels. The AAA and ASHA each have professional certifications for audiologists: *American Board of Audiology (ABA) certification* through AAA, and the *Certificate of Clinical Competence in Audiology (CCC-A)* through ASHA. In addition, each of these organizations can award accreditation to academic programs who meet a set of standards; the Accreditation Commission for Audiology Education (ACAE) associated with AAA, and the Commission on Academic Accreditation (CAA) associated with ASHA. Another professional organization, American Doctors of Audiology (ADA), was originally established in 1977 as the Academy of Dispensing Audiologists (ADA) in order to directly support the needs of audiologists dispensing of hearing aids. They later changed their name to the Academy of Doctors of Audiology, and focuses on the needs of audiologists in private practice or who wish to establish a private practice. Finally, recognition should be given to the national student organization for those interested in audiology, called Student Academy of Audiology (SAA). The SAA is devoted to audiology education, student research, professional requirements, and networking of students enrolled in audiology doctoral programs (AuD and PhD) Most university programs have local student chapters of SAA that are part of the national organization.

What Do Audiologists Do?

Audiologists provide a variety of services to meet the needs of persons with hearing and balance problems. As mentioned earlier, audiologists are involved with identification (screening), assessment, treatment, and prevention. Audiologists might wear different hats or many hats, such as those of a diagnostician, therapist, counselor, consultant, preceptor, team leader, advocate, business person, researcher, or teacher. An audiologist's role as a

teacher might involve being an AuD student preceptor, or providing in-service training sessions or case study presentations to other hospital staff, medical students, residents, and fellows. They might develop brochures or workshops for consumers or industry on the effects of hearing loss or its prevention and treatment. They might lead an aural rehabilitation group therapy session with adults who have hearing loss. They might be asked to provide input on a treatment plan for those receiving cochlear implants or ototoxic medications, or patients with vestibular disorders, tinnitus, head- injury or other speech-language disorders, and/or for a child's school-based educational plan. Audiologists must be able to assess and treat patients of all ages, including, for example, newborns and patients with a variety of disabilities, and must be culturally and linguistically sensitive in their selection of tests, counseling, and treatment.

Audiologists working in hospitals or clinics spend a good deal of their time planning, performing, and interpreting diagnostic tests; usually this is followed by some patient counseling, consulting with the physician, writing a report for the patient's chart, and filling out the billing information. In many cases, the audiologist seeks additional services for the patient. Most patients being seen for an assessment will receive a basic audiologic test battery, including pure-tone audiometry, speech tests, immittance tests, and otoacoustic emissions. When appropriate, advanced tests are scheduled, such as ABR or central auditory processing. Audiologists are often involved with vestibular testing and facial nerve testing. Audiologists must keep up with technological advances and learn to incorporate new equipment and tests into their practice.

Audiologists are experts in hearing aid fittings. They determine hearing aid candidacy, perform hearing aid fittings, and verify and validate the fitting and benefit. They make the ear impression, order the hearing aid from a selected manufacturer, handle the sales transaction, and provide the necessary orientation, counseling, and follow-up services. Audiologists also are knowledgeable about other assistive listening devices, such as FM or infrared amplifying devices, personal listening devices, amplified telephones, and/or alarms for those who are deaf. Audiologists may also work with otologists and their patients who have been fit with a bone-anchored hearing aid (BAHA). Also, of course, the audiologist may work with patients who are being considered or have received a cochlear implant.

In many situations, audiologists are part of specialty teams consisting of physicians, nurses, and speech-language pathologists, working with patients who have cleft-palate, cystic fibrosis, childhood hearing loss, or cochlear implants. Many audiologists are also involved with newborn hearing screening and work closely with pediatric nurses and trained volunteers or other nonaudiologist hearing screening staff. Audiologists also refer patients to a number of other professionals, including pediatricians, psychologists, rehabilitation counselors, geneticists, and social workers.

Audiologists use established and emerging technologies as tools to facilitate their patient care; however, it is important to realize that audiologists are the most knowledgeable of all professionals regarding the effects of hearing loss on communication and how to improve the quality of life for individuals and families who are dealing with hearing loss. Counseling, treatment, and extended rehabilitation are very important and rewarding aspects of an audiologist's role (Hawkins, 1990). The humanistic characteristics that are important skills of audiologists are described thoroughly by DeBonis and Donohue (2004), and include such things as listening, respect for the client's beliefs, understanding the feeling of the patient and how the hearing loss impacts the patient's life, styles of clinician-patient interactions, and collaboration with the patient and other professionals.

The AAA and ASHA have each developed a document called the *Scope of Practice*, which describes those services that are considered appropriate for audiologists. These documents are available on the respective websites, and are periodically updated to reflect changes in the profession. The Scope of Practice defines a wide range of activities in which audiologists may engage; however, it does not imply that all audiologists have the necessary knowledge and skill to perform all of the activities; therefore, every audiologist should only perform those activities that they feel they are adequately trained to do, or obtain the necessary training should something unfamiliar be

required as part of their job. In addition to all of the activities mentioned in the preceding sections, here are some other activities considered within the scope of practice (see AAA and ASHA websites for details of the scope of practice in audiology):

- Otoscopic examination of the external ear
- Screening of speech, language, orofacial, and cognitive disorders
- Identification of high risk factors associated with hearing, speech, or balance problems
- Cerumen management (consult state licensure limitations).
- Perform and interpret tests of sensory and motor evoked potentials, including electromyography of facial nerve function, and intraoperative monitoring
- Perform tests of vestibular function, including electronystagmography, videonystagmography, balance platform testing, and rotary chair testing
- Evaluation of auditory processing disorders
- Cochlear implant mapping
- Noise measurements and consultations regarding environmental modifications that might impact hearing and communication
- Tinnitus evaluation and treatment
- Design and conduct audiologic research

On a final note, the audiology scope of practice will change or some activities will take on less importance as new techniques emerge, current techniques go by the wayside, or other specialists reclaim the turf. For example, the use of ABR to diagnose 8th nerve tumors has been supplanted, to a large extent, by better imaging techniques, such as contrast CT and MRI scans. As another example, some audiologists are involved with intraoperative monitoring (by virtue of their experience with ABR), which may often involve evoked potential measures of spinal nerves during back surgery; and it is conceivable that this type of work may be subsumed by other specialists in the future. Finally, although a case may be made for vestibular assessment based on its relation to the auditory system, it remains to be seen if audiologists will continue to provide this service.

Membership Demographics and Work Settings

According to the ASHA (2011), at the end of 2011, there were 11,897 ASHA certified audiologists (and 130,997 speech-language pathologists). Males comprise 17.4% of audiologists (compared with 4.0% of speech-language pathologists). Approximately one quarter of the ASHA membership is 55 years of age or older (29.4% of audiologists, 25.2% of speech-language pathologists). Only about 7% of audiologists and speech-language pathologists identify themselves as members of a racial or ethnic minority.

Audiologists have the opportunity to work in a variety of settings. The majority of today's audiologists work in private practice, otolaryngologists' practices, community hospitals or other clinics, and Veterans Administration hospitals; others work in public schools, rehabilitation centers, nursing homes, industry, or research. Private practice as a work setting for audiologists grew rapidly after the 1980s, primarily driven by the change in ASHA that allowed audiologists to dispense hearing aids. Prior to that time, most audiologists were employed in hospitals and clinics.

The interest and growth in private practice has also been fueled by the transition to the AuD degree, which may bring greater awareness and respect from consumers, similar to an optometrist. In addition, there appears to be a trend for those in private practice, especially owners, to make a higher salary. Audiologists contemplating private practice must become knowledgeable about marketing and business practices, and often these types of courses and experiences are not part of an AuD curriculum. In addition, as more private practices became established and lucrative, larger corporations (e.g., Sonus, HearEx) were formed, and these corporations began to buy out those in private practice or hire audiologists to work in franchises or practices owned by the corporations.

The AuD degree may also have a positive effect on the demand for audiologists by hospitals, where the advanced education and better training of today's audiologist can provide better and more comprehensive patient care. The hospital setting is an attractive choice for many audiologists, especially for those who are not so much interested in the business side of audiology. Hospitals provide a stimulating work environment with opportunities to work with other professionals. Audiologists in hospitals see a variety of interesting cases that need medical management, as well as audiological management, and are the perfect place to perform all of those advanced audiological procedures and provide differential diagnoses. In addition, hospitals provide opportunities to work with cochlear implant teams, newborn hearing screening programs, and intraoperative monitoring, to name a few. Many hospitals and university clinics also dispense hearing aids, and it is likely that this will increase in popularity. Indeed, the times are changing, and as the AuD becomes the standard for practicing clinical audiology, it will be interesting to see how the trends in work setting and salaries change over the next decade.

Synopsis 12–1

- Audiology is a discipline that focuses on the study of normal hearing and hearing disorders. An audiologist is a licensed professional who practices audiology. Otology is the medical discipline related to hearing disorders, and is practiced by otologists. Audiology in the United States had its beginnings just after World War II.

- The American Academy of Audiology (AAA) and the American Speech-Language-Hearing Association (ASHA) are the two main professional organizations serving their audiologist members. The AAA is entirely run by and for audiologists, whereas ASHA also has a large speech-language pathology membership.

- Audiologists are educationally and clinically prepared to work in most settings and perform most audiological services; however, some audiologists may choose to focus on specific areas/subspecialties, such as pediatric audiology, geriatric audiology, hearing aid dispensing audiology, educational audiology, military audiology, industrial audiology, forensic audiology, intraoperative monitoring specialist, as well as work in academia or research.

- A professional doctorate (AuD) is required to practice clinical audiology. The AuD is obtained by successfully completing a 4-year graduate degree, passing the national examination in audiology, and obtaining an audiology license from the state in which they reside. Professional accreditation is usually obtained as well; CCC-A certification by ASHA and/or ABA certification by AAA.

- Some key developments in audiology include: immittance measures (early 1970s), ABR (late 1970s), HA approval for audiologists to dispense hearing aids (1979), OAE (1980s), AAA founded (1988), and digital hearing aids (1990s).

- The national student organization for future doctoral level audiologists is called Student Academy of Audiology (SAA). Most doctoral audiology programs have local chapters of SAA, many of which encourage undergraduates to participate.

- Audiologists perform a variety of diagnostic tests for hearing and balance function from a culturally and ethnically sensitive perspective, and a large number of audiologists dispense hearing aids. Audiologists also engage in counseling, teaching, business practices, newborn hearing screening, precepting AuD students, and/or consulting. Audiologists may find themselves performing cerumen management, tinnitus evaluations, intraoperative monitoring, neuromuscular assessment of facial nerve function, and/or assessment and mapping of cochlear implants.

- The majority of audiologists work in hospitals or university clinics, private practice, and ENT practices; others work in industry, schools, rehabilitation centers, universities, industry, or research.

References

DeBonis, D. A., & Donohue, C. L. (2004). *Survey of audiology*. Boston, MA: Pearson Allyn and Bacon.

Hawkins, D. B. (1990). Technology and hearing aids: How does the audiologist fit in? *American Speech-Language-Hearing Association, 32,* 42–43.

Katz, J. (Ed.). (2002). Clinical audiology. *Handbook of clinical audiology*. Baltimore, MD: Lippincott Williams & Wilkins.

Martin, F. N., & Clark, J. G. (2003). *Introduction to audiology*. Boston, MA: Allyn & Bacon.

13

Brief History of Audiology in the United States

James Jerger and Cheryl DeConde Johnson

Historical Overview

The history of modern audiology in the United States begins in 1922 with the fabrication of the first commercial audiometer, the Western Electric 1-A by Harvey Fletcher and R. L. Wegel. Harvey Fletcher was one of the true pioneers of research in speech communication. His early studies at the Bell Telephone Laboratories in New Jersey set the stage for what later became the concept of the articulation index and, more recently, the speech intelligibility index. The 1-A audiometer was hardly portable, but subsequent models were smaller and lighter. They were sold mainly for use in otolaryngology practices.

The first genuine audiologist in the United States was undoubtedly Cordia C. Bunch. As a graduate student at the University of Iowa, late in World War I, Bunch came under the influence of Carl Seashore, a psychologist who was studying the measurement of musical aptitude, and L. W. Dean, an otolaryngologist. Together, they stimulated Bunch's interest in the measurement of hearing. Over the 2 decades from 1920 to 1940, Bunch car-

ried out the first systematic studies of the relation between types of hearing loss and audiometric patterns as he pursued an academic career, first at the University of Iowa, then at Johns Hopkins University, next at Washington University and Central Institute for the Deaf in St. Louis. These pioneering efforts were published in a slender volume entitled *Clinical Audiometry* which is now a classic in the field.

In 1941, Bunch accepted an offer from the School of Speech at Northwestern University to come to Evanston as research professor in education of the deaf and to teach courses in hearing testing and hearing disorders. There he met and did a bit of mentoring of a young faculty member in speech science, Raymond Carhart. In June of 1942, Bunch unexpectedly died at the age of 57. In order to proceed with the course, the Northwestern administration tapped Carhart to teach it. The rest, as they say, is history. Carhart told me, years later, that no single person had more influence on his career than C. C. Bunch.

During World War II, Carhart served in the Army Medical Corps as a captain and was assigned to head a unit at Deshon General Hospital in Butler,

Pennsylvania, whose mission was to rehabilitate returning soldiers who had sustained hearing loss during military service. Although Carhart initiated an ambitious auditory training program, his principal rehabilitative weapon was the hearing aid, then a fairly bulky device about the size of a package of cigarettes, which was worn in the pocket or in a holder suspended around the neck. It was connected by a thin wire to a transducer mounted in a fully occluding earmold. Carhart's task was to devise a set of procedures upon which to base a rational decision about which of several possible hearing aids to dispense to the serviceman. To accomplish this, he virtually invented, from scratch, what we now know as speech audiometry. He adapted the earlier work at the Harvard Psychoacoustic Laboratory on spondee and phonemically balanced (PB) word lists into the concepts of the speech reception threshold (SRT) and the maximum PB score (PB_{max}).

Over the next 5 decades, audiology evolved along seven distinct paths: (a) a diagnostic path, (b) a rehabilitative path, (c) a pediatric path, (d) an auditory processing disorder (APD) path; (e) a hearing conservation path; (f) a tinnitus evaluation and therapy path; and (g) an educational audiology path. In the following sections, we have attempted to trace the major developments in each of these paths over the past half century.

The Diagnostic Path

One of the earliest diagnostic test procedures, over and above the conventional tests for air and bone conduction threshold sensitivity, was the alternate binaural loudness balance test (ABLB). Edmund Prince Fowler devised and developed this test in the late 1920s and 1930s as a procedure for comparing suprathreshold loudness at the two ears. It often revealed that, in spite of unilateral threshold hearing loss, loudness in the bad ear was achieved by suprathreshold sounds at the same intensity in the two ears, a phenomenon which came to be called *loudness recruitment*. Fowler used the ABLB procedure to explore patients with

unilateral otosclerosis but did not learn very much that was useful. Later, however, the technique was used to great advantage in differentiating Ménière disease from acoustic tumor.

In 1946, Otto Metz of Denmark developed the first viable middle ear impedance bridge. Metz built a fairly unwieldy gadget, principally to detect contraction of the middle ear muscles. Using the device, Metz was able to demonstrate loudness recruitments as a reduction in the sensation level of the tone eliciting a reflex contraction of the stapedius muscle.

One might view 1948 as the birth of site-of-lesion testing. In England, Dix, Hallpike, and Hood published a paper in the Proceedings of the Royal Society of Medicine, in which they showed that one could differentiate unilateral loss due to Ménière disease from unilateral loss due to acoustic tumor using Fowler's ABLB test. Patients with Ménière disease showed partial or complete loudness recruitment, especially for high frequencies, but patients with acoustic tumor did not. C. S. Hallpike went on to study vestibular disorders and is well remembered for the Hallpike maneuver in vestibular assessment.

The 1948 publication by Dix, Hallpike, and Hood stirred a good deal of interest in the loudness recruitment phenomenon as a means of differentiating cochlear from retrocochlear site of disorder. The principal problem with ABLB was the fact that it could only be used effectively in patients with unilateral loss. How, people asked, can we detect loudness recruitment in patients with bilateral losses? Is there another way of getting at the apparent abnormal growth of loudness? In Switzerland, Professor E. Lüscher reasoned that, if loudness was growing too rapidly with intensity, then the difference limen for loudness (the smallest detectable loudness) must be smaller than in a normal ear. Could one then detect this by measuring the intensity difference limen at suprathreshold levels? He enlisted the aid of a young assistant with a background in electrical engineering, a Polish immigrant to Switzerland named Jozef Zwislocki. Together they crafted a device to measure the smallest detectable modulation in the amplitude of a continuous pure tone. They then applied it to patients in Lüscher's ENT clinic. Most patients with sensorineural loss did, indeed, show amplitude modulation thresholds well below the values characterizing normal ears at comparable sensation levels. Lüscher and Zwislocki suggested this as an "indirect" measure of the loudness recruitment phenomenon. Their findings created worldwide interest in how one might detect the presence of loudness recruitment indirectly and, thereby, facilitate the distinction between sensory and neural lesions of the auditory system.

In the same year, 1948, John Gaeth, at Northwestern University, studied word recognition in an elderly cohort, and concluded that you could not fully explain all of the word recognition scores from the audiogram alone. Something else seemed to be reducing PB_{max} scores in some elderly individuals. He named the phenomenon "phonemic regression." Five decades later, many still find this concept difficult to accept but we now know that, in addition to the undeniably important audibility factor, there are age-related changes in frequency resolution, temporal resolution, cognition, and central auditory processing.

In Italy, in the early 1950s, a group of investigators led by Ettore Bocca were approaching central auditory processing problems from a different direction, the study of neurological patients with temporal lobe disorders. These investigators, especially Antonelli and Teatini, showed that, while these patients had no difficulty understanding simple speech in either ear, when the listening task was made more difficult, either by low-pass filtering or temporal speeding, performance on the ear contralateral to the affected side of the brain was noticeably poorer than performance on the ipsilateral ear. They called their measures "sensitized speech audiometry." Their findings stirred great interest, especially among American investigators seeking a better understanding of the effects of brain lesions on auditory perception. Many of our current tests for auditory processing disorders derive from this early work by the pioneering Italians.

In 1958, Dan Geisler, then at the University of Chicago, using an early digital computer, discovered what we now call the middle-latency auditory evoked potential. He noted a consistent positiv-

ity in the latency region of 30 to 40 ms, which we now call Pa. This was the first in the family of computer-averaged auditory evoked potentials to be described. It was later studied at great length by Robert Goldstein and his students, first at Jewish Hospital in St. Louis, and later at the University of Wisconsin at Madison.

In that same year, 1958, Carhart and Jerger published results on what later came to be called tone decay or abnormal adaptation. From 1953 to 1954, Jerger was running subjects for his dissertation research on intensity discrimination using the quantal psychophysical method. He presented a continuous tone at 20 dB SL, upon which there were superimposed intensity increments that the subject was asked to detect. Jerger recruited Ray Carhart as a subject for the experiment because he had a deep notch at 4000 Hz due to an aspirin regimen he was under. After the session, Carhart reported that, although he continued to hear the increments, the continuous carrier tone promptly faded away entirely. After a few minutes into the trial he could not hear the continuous tone at all. Jerger and Carhart pursued this interesting observation with some acoustic tumor patients and found that they showed the same phenomenon to a remarkable degree. These findings led to the various tone decay and reflex decay tests that are still in use today.

Based on his work with short intensity increments, Jerger modified the classical quantal method down to the presentation of 20 increments of exactly 1 dB superimposed on a continuous tone at 20 dB SL, and called this test the short-increment sensitivity index or SISI test. The bottom line was that patients with cochlear lesions could detect the increments with ease, especially at high frequencies, but patients with 8th nerve problems, or with conductive loss, could not. It was one of several tests that worked moderately well but was ultimately supplanted by the ABR.

The automatic audiometer was invented by Georg von Békésy during his time in Stockholm after he fled Hungary before World War II. But it received little clinical attention until the Grason-Stadler Co., in the late 1950s, produced a commercial instrument, the venerable E-800. Northwestern bought one of the first units and Jerger ran some 400 patients through the procedure. In Békésy's original instrument, the test tone was on continuously, but on the E-800 there was the option of periodically interrupting the continuous test tone. Based on an earlier suggestion by Peter Denes, Jerger thought it might be useful to test in both the continuous and interrupted modes. This resulted in the four Békésy types: Type I in normal listeners and conductive losses, Type II in cochlear losses, and Types III and IV in 8th nerve disorders. Later, Gilbert Herer added a Type V, in which the continuous trace runs well above the interrupted trace, a sure sign of functional and malingering losses.

In 1963, Zwislocki tried to improve on the Otto Metz impedance bridge by adding a way to measure resistance as well as compliance, and by making the instrument much smaller. The only problem was that it took a three-handed person to carry this out. You needed one hand to hold the instrument in the ear canal, a second hand to move the compliance plunger in and out, and a third hand to turn the resistance adjuster. The device never really caught on clinically, but it served the important function of arousing great interest in the possibilities of impedance audiometry (later called "immittance audiometry") in the United States.

What we now call the N1-P2 complex, occurring in the 100 to 250 ms latency range, was the second auditory evoked potential to be identified. Hallowell Davis, working at the Central Institute for the Deaf, called it the vertex potential because it was largest at the CZ or vertex electrode. Davis and his colleagues spent many years attempting to exploit the vertex potential as a test of hearing in infants and other difficult to test children. But it never really worked too well, largely because of the labile state of the young brain.

In 1970, the first really usable instruments for measuring middle ear impedance characteristics and acoustic reflex measurement were produced by the Madsen Company in Denmark. Jerger was at the Baylor College of Medicine in Houston at the time and managed to acquire one of the earliest of the ZO70 instruments. Following Bunch's example, Jerger simply had his audiologists run every patient through the procedure. After some 400 cases had been tested, the clinical value of impedance testing became evident. Absolute impedance measures, which had been the driving force behind the development of these instruments, turned out to be the least interesting data. The real value was in exploring tympanograms and the stapedius muscle reflex. Jerger's 1970 publication on all of this, in the AMA *Archives of Otolaryngology*, continues to be a frequently cited reference 35 years later.

Few test procedures have had the same profound effect on audiological practice as the auditory brain stem response (ABR). It has truly revolutionized diagnostic evaluation. Gone today are the SISI, ABLB, and Békésy-type audiograms. They have been replaced by a single powerful tool that objectively differentiates cochlear loss from 8th nerve disorders with high sensitivity and acceptable specificity. Donald Jewett stumbled upon this response almost by accident. He was looking at later evoked responses when he noticed what appeared to be repeatable bumps in the first 10 ms after stimulus onset. Previous investigators missed them because it was the fashion to band-pass filter the EEG rather narrowly around the frequency region of interest, which for the middle and late responses was well below 100 Hz; thus, activity in the 500 to 1000 Hz range, where the ABR response is maximal, was, in effect, discarded (filtered out). But no one told Jewett that you were supposed to filter so narrowly, and he had a much wider filter setting, which allowed the ABR peaks to be viewed. Clearly, the ABR has had a tremendous effect on diagnostic evaluation in our field.

The successful recording of evoked and spontaneous emissions from the inner ear, by David Kemp in 1978, set off a flurry of activity around the world. It seemed that here, at last, we might have a truly objective method for measuring degree of hearing sensitivity loss without the need for active cooperation from the person being evaluated. As luck would have it, otoacoustic emissions (OAEs) turned out to be too sensitive: They are so sensitive to the status of the outer hair cells that they drop out altogether when degree of loss exceeds 40 to 50 dB HL. However, this did set the stage for their use in newborn hearing screening. Also, as so often happens in our field, other applications of the OAEs have turned out to be even more interesting and valuable.

One such application, the efferent suppression of OAEs, first described by Lionel Collet and his colleagues in France, continues to show great promise in the evaluation of central auditory processing, especially at the low brainstem level. Ever at the forefront of innovation, Charles Berlin and his colleagues at the Louisiana State University Medical Center pioneered the clinical applications of efferent suppression.

The Rehabilitative Path

Throughout much of the history of modern audiology, the principal rehabilitative weapons have been: (a) the wearable hearing aid, (b) auditory training, and (c) the cochlear implant. Their paths have been interestingly intertwined.

Hearing Aids

The wearable hearing aid was made possible by the invention and systematic improvement of the miniature vacuum tube in the 1930s. The filaments of the tubes were heated by a 1.5-volt A battery, and the plate biased by a 22 to 30-volt B battery. These aids, about the size of a package of cigarettes, could be worn in the shirt pocket or in a cloth pocket suspended from the neck. They were connected by a thin wire to a small transducer, curiously referred to as a receiver, mounted in the ear canal by a totally occluding earmold. Such aids were made available to the aural rehabilitative programs of the various services during and after World War II and were widely distributed to returning servicemen.

The military programs generated a longstanding debate, which at times became quite contentious, over what might be called the philosophy of fitting a hearing aid. On the one hand were the exponents of hearing aid selection, a proce-dure promoted most notably by Ray Carhart and his many students. The rationale here was that the audiologist must seek, through objective testing of speech understanding, the hearing aid that best matches the unique shape and degree of the serviceman's loss. This was achieved by manipulation of gain and tone control of each of several candidate aids in search of optimal word intelligibility. Carhart adapted, for this purpose, the spondee and PB word lists developed at the Harvard Psychoacoustic Laboratory during the war. The underlying assumption of the hearing aid selection procedure was that individuals differed in the unique details of their losses, and that the best aid was the aid that complemented the shape of the loss, especially in terms of its frequency response. In future years this came to be called selective amplification.

As early as 1946, however, an alternative philosophy emerged from two sources: (a) the British MEDRESCO hearing aid, and (b) the *Harvard Report*. The MEDRESCO aid was developed by British engineers to meet the needs of the nascent National Health Service. They were convinced that a single, relatively flat frequency response was sufficient for most hearing impaired individuals; thus, they allowed for only minimal adjustment of the tone control of the aid.

The *Harvard Report* was generated by a group of scientists working on the National Defense Research Council (NDRC) Aural Rehabilitation Project at Harvard University during the last years of World War II. They tested a number of hearing impaired individuals with a master hearing aid, in which the frequency response could be manipulated over a wide range. Their report, published in 1946, concluded that selective amplification was of little value. A uniform (flat) frequency response almost always yielded the best speech understanding scores; thus, elaborate selection procedures were not warranted. For the next decade, lively debate ensued between proponents of the two conflicting philosophies. Traditionalists continued to carry out hearing aid selection testing in the Carhart manner, whereas others pushed for reform, but usually to little avail. It must be said, however, that the physical characteristics of the aids of that era did not permit very precise control over the frequency response of any aid. In retrospect, it is doubtful that either side could have amassed very much hard evidence in support of its position.

In the early 1950s, the transistor was developed and its value in the design of wearable aids was immediately apparent. Transistors were certainly smaller than miniature vacuum tubes, but the main advantage was the elimination of the need for the bulky, high voltage B battery. Transistors could manage the same amplification when powered only by a small 1.5-volt A battery. This additional miniaturization made it possible to move the amplifier unit from the shirt pocket to a location over and behind the auricle, the behind-the-ear unit, and ultimately into the ear canal itself. Miniaturization also made bilateral fittings feasible, permitting for the first time the capability of exploiting the several advantages of two-eared hearing.

But no engineering advance in the past half century has had greater impact on the wearable hearing aid than the advent of digital signal processing. With this breakthrough, for the first time, it was possible to really manipulate the fine grain of the frequency response of an aid in order to match it to the shape of the audiometric contour. This capability, combined with digital compression/expansion and various adaptive algorithms, fueled a resurgence in the interest in selective amplification as the best way to fit hearing aids. At the same time, studies by David Pascoe and Margo Skinner at Washington University, by Larry Humes at Indiana University, and by many other investigators have emphasized the critical impact of the exact degree and configuration of high frequency sensitivity loss on speech understanding. These two forces have lent such strong support to the philosophy of selective amplification that it became the virtual rule in hearing aid fitting. At the same time, the laborious testing characterizing Carhart's original concept of hearing aid evaluation gave way to emphasis on fine tuning a smaller number of aids, with heavy reliance on the real-ear measurement of their physical characteristics.

Confluent with advances in digital signal processing, microphone technology has advanced to a point permitting the development of a truly directional microphone, in which directivity patterns favoring input from a particular direction have been implemented. Although there have been voices of dissent, the available evidence seems to favor the use of directional microphones in most listening situations involving competing speech or noise.

In the months and years to come, it is certain that continuing advances in hearing aid technology will broaden our rehabilitative capabilities. Indeed, we are already seeing aids that learn the client's preferred volume setting and switch among programs for quiet listening, music, listening to speech alone, and listening to speech in a noisy background. Also, there are aids that will automatically switch to the directional mode when background noise is detected, aids that can be recharged, and even aids that can be individually programmed to suit a particular lifestyle.

Auditory Training

Attempts to exploit the residual hearing of severely and profoundly hearing-impaired persons have a history much longer than audiology. Long before there were audiometers and hearing aids, educators of the deaf were at the front lines of auditory training, using whatever tools were available. Alexander Graham Bell, inventor of the telephone and founder of the AG Bell Association, took a special interest in the possibilities of auditory training because of his wife's hearing loss. He was a strong proponent of the aural approach and lent his considerable reputation to its promulgation in the last quarter of the 19th century. Another early supporter of systematic training in listening was Max Goldstein who founded the world-famous Central Institute for the Deaf in St. Louis.

But it was the advent of World War II, and the military aural rehabilitation programs, that mark the beginning of the modern era in auditory training. At Deshon General Hospital, Ray Carhart developed an 8-week individualized therapy program emphasizing critical listening, precise and rapid recognition of phonetic elements, reestablishment of the recognition of familiar noises, and training in auditory discrimination under adverse listening conditions. Similar programs were initiated at other centers as the war wound down. The programs were popular with the veterans who experienced the programs, but after the war enthusiasm for auditory training as a supplement to hearing aid use slowly waned. There were a number of reasons for this decline; the two most important were lack of third-party reimbursement for such training and lack of empirical evidence of its efficacy. Dedicated professionals like Mark Ross, who as a World War II veteran passed through a wartime program, and Norman Erber continued to research and develop training programs, but, across the field, interest in auditory training continued to wane.

Beginning in the 1980s, however, renewed broad interest in auditory training was stimulated by two research thrusts: (a) maximizing the value of cochlear implants, and (b) carefully controlled efficacy studies. The impact of cochlear implants on the resurgence of auditory training is amplified in the next section. Relative to efficacy, a ground-breaking study at Walter Reed Army Hospital by Brian Walden and colleagues in 1981 demonstrated the value of a comprehensive analytic auditory training program emphasizing a consonant discrimination in young hearing impaired adults. In 1996, Patricia Kricos and Alice Holmes reported results of a very well-controlled study in which they compared the efficacy of a bottom-up analytic approach with a more top-down synthetic approach to auditory training. In 2005, however, Robert Sweetow and Catherine Palmer carried out a comprehensive review of the auditory training literature and found very little convincing evidence of genuine efficacy.

Interestingly, both Walden et al. and Kricos and Holmes questioned the value of an analytic approach in the case of elderly hearing aid users. Since elderly persons are the majority of hearing aid users, this conclusion, based on careful research, has been of more than passing interest to the developers of auditory training programs. Some developers have suggested that, over the years, Carhart's emphasis on "critical listening" and "precise and rapid recognition of phonetic elements" has led to an overemphasis on an analytic approach as opposed to a more synthetic approach to audi-

tory training. Perhaps, they reasoned, an auditory training regimen that focused on consonant discrimination drills is likely to be less effective with elderly persons than a more synthetic approach that emphasizes coping strategies, development of good listening habits, concentration on the meaning of messages, and nonverbal and situational cues, which can lead to improved communication efficiency.

Much of the current enthusiasm for auditory training derives from relatively recent studies of neural plasticity, especially in the auditory system, by neuroscientists. There is convincing evidence that concentrated auditory stimulation can alter neural activity throughout the auditory system. Moreover, Kelly Tremblay and her colleagues have shown that neurophysiological changes produced by auditory training actually generalize to other stimuli not specifically targeted for training. Tremblay and Nina Kraus have even shown changes in the P1, N1, and P2 components of the auditory evoked response after systematic auditory training.

In summary, auditory training flowered immediately after World War II, and then faded almost from sight for the next 3 decades. Within the past 2 decades, however, we have seen a strong resurgence of research and the clinical application of auditory training, influenced greatly by its successful use in cochlear implant rehabilitation and by the demonstration of neural plasticity in the auditory system. In their excellent historical review, Kricos and Holmes make a profound point:

It is clear that auditory training may be the most powerful, underutilized, and not completely understood tool in the audiologist's armamentarium.

Cochlear Implants

Cochlear implants in the United States were pioneered in the early 1960s by F. Blair Simmons at Stanford University, William House at the House Ear Institute in Los Angeles, Michael Merzenich and Robin Michelson at the University of California at San Francisco (UCSF), and Donald Eddington at the University of Utah. Early models were essentially single-channel devices, employing a unitary implanted electrode that provided virtually no "place" or spectral information. But to many people's surprise, just the information in the temporal envelope seemed to provide useful cues for speech understanding in severely and profoundly hearing impaired individuals. These early successes encouraged the development of multichannel devices. One of the most successful devices has been the Nucleus system, originally developed by Graeme Clark and his team at the University of Melbourne, Australia. Another successful device is the Clarion unit, developed as a result of scientific effort led by Michael Merzenich at UCSF.

The progress of cochlear implants over the past 3 decades has been truly remarkable. The early systems were essentially aids to lipreading. Few users could maintain a conversation without the aid of visual cues. But as the number of electrodes increased, and speech coding strategies became more sophisticated, performance in the auditory only condition has improved severalfold. It is now quite reasonable to expect that a suitably chosen candidate will be able to converse easily over the telephone. Thirty years ago few people would have predicted that this level of performance would ever be attainable.

While the importance of successful surgical placement of the electrodes within the cochlea cannot be overestimated, the major share of the credit for the present status of cochlear implants must surely go to those researchers who have patiently and methodically improved the speech coding strategies, and to the audiologists who have provided the lengthy, often tedious, aural rehabilitation sessions so critical to the successful use of cochlear implants.

Indeed, the steady rise of cochlear implants has been responsible for much of the resurgence of interest in auditory training. Very early in the history of cochlear implants it became increasingly clear that their efficacy was enhanced by a program of systematic auditory training following implantation. Audiologists had long paid lip service to the idea that the value of a wearable hearing aid could be enhanced by auditory training, but only a few (Elmer Owen at UCSF, for example) pursued the

possibilities vigorously. But from the very first patient implanted with a single-channel device, the dramatic value of a rigorous program of postsurgical aural rehabilitation was evident. The success of the auditory training programs developed to meet this need have, quite appropriately, sparked a resurgence of interest in all applications of systematic auditory training. Robert Sweetow, at UCSF, has employed the sophisticated possibilities inherent in modern computer technology to develop self-paced and self-administered auditory training programs. Such an approach promises to make efficient auditory training procedures available to a wide array of hearing impaired individuals.

Finally, space does not permit a detailed account of the historic contributions of audiologists to tinnitus therapy, to educational audiology, and to industrial monitoring, and those interested in this area are directed to other sources.

The Pediatric/Screening Path

Individuals who worked with hearing impaired and deaf children were long aware of the critical importance of early detection of loss for subsequent language development and academic achievement; thus, efforts to screen young children for hearing loss have a long history, but the behavioral tools available for screening in the early years of the profession were not totally satisfactory. The behavioral tools included observation of head turning in response to common environmental sounds and conditioning paradigms that ranged from simple to complex. Two persistent problems plagued these approaches. First, one could not always be sure of the reliability of the child's behavioral responses, and, second, screening children in the important age range from 0 to 3 years was always a bit dicey. But the advent of the ABR and OAEs opened up the playing field substantially. These two techniques made it possible, for the first time, to screen babies literally from the moment of birth, with techniques whose reliability could be tested and affirmed. It seemed that the screening of all babies born in the United States, that is, genuine universal screening, might indeed be feasible.

The single individual who has had the greatest impact on the concept of universal screening of all newborn babies is certainly Marion Downs of the University of Colorado. She founded the first screening program in Colorado in 1962, and she has never ceased to push for universal screening of every newborn baby. Few people have been so devoted to an audiologic cause.

Because of independence of a person's state, the ABR seemed a likely candidate for screening babies of all ages, but it was not until the publication of a seminal paper by Kurt Hecox and Robert Galambos in 1971 that the value of ABR in the evaluation of the pediatric population began to be accepted by the pediatric audiologic community. Nowadays, it is difficult to imagine the evaluation of newborns, infants, and young children without ABR, but before this important paper appeared, behavioral techniques, many of extremely questionable validity, were the rule. The paper by Hecox and Galambos stirred the pot, and the extraordinary value of ABR in the evaluation of infants and young children soon became evident. Nevertheless, it was difficult to reconcile the magnitude of universal individual screening with what was perceived to be the excessive cost of individual ABR testing. The false positive rate was low, but the ABR procedure was perceived to be too expensive for widespread use.

A more likely candidate appeared on the scene with the advent of transient otoacoustic emissions (TEOAEs). A series of pioneering studies at the Women and Infants Hospital of Rhode Island by a team led by Karl White of Utah State University and Thomas Behrens of the U.S. Department of Education showed that TEOAEs could be used to screen babies quite successfully, and at moderate cost. The only problem here was the perception that the false positive rate of TEOAE screening (variously estimated at 10 to 20%) was prohibitive. Well, if ABR had a low false-positive rate but was too expensive, and TEOAE had a high false positive rate but was less expensive, then the idea quickly took hold that the ideal solution was a two-stage process in which TEOAEs are used on every baby in the first stage, and ABR is used in the second stage, but only on those babies who fail the first stage. All of this led to an NIH Consen-

sus Conference on Newborn Screening in 1993, in which just such a two-stage program for screening was recommended. At this writing, universal screening programs based on this and similar models have now been successfully organized in 37 states. We can count this as one of the major achievements of our profession.

The Auditory Processing Disorder Path

In the late 1940s, Helmer Myklebust opened a diagnostic children's hearing clinic at Northwestern University's School of Speech and encouraged parents, pediatricians, and other professionals to refer children suspected of possible hearing loss. The primary presenting symptom that brought children to the clinic, and indeed to most hearing care professionals in that era, was "not talking" (i.e., failure to develop speech appropriate to the child's chronological age), an inevitable consequence of moderate to severe hearing loss. Myklebust found such losses in the majority of the children referred to the clinic. But he also noted that many of the children referred for lack of appropriate speech development had no obvious hearing loss. Myklebust thought that some of these children might have a form of mild auditory agnosia. His descriptions of these children still resonate today:

One of their fundamental difficulties is that they cannot listen; therefore, they cannot direct their attention selectively to an expected sound. To them the auditory environment does not consist of many individual sounds to be used as the immediate situation demands. Their auditory world is conglomerate; all sounds having equal importance and all being foreground sounds simultaneously.

To fit these children into a coherent framework, Myklebust introduced the term *auditory disorder* as a descriptor covering not only peripheral hearing loss but problems at higher levels in the auditory system, especially as they affected language development. He then developed a systematic behavioral approach to the differential diagnosis of such disorders.

A number of audiologists in the United States thought that the development of sensitized speech testing by the Italians under Bocca in the 1950s had important implications for the diagnosis of such central auditory disorders. The work of the Italians had been based on patients with temporal lobe tumors, but the intuitive leap to the assessment of persons with auditory complaints, but lacking hard neurological signs, was irresistible. Several investigators set out to devise difficult or sensitized speech audiometric tasks. Chief among these were tests involving dichotic listening. The work on ear and hemisphere asymmetries by Brenda Milner and Doreen Kimura, at McGill University in Montreal, generated an interest in the development of dichotic listening tests that might prove useful in evaluating adults with brain lesions, and by extension, children with auditory disorders.

Over the next 2 decades, a number of dichotic tests or test batteries were developed for clinical use. In 1962, Jack Katz developed the staggered spondee word (SSW) test. In this test, a pair of spondee words is presented dichotically, but the second syllable of one word overlaps the first syllable of the other. Scoring and interpretation of the SSW are complex.

In 1977 Jack Willeford developed a dichotic sentence test using natural sentences. During this same period, Charles Berlin and colleagues developed a dichotic test procedure based on consonant–vowel nonsense syllables. Copies of the Berlin tapes were widely used worldwide for the next 3 decades. During the 1970s, Susan and James Jerger modified the Synthetic Sentence Identification (SSI) paradigm by adding either an ipsilateral (SSI-ICM) or a contralateral (SSI-CCM) competing message.

It should be emphasized that virtually all of this early development of dichotic testing was focused on the study of adults, usually with *verified brain lesions*. Beginning in the late 1970s, however, interest turned toward children. Could sensitized speech tests, and especially dichotic testing, be used to evaluate children suspected of auditory processing disorder (APD)? Although dichotic tests have played a major role in APD assessment, other approaches have included low-pass filtering, compressed or speeded speech, temporal and frequency patterning, and gap detection.

During the 1980s, the idea that some children might have particular problems with the processing of auditory input in spite of normal sensitivity spread rapidly. Although Myklebust had raised the issue 3 decades earlier, the burgeoning societal interest in reading problems, language delay, learning disability, and attention deficit disorder stimulated a widespread rebirth of the concept. Historically, one can discern the development of two dissimilar approaches to the concept of auditory processing disorder; one might be called the "audiologic" approach, and the other the "psychoeducational" approach.

The audiologic approach built on the earlier observations that persons with brain injury affecting the auditory central nervous system exhibited certain behaviors; ergo, if tests revealed these same behaviors, then a link to brain injury was established. Several investigators set out to devise tests of the desired behavior appropriate for children. Based on the model of dichotic listening, Robert Keith developed two dichotic test procedures, one employing competing words, the other competing sentences. His SCAN procedures for both adults and children have been widely used in pediatric evaluation. Willeford's battery, including his competing sentences test, and Katz's SSW procedure have also been widely applied to children with apparently poor listening skills. In 1983 Jerger, Jerger, and Abrams developed the Pediatric Speech Intelligibility (PSI) test, a word-and-sentence-based test procedure, involving both ipsilateral and contralateral competing messages, for use with very young children. The rationale for most of these procedures might be summarized as follows: If persons with known injury to the auditory nervous system perform in a characteristic way on these tests, then if a child performs in that same characteristic way, an injury to that same part of the auditory nervous system may be assumed. The validity of this rationale has only rarely been tested in children.

The psychoeducational approach, on the other hand, is built on the premise of a set of primary auditory abilities that are measurable by appropriate techniques. This approach is illustrated by the auditory skills subtests of the 1974 Goldman, Fristoe, Woodcock Scale. This instrument posited four dimensions of auditory perceptual processing:

- Auditory discrimination
- Auditory memory
- Auditory selective attention
- Sound-symbol association

Other investigators have suggested additional dimensions, but they are all variations on the theme of hypothesized discrete perceptual processes.

The idea that auditory processing ability underlies other basic abilities, such as language development and reading, was a natural outgrowth of the consideration that, if learning is based on language, and if language is learned primarily through the auditory modality, then it is reasonable to suppose that problems in auditory perceptual processing could lead to problems in language acquisition and to subsequent learning disability. Christine Sloan was an early advocate of this position. Paula Tallal and her colleagues were among the first to investigate the area systematically. Their early studies of children with language delay suggested that some showed specific difficulty in responding to rapidly changing stimuli, whether the stimuli were verbal or nonverbal. Here was a suggestion that the number of primary auditory perceptual abilities underlying the auditory processing abilities which, in turn, underlie successful language development, may be limited in number. Tallal and colleagues have developed sophisticated techniques for evaluating and treating disorders of rapid auditory processing or RAP.

Recently, a group of Australian investigators, led by Sharon Cameron, suggested that a different unitary aspect of auditory perception, the ability to differentiate spatially dissimilar foreground and background sounds, might be present in a high proportion of children at risk for APD. This is eerily reminiscent of Myklebust's original description quoted above.

Gradually, the initial emphasis on auditory processing has, in some circles, become an empha-

sis on language processing. People whose primary interest is childhood language disorders, particularly their management, emphasize that auditory processing is only one component of the processing of language in difficult acoustic environments. In other words, factors other than auditory perceptual disorder may contribute to what many have identified as symptoms of APD, and they may interact with auditory perceptual disorders to complicate language processing.

The Hearing Conservation Path

The effects of excessive noise on hearing had been recognized virtually since the birth of the industrial age. Early writers described the deafness of weavers, due to the impact noises created by looms and the deleterious effects on hearing of the great artillery battles of World War I, but it was not until World War II, and its tremendous toll on hearing, especially from aircraft noise, that the armed services of the United States addressed the issues of hearing conservation with a series of regulations defining noise exposure as a hazard, setting forth conditions under which hearing protection must be employed, and requiring that personnel exposed to potentially hazardous noise be monitored audiometrically. The introduction of jet aircraft into both the Air Force and the Navy in the late 1940s, generating high levels of broad-spectrum noise, was an important factor driving interest in hearing protection. Early research studies of the effects of noise on the auditory system were carried out in the 1940s and 1950s at the Naval School of Aviation Medicine, in Pensacola, Florida. Similar research programs were established at the Navy submarine base in Groton, Connecticut, and at the Navy Electronics Laboratory in San Diego, California.

Early in the 1950s the National Research Council of the National Academy of Sciences formed a Committee on Hearing and Bioacoustics (CHABA), to study and make recommendations to the Armed Services concerning the intense jet engine noise on the flight line and the aircraft carrier deck. This led to the now famous NRC publication, "Biological

Effects of Noise Exploratory Study" (the BENOX report), which, for the first time, summarized what was known about the effects of intense noise exposure on humans, including hearing loss, aural pain, psychological effects, communication problems, disorders of spatial orientation and other effects on the central nervous system. The BENOX report had a major effect on subsequent efforts to establish standards for the protection of human hearing.

Interest in hearing conservation in the civilian sector was promoted by the 1970 amendment to the Walsh-Healy Public Contracts Act of 1936, which mandated that holders of certain public contracts must assure the health and safety of their workers against all hazardous conditions. The Williams-Steiger Occupational Health Act of 1971 established the Occupational Safety and Health Administration (OSHA) which published in 1983 its guidelines, including standards for maximum allowable noise environments, procedures for noise abatement, and protection of workers' hearing. Many audiologists have played key roles in the design and implementation of industrial audiometric monitoring mandated by the OSHA regulations.

Tinnitus Evaluation and Therapy Path

Tinnitus researcher Gary Jacobson, of Vanderbilt University, has estimated that there may be as many as 40 million individuals suffering from tinnitus in the United States. Perhaps 7 to 8 million of these people are so bothered by the ringing noise that they seek medical attention. Yet few audiologists have engaged in systematic research on the topic. James Henry, of the National Center for Research in Auditory Rehabilitation (NCRAR) in Portland, Oregon, has traced the history of efforts to evaluate and treat tinnitus over the past several decades. He notes that, as early as 1821, Jean Marc Gaspard Itard, Chief Physician at the National Institute for Deaf Mutes in Paris found that, in his pupils, tinnitus could often be treated with a masking sound and that the pitch of the tinnitus was linked to the pitch of the most effective masking sound.

In recent years many individuals have attempted to quantify tinnitus by asking the sufferer to match the loudness and pitch of the subjective percept with the frequency and intensity of an objective stimulus. As early as the 1930s Edmund Prince Fowler (of audiogram fame) found that when patients were asked to match the loudness of their tinnitus to the intensity of a pitch-matched pure tone, the apparent sensation level of the match was in the 5 to 10 dB range. He concluded that tinnitus was an "illusion" that tended to be exaggerated by the patient. There is a considerable history of attempts to match tinnitus to a specific frequency on the audiometer, but a fundamental problem with this approach is that while some tinnitus sufferers hear a "ringing" tone, others hear a sound more accurately described as either a narrow or broadband noise; thus, matching to the pitch of a pure tone is not always feasible. Pioneers in tinnitus evaluation over the past 3 to 4 decades have included Victor Goodhill at UCLA, Jack Vernon, Robert Johnson, and Mary Meikle at the Oregon Health Sciences University Hearing Research Center, Richard Tyler at the University of Iowa, M. J. Penner, at the University of Maryland, and Aage Moller at the University of Texas at Dallas.

In the continuing effort to quantify the actual handicap related to this elusive phenomenon, a number of investigators have turned to the development of questionnaires. Those in current use include the Tinnitus Handicap Questionnaire, developed by Kuk, Tyler, and Russell; the Tinnitus Handicap Inventory, developed by Newman and Jacobson; and the Tinnitus Cognitions Questionnaire, developed by Wilson and Henry.

Harald Feldman, of Germany, is credited with the first observation that tinnitus could be relieved by purposely masking it with an external sound. He reported a success rate of 89% by the use of a tinnitus masker. Subsequent research on this topic has demonstrated that either specific devices known as tinnitus maskers, or actual hearing aids are helpful to many tinnitus sufferers. In recent years treatment options for tinnitus have expanded dramatically. Drug treatment includes antidepressants, acamprosate, zinc, gabapentin, antioxidants, vitamins, herbs, minerals, and melatonin. Another treatment approach has been cognitive therapy. The Tinnitus Retraining program of Jastreboff, and the Tinnitus Activities treatment of Tyler, Gogel, and Gehringer are particularly noteworthy. Although investigators from many disciplines contribute to our understanding of tinnitus and its treatment, audiologists will play an increasing role in this area in the years to come.

Educational Audiology Path

The history of what we now call educational audiology can be traced back to those eighteenth and nineteenth century educators of the deaf who eschewed signing in favor of an aural approach. Before the advent of electronic amplification, intervention was limited to training in lipreading and the use of a diversity of mechanical aids ranging from speaking tubes to an incredible amplifying chair. But within the constraints of these limited resources, dedicated teachers in the classroom environment worked valiantly to develop communication skills in severely hearing-impaired children.

In the modern era one of the earliest educational audiologists was Moe Bergman, now a distinguished elder statesman of audiology at Tel Aviv University in Israel. In the 1930s, at the depth of the economic depression in America, Bergman was employed in the New York City school system as a speech correctionist. As part of a project to collect data on the prevalence of various speech disorders in the schools he used an early Western Electric 6B portable audiometer to screen for hearing loss. This schoolroom project led him to an interest in the educational needs not only of severely impaired children, but those with mild and moderate losses as well. He went on to found the New York VA Audiology Clinic, the first in the Veterans Administration system, then to an outstanding career at Hunter College of the City University of New York, before finally emigrating to Israel. Today educational audiologists work in school systems throughout the United States. They are well served professionally by the Educational Audiology Association (EAA).

Ann Mulholland is credited as the first person to use the term "educational audiology" in 1965.

The concept of educational audiology as a discipline began in 1966 when Frederick S. Berg generated the first known grant to train professionals to work with children with hearing losses in the public school system at Utah State University. He continued to receive Department of Education support for the MA level training until 1970. During this period, Berg and Fletcher published *The Hard of Hearing Child* (1970) which helped foster the concept of educational audiology on a national basis. With interest in educational audiology expanding, a doctoral program was added in 1979 and a specialist degree in 1986.

During the developmental period between 1970 and 1979, Berg wrote another book, *Educational Audiology: Hearing and Speech Management* (1976). This book helped to further the concept of educational audiology as one focused on the importance of hearing and listening skills, speech and listening training, and advancements in hearing technology for children in regular school classrooms. The model promoted the concept of the resource specialist for hard of hearing children in contrast to the traditional teacher of the deaf in a special classroom by emphasizing audiometry assessment, hearing aid evaluation and management, communication training, educational evaluation and training, and environmental evaluation and adjustments. By integrating conventional aspects of clinical audiology with components of deaf education, a definition of educational audiology evolved:

Educational audiology seeks to isolate the parameters of hearing impairment, to identify the deficiencies rising from hearing disability, to relate these to the unique characteristic of individuals, and to develop educational programs specifically for hard of hearing children.

The model of educational audiology continued to progress with the influence of many others. Multiple publication of guidelines and position statements by ASHA (Audiology Programs in Educational Settings for Hearing-Impaired Children, 1976; Audiology Services in the Schools, 1983; Audiology Service in the Schools, 1993; Guidelines for Audiology Service Provision in and for Schools, 2002) and EAA have further defined educational audiology.

In 1983, a doctoral student at Utah State University, Ann Wilson-Vlotman, surveyed all known educational audiologists in the United States. This survey revealed a strong interest in forming a national group of professionals in educational audiology. On November 18, 1983, during the annual ASHA convention, EAA was formed with eight members: Fred Berg, Jim Blair, Dorinne Davis, Bill Johnson, Alice Kreisle, Marvin Pekny, Sherry Press Redler, and Debra Smith. The Educational Audiology Association (EAA) is a professional membership organization of audiologists and related professionals who deliver a full spectrum of hearing services to all children, particularly those in educational settings. "The mission of the Educational Audiology Association is to act as the primary resource and as an active advocate for its members through its publications and products, continuing educational activities, networking opportunities, and other professional endeavors" (http://www.edaud.org).

Fred Berg was elected the first president serving from November 1984 through December of 1985. The association's constitution and bylaws were approved in 1985 and the association was formally incorporated in March 1985.

The association met annually during or before the ASHA Convention each year until 1998 and later periodically during Audiology Now. Meetings were also often held in conjunction with the Alexander Graham Bell Association Convention in even-numbered years.

In June, 1991, EAA joined the Academy of Rehabilitative Audiology at their Summer Institute at Beaver Run Resort in Breckenridge, Colorado, for its first major conference. A large portion of the program was devoted to issues of concern to educational audiologists. Since then, EAA has hosted its own summer conferences every other year in varying sites around the country offering professional development and networking opportunities.

Concluding Remarks

Although this brief review has traced seven distinct paths in which the profession of audiology has developed over the past half century, it is interesting to observe the degree to which these paths have interacted. We see the fruits of progress in the diagnostic path reflected in the development of APD testing, the impact of advances in electroacoustics and electrophysiology on universal screening procedures, the influence of cochlear implant advances on auditory training, and the influences of all on intervention with amplification, hearing conservation, tinnitus therapy, and audiology in the educational setting. These are, we believe, hallmarks of a robust and growing profession with a remarkable history.

Suggested Readings

Berg, F. (1976). *Educational audiology: Hearing and speech management*. New York, NY: Grune & Stratton.

Berg, F., & Fletcher, S. (1970). *The hard of hearing child*. New York, NY: Grune & Stratton.

Blair, J., & VonAlmen, P. (1991). Historical growth of educational audiology and the Educational Audiology Association. *Educational audiology monograph (2), 1*, ii–iii. Educational Audiology Association: http://www.edaud.org.

Cacace, A., & McFarland, D. (1998). Central auditory processing disorder in school-aged children: A critical review. *Journal of Speech, Language and Hearing Research, 41*, 355–373.

Hall, J. (2007). *New handbook of auditory evoked responses*. Boston, MA: Allyn & Bacon.

Jerger, J. (1973). *Modern developments in audiology*. New York, NY: Academic Press.

Jerger, S., & Jerger, J. (1981). *Auditory disorders: a manual for clinical evaluation*. Boston, MA: Little, Brown and Company.

Kricos, P., & Holmes, A. (2007). *From ear to their: A historical perspective on auditory training. Seminars in Hearing, 28*, 89–98.

Mueller, H., & Hall, J. (1998). *Audiologists' desk reference* (Vols. I and II). San Diego, CA: Singular.

Silman, S., & Silverman, C. (1991). *Auditory diagnosis: Principles and applications*. San Diego, CA: Academic Press.

Watson, L., & Tolan, T. (1949). *Hearing tests and hearing instruments*. Baltimore, MD: Williams & Wilkins.

Glossary

1B1G trace Vanhuyse tympanogram classification, used with higher frequency probe tones, in which there is one change of direction (e.g., peak) on the B (susceptance) trace and one change of direction on the G (conductance) trace

3B1G trace Vanhuyse tympanogram classification, used with higher frequency probe tones, in which there are three changes of direction (e.g., peaks or troughs) on the B (susceptance) trace and one change of direction on the G (conductance) trace

3B3G trace Vanhuyse tympanogram classification, used with higher frequency probe tones, in which there are three changes of direction (e.g., peaks or troughs) on the B (susceptance) trace and three changes of direction on the G (conductance) trace

5B3G trace Vanhuyse tympanogram classification, used with higher frequency probe tones, in which there are five changes of direction (e.g., peaks or troughs) on the B (susceptance) trace and three changes of direction on the G (conductance) trace

absolute refractory period minimal period of time needed for a neuron to recover before it can respond again (about 1.0 ms), imposing restrictions on the discharge rate (1,000 discharges per second)

AC IA (with insert earphone) = 55 dB the suggested minimum amount of interaural attenuation used in making decisions about air conduction masking for pure tones when using insert earphones

AC IA (with supra-aural earphone) = 40 dB the suggested minimum amount of interaural attenuation used in making decisions about air conduction masking for pure tones when using supra-aural earphones

acoustic neuroma benign tumor involving the 8th cranial nerve; also known as vestibular schwannoma due to its common origin being on the vestibular portion of the 8th cranial nerve

acoustic reflex involuntary contraction of the stapedius muscle and tensor tympani muscle when stimulated by loud sounds that reduce the vibration of the ossicles; also called the middle ear reflex or the stapedial reflex (because the stapedius muscle is mostly involved in humans)

acoustic reflex decay (ARD) an inability of the acoustic reflex to sustain contraction during a 10-s tonal stimulation at 10 dB above the acoustic reflex threshold; abnormal acoustic reflex decay is defined as more than 50% return of the acoustic reflex toward baseline within 5 s, and is suggestive of an 8th nerve tumor

acoustic reflex threshold (ART) the lowest intensity level (in 5 dB steps) of a reflex eliciting tone that produces a repeatable acoustic reflex (e.g., greater than or equal to 0.02 mmhos)

acoustics study of the physical properties of sounds in the environment and how they travel through air

acquired hearing loss hearing loss that occurs due to injury or disease that is not of genetic or congenital origin

active cochlear process physiological process present in a healthy normal cochlea related to the motility of the outer hair cells, and which is responsible for enhanced displacement of the traveling wave, good sensitivity, and relatively sharp frequency selectivity (tuning)

acute disorder a disease that is in its initial stage; usually comes on suddenly and lasts a relatively short duration

acute otitis media inflammation (infection) of the fluid in the middle ear

adaptation ability of the 8th nerve fibers to sustain adequate neural information; normally characterized by a higher discharge rate at the onset of the stimulus and then settles down to a steady state; abnormal adaptation, found in 8th nerve disorders, is characterized by a relatively normal onset discharge response, but the discharge rate is not able to settle into a normal steady state (keeps declining)

admittance (Y) the amount of applied energy that flows through a system; measured in millimhos (mmhos); reciprocal of impedance

admittance of the middle ear (Y$_{tm}$) the measure of admittance during tympanometry that is representative of the middle ear (after removing the admittance due to the ear canal); the difference between overall admittance (Y) and the ear canal admittance (V$_{ec}$); also called peak compensated static acoustic admittance

afferent auditory neurons nerve fibers that carry impulses from the sensory organs (peripheral) toward the brain (central); approximately 31,000 afferent auditory neurons come from each cochlea

affricates a type of speech sound created by the transition of a stop into a fricative

air–bone gap the difference in pure-tone threshold obtained by air conduction (AC) and bone conduction (BC); represents amount of hearing loss related to involvement of the conductive parts of the ear (outer and middle)

air conduction (AC) testing mode of sound presentation through earphones; stimulates the entire auditory system

American Board of Audiology (ABA) Certification professional certification available for audiologists through the American Academy of Audiology

American Academy of Audiology (AAA) professional organization of audiologists; offers accreditation to academic programs (ACAE) and professional certification for audiologists (ABA certification)

aminoglycosides antibiotic drugs that are associated with hearing loss (cochleotoxic) and/or balance disorders (vestibulotoxic)

amplitude characteristic of a waveform that is related to its magnitude or size

ampulla (plural = ampullae) bulbous region near the anterior end (near the vestibule) of each semicircular canal; houses the crista ampullaris

anotia complete absence of the auricle

ANSI (American National Standards Institute) a committee of specialists that develops standards; responsible for standards related to audiologic test equipment and recommended procedures for hearing testing

antihelix ridge of cartilage that runs along the central portion of the auricle; parallel to the helix

antimalarial drugs used to prevent malaria, e.g., quinine and chloroquine

antinodes property of resonance whereby two interacting tones combine

antitragus small cartilaginous flap at the top of the earlobe and at the end of the antihelix; opposite to the tragus

aperiodic vibration sound wave in which the pattern of vibration does not regularly repeat itself over time; also known as noise

area ratio advantage one of the middle ear mechanical amplification methods due to the larger size (area) of the tympanic membrane compared with the oval window

articulation or audibility index (AI) prediction of the amount of the acoustic information (scale of 0–1) of speech that is available to the listener; basic principle is that as less of the speech spectrum becomes audible (by externally filtering or by the presence of a hearing loss) speech intelligibility gets poorer in a predictable way; later revised and renamed the speech intelligibility index (SII)

articulators oral and nasal components of movement during shaping of speech sounds (e.g., tongue, lips, velum, jaws)

ascending method procedure in which thresholds are obtained by raising the level from inaudible to audible; opposite of descending method

ASHA (American Speech-Language-Hearing Association) professional organization of audiologists and speech-language pathologists; offers accreditation to academic programs (CAA)

and professional certification for audiologists and speech-language pathologists

asymmetric significant difference in the hearing loss between the two ears

atresia (atretic ear) congenital absence of an external auditory canal

attenuation rate the amount that a filter reduces certain frequencies; slope of the curve in a filter above and below the cutoff frequencies, specified as dB per octave

AuD (Doctor of Audiology) degree designator commonly used for the professional doctorate in audiology; minimum degree needed to practice clinical audiology

audiogram the graph used in audiometry to plot the patient's pure-tone thresholds

audiologist a professional who has the appropriate degree and license in his state to practice audiology; typically certified by a professional board (American Academy of Audiology and/or American Speech-Language-Hearing Association)

audiology discipline that focuses on the scientific study and clinical practice related to hearing and hearing disorders

audiometer electronic or computer-based instrument used for many of the behavioral hearing tests performed in audiometry

audiometric pertaining to measures made with audiometry

audiometry assessment of a person's responses to sounds

auditory brainstem response (ABR) physiological test used in audiology for documenting auditory sensitivity in difficult-to-test populations or for assessment of 8th nerve tumors; series of auditory evoked potentials from the 8th nerve and brainstem auditory pathways that occur within the first 10 ms after stimulus onset and measured with small disk electrodes placed on the surface of the head

auditory dyssynchrony condition where 8th nerve neurons do not fire with normal synchrony; also known as auditory neuropathy; characterized by the absence of auditory brainstem responses and the presence of normal otoacoustic emissions

auditory evoked (electroacoustic or electroneural) responses electrical potentials evoked by sound; include the auditory brainstem responses, middle latency responses, late latency responses, and otoacoustic emissions; used to assess and screen for auditory function in difficult-to-test populations and/or to differentially diagnose type and locations of some hearing disorders

auditory nerve portion of the 8th cranial nerve consisting of nerve fibers from the cochlea

auditory neuropathy see auditory dyssynchrony

auditory processing disorder (APD) reduced ability to process or use auditory information when it is presented in more degraded types of listening situations; pure-tone thresholds are typically normal; sometimes called central auditory processing disorders (CAPD)

aural fullness reported sensation of pressure in the ear; can occur with inner or middle ear disorders

auricle cartilaginous portion of the outer ear that is attached to the lateral surface of the temporal bone

auricular pertaining to the auricle

auricular hematoma internal bleeding within the auricle; like a bruise

automatic audiometer an audiometer with the capability of automatically changing the signal level based on the response of the patient; Békésy audiometry

automatic gain control (AGC) circuitry that automatically maintains the level of a signal; used to maintain immittance probe tone at 85 dB SPL in the ear canal; used in hearing aids to adjust the gain depending on the changes in signal level

band-pass filter a filter that transmits (passes) a range of frequencies between some selected high and low frequency cutoffs (at 3 dB down points), and excludes those above and below the cutoff frequencies at a specified attenuation rate

band-reject filter a filter that excludes (rejects) a range of frequencies between some selected high and low frequency cutoffs (at 3 dB down points), and transmits (passes) those above and below the cutoff frequencies at a specified attenuation rate

barotrauma middle ear disorder caused by sudden change in external air pressure; results in a mismatch in pressure between that in the ear canal and that in the middle ear spaces

basilar membrane portion of the membranous labyrinth that supports the organ of Corti; attaches from the osseous spiral lamina to the outer wall of the bony labyrinth; separates scala media from scala tympani; important for the transduction of sound in the cochlea through the generation of the basilar membrane traveling waves

BC IA = 0 dB the suggested minimum amount of interaural attenuation used in making decisions about bone conduction masking for pure tones

behind-the-ear hearing aid (BTE) curved hearing aid that is worn behind the ear (or one on each ear) and coupled to the earmold in the ear through a tube

Bel unit of sound intensity or pressure expressed as the logarithm of a ratio scale relative to a specified reference value; Bels are too large for use in hearing measures (see decibel)

BiCROS (bilateral CROS) bilateral CROS type of hearing aid fitting used when one ear has poor hearing and the better ear has a mild to moderate hearing loss; a microphone is placed on the poorer hearing ear and a complete hearing aid is placed on the better hearing ear; all sounds are amplified and channeled into the better hearing ear

bilateral pertaining to both sides or to both ears

binaural hearing simultaneous use of both ears in hearing

Bing test a tuning fork test in which the tuning fork is placed on the mastoid and the patient is asked to indicate if the sound changes when occluding the ear by pushing in on the tragus

binomial distribution a statistically derived table of probabilities, made popular by Thornton and Raffin (1978), to interpret critical differences (95% confidence intervals) between two word recognition scores; reflects the variability (standard deviation) of scores as a function of the number of test items

biological battery role of the stria vascularis in maintaining the endocochlear potential (EP) for the scala media

body aid a relatively large square or rectangular hearing aid worn on the body; the sounds are delivered by an electrical cord to the receiver/earmold, which is placed in the ear

bone-anchored hearing aid (BAHA) hearing aid that is surgically implanted by an otologist into the mastoid area behind the ear; useful for hearing losses with good bone conduction thresholds

bone conduction (BC) testing mode of sound presentation through a bone oscillator used in pure-tone audiometry; delivers vibration directly to the inner ear through vibrations in the temporal bone, which essentially bypasses the conductive (outer and middle ear) portions of the auditory pathway; provides a measure of the sensorineural component of a hearing loss

bone conduction vibrator a transducer which has a hard plastic casing that is set into vibration by pure tones; used in pure-tone audiometry for bone conduction (BC) testing, and usually placed behind the ear on the mastoid portion of the temporal bone; also called a bone conduction oscillator

bony labyrinth series of canals within the petrous portion of the temporal bone that houses the inner ear

carboplatin antineoplastic cancer-treating chemical agent; can cause hearing loss

Carhart's notch mild decline in the bone conduction threshold at 2000 Hz often seen with otosclerosis

carrier phrase a short sentence, such as, "Say the word____," often used prior to the test word in word recognition score testing

CCC-A (Certificate of Clinical Competence in Audiology) professional certification available for audiologists through the American Speech-Language-Hearing Association

center frequency frequency at the center of a filter where the maximum sound is delivered

central auditory disorders pathologies and/or processing that involve the central auditory system

central auditory (or vestibular) system part of the auditory system that includes the neural pathways and nuclei in the brainstem and cortical areas; excludes the peripheral auditory structures

cerebellar-pontine angle (CPA) region of the brain where the 8th nerve exits the internal auditory canal and the brainstem; formed by the area between the cerebellum, pons, and internal auditory canal; site of 8th nerve tumors

cerumen waxy substance produced by glands in the external auditory canal that helps protect, lubricate, and clean the canal; also called earwax

characteristic frequency the frequency where the basilar membrane or auditory nerve fiber is most sensitive; most sensitive point of a tuning curve

chemotherapeutic (neoplastic) agents cancer-treating chemical drugs

cholesteatoma benign tumorlike mass that invades middle ear space; formed by deposits of squamous epithelia that become keratinized and infected; often secondary to retracted tympanic membrane from poor eustachian tube function

chronic disorder persistent condition over a long period of time

chronic otitis media persistent middle ear condition with thickening fluid remaining in the middle ear for an extended time; infections may reoccur and hearing loss may be present

cisplatin cancer-treating chemical agent; can cause hearing loss

Claudius cells support cells within the organ of Corti; located next to the Hensen cells along the outer edge of the organ of Corti

clinical masking the process of putting noise into the non-test ear while measuring thresholds in the test ear

closed-head injury nonpenetrating trauma to the skull

closed-set speech materials in which patients select from a list with which they are familiarized or is visually available to them

cochlea the part of the inner ear involved with hearing; houses the organ of Corti

cochlear aqueduct narrow bony canal of the inner ear that connects the perilymph of the bony labyrinth with the cerebral spinal fluid

cochlear implant (CI) biomedical device with an electrode array inserted into a nonfunctional cochlea to electrically stimulate neurons of the cochlear nerve

cochlear implant mapping computer software, designed by manufacturers of cochlear implants, and used by audiologists to maximize the patient's use of the electrode array for communication

cochlear nerve portion of the 8th cranial nerve consisting of nerve fibers from the cochlea

cochlear nucleus (CN) collection of cell bodies in the lateral pontine region of the brainstem that connects to the 8th cranial nerve fibers associated with the cochlea

cochlear otosclerosis a type of otosclerosis (otospongiosis) in which the bony growth invades the inner ear and destroys hair cells

collapsed canals a temporary closing off of the ear canal that can occur in some individuals with reduced elasticity in the cartilaginous portion of the external ear canal and due to pressure exerted by supra-aural earphones

commissure nerve fibers that provide interconnections between two sides of the brain; as in commissure of Probst and commissure of the inferior colliculi of the auditory pathways in the brainstem

compensated tympanogram a way to display a tympanogram whereby the instrument automatically removes the component of admittance related to the ear canal (as measured at +200 daPa) and only graphs the admittance characteristics of the middle ear

completely-in-the-canal (CIC) a hearing aid in which all the components reside in a casing that fits completely in the ear canal; smallest of the custom hearing aids

complex periodic vibration nonsinusoidal sound wave in which the vibratory pattern is composed of more than one tone and which repeats itself as a function of time; also known as complex periodic tone

compression non-linear amplifier gain that is part of most hearing aids; adjusts the gain dependent of the amount of input

computer-based audiometry audiometric hearing tests in which a computer is used to generate and control the signals; can also record patients' responses, automatically analyze and print the results, and track patient databases

concha the bowl-shaped indentation of the auricle just before the entrance (meatus) to the external auditory canal

condensation the phase of a waveform that is associated with an increase in the density of air molecules, which corresponds to an increase in sound pressure

conditioned-play audiometry an audiometric technique used for testing children 2 to 4 years old; procedure employs play techniques such as putting a toy in a bucket when they hear the sound

conductance (G) the part of the admittance that is related to the frictional component; conductance is characterized by the force and velocity being in-phase with each other

conductive hearing loss hearing loss due to involvement of the outer and/or middle ear; characterized by an air–bone gap of more than 10 dB and bone conduction thresholds within normal range

congenital hearing loss hearing loss present at birth due to pre- or perinatal events

connexin-26 genetic protein mutation during embryologic development; common cause of congenital hearing loss

consonants parts of speech that generally contribute to speech intelligibility; generally lower in intensity and higher in frequency than vowels; precede and follow vowel sounds to construct meaningful parts of speech; may be periodic or aperiodic

continuous spectrum amplitude spectrum that involves a continuous line to indicate that there are infinite frequencies that are present over the specified range

contralateral acoustic reflex acoustic reflex obtained from the ear on the opposite side from the ear being stimulated; due to the contralateral pathway of the bilateral acoustic reflex

corneoretinal potential electrical potential from the eyes; surface electrodes around the eyes are used to measure eye movements (nystagmus) during vestibular testing with electronystagmography

corpus callosum prominent band of nerve fibers that connects the two hemispheres of the cortex

count-the-dots audiogram a simpler method to represent the acoustic weightings from the articulation/speech intelligibility index as dots on an audiogram; a specified number of dots are used to represent the speech banana, weighted more heavily at 2000 and 4000 Hz regions; useful tool to let patients know how much of the speech sounds they may be missing

crista (plural = cristae) sensory organ of the semicircular canals that responds to angular accelerations of the head; located in the ampulla within the membranous labyrinth of each semicircular canal; also called crista ampullaris

critical differences table used to compare two word recognition scores to determine if they are significantly different from each other (95% confidence interval), based on a binomial distribution

CROS (contralateral routing of signals) hearing aid type of hearing aid fitting used as an option with unilateral hearing loss; a microphone is placed on the poorer hearing ear and the sounds are channeled into the better hearing ear fit with an open-fitting-type earmold

cross-hearing the amount of a signal presented to one ear that can be heard in the non-test ear when the interaural attenuation is exceeded

cross-links microfilaments that interconnect the stereocilia of each inner and outer hair cell; well-developed cross-links of the outer hair cell stereocilia keep them well organized and rigid

cubic difference tone most prominent distortion product tone associated with the nonlinearity of the basilar membrane; occurs at frequencies equal to 2f1–f2

cupula gelatinous membrane within the crista; stereocilia and kinocilium of the sensory hair cells are embedded in the cupula and are bent with deflections of the cupula during angular accelerations

curved membrane advantage one of the middle ear mechanical amplification methods resulting from the cone shape of the tympanic membrane, which tends to focus its movement in such a way that it moves the malleus with more force than if the tympanic membrane was flat

custom hearing aids hearing aids worn in the concha or ear canal that have all of the components built inside of the earmold, e.g., in-the-ear (ITE), in-the-canal (ITC), and completely-in-the-canal (CIC)

cutoff frequency upper and/or lower frequencies where the filter begins to be attenuated; defined as the frequency that is 3 dB less than the frequency with the highest amplitude

cycle pattern of movement as an object goes through its full range of motion one time

cytomegalovirus (CMV) a common viral infection with mild flulike symptoms; primary cause of congenital progressive hearing loss when fetus is exposed to virus in utero

damage risk criteria industrial standards that limit the amount of noise exposure workers can be exposed to in a 24-hr period without the risk of noise-related hearing loss

Davis Battery Theory a theory, first postulated by Davis (1965), stating that the 120–140 mV electrical potential between the endolymph and the inside of the hair cells acts like the voltage of a battery, and this serves as the force that drives the ionic current into the hair cell that is modulated by changes in resistance due to the bending of the stereocilia

dB intensity level (dB IL) intensity (in dB) of a sound that is referenced to the standard reference value for intensity (10^{-12} w/m^2); dB IL implies that 10^{-12} w/m^2 is in the denominator of the dB formula for intensity measures

dB sound pressure level (dB SPL) pressure (in dB) of a sound that is referenced to the standard reference value for pressure (20 µPa); dB SPL implies that 20 µPa is in the denominator of the dB formula for pressure measures

decibel (dB) unit of sound intensity or pressure that is 1/10 of a Bel

decibels hearing level (dB HL) decibel scale in which the reference value is the minimum sound pressure level standards for normal hearing as a function of frequency, where 0 dB HL at any frequency represents the lowest level for normal hearing

decibels of sensation level (dB SL) decibel scale in which the reference value is the patient's own threshold

degree of hearing loss one of the parameters used in describing audiograms; refers to the amount of hearing loss; slight, mild, moderate, moderately severe, severe, and profound

Deiter cells support cells within the organ of Corti that have outer hair cells sitting on top of them; each Deiter cell also has a phalangeal process that extends to the upper surface of the outer hair cells and fills in the gaps; also called outer phalangeal cell

descending methods procedure in which thresholds are obtained by lowering the level from audible to inaudible; opposite of ascending method

desynchronize the disruption of the synchronized firings normally present in the auditory nerve; underlying cause of the disorder auditory dyssynchrony (auditory neuropathy)

diagnostic (clinical) audiometer electronic or computer-based instrument capable of performing a variety of tests, including pure-tone audiometry (with masking), speech, and other special tests; must conform to standards of operation as specified by American National Standards Institute (ANSI)

differential diagnosis analyses of different tests to determine the type and/or location of a disorder (determine which part or parts of the ear are affected)

diffraction bending or scattering of a sound wave as it encounters an object, opening, or different medium

digital conversion a means of converting electrical signals from the microphone into digital information (analog to digital converter) or digital information into electrical/acoustic signals to the hearing aid receiver (digital to analog converter) in order to allow for computerized signal manipulation and application of different processing algorithms

digital hearing aid hearing aids that use computer-based technology (digital) to process sounds

disarticulation separation of the ossicular chain or break in one of the ossicles; also called ossicular discontinuity

discharge rate the number of discharges per second that a neuron produces in response to a specified sound

distal away from the origin or center of a structure or nerve; opposite of proximal

distortion product otoacoustic emissions (DPOAEs) type of otoacoustic emissions evoked by two closely spaced pure tones (f1/f2 = 1.22) to produce distortion tones in the cochlea, the largest of which is the cubic difference tone (2f1–f2); measured by signal averaging of the acoustic signals generated by the ear and picked up by a sensitive microphone in the ear canal

Doctor of Audiology (AuD) professional doctorate which is the entry-level degree to practice clinical audiology

ductus reuniens small channel connecting the membranous labyrinth of the vestibular organs and the cochlea

dynamic range the difference in decibels between the patient's hearing threshold and an uncomfortable listening level for tones or speech

earhook part of the behind-the-ear (BTE) hearing aid that hangs (hooks) over the auricle onto the ear and connects to tubing that leads to the earmold

earlobe noncartilaginous lower portion of the auricle; traditional location for decorative earrings

early hearing detection and intervention (EHDI) synonymous with hearing screening and implies a comprehensive strategy of detection and follow up

early-onset genetic hearing loss hearing loss due to genetic factors that manifests during the infant–toddler stage

earmold custom-made earpiece that is attached to a behind-the-ear (BTE) hearing aid

earmold impression ingredients are mixed and inserted partially into a patient's ear to form a custom shape for the hearing aid or earmold; the impression is sent to the manufacturer to form the permanent earmold or casing for the hearing aid

effective masking levels a calibrated amount of narrow-band noise that provides a threshold shift to a corresponding dB HL for a tone centered within the noise

efferent neurons nerve fibers that carry impulses from the brain (central) toward the sensory organs (peripheral)

effusion accumulation of fluid into a cavity; middle ear effusion occurs from the extraction of fluid from the mucous lining of the middle ear cavity

electroacoustic analysis measurements of a hearing aid in a special test box to determine whether the hearing aid meets certain performance requirements, set by the American National Standards Institute (ANSI)

electronystagmography clinical tests of vestibular function based on recordings of the corneoretinal potential and nystagmus that is induced by various conditions

endocochlear potential (EP) +80 mV electrical potential (charge) in the endolymph of the scala media due to the high concentration of potassium (K^+); maintained by the stria vascularis

endolymph fluid in the membranous labyrinth that has a relatively high potassium (K^+) concentration and low sodium (Na^+) concentration; ionic composition similar to that of intracellular fluid; therefore, endolymph is unique as an extracellular fluid

endolymphatic duct and sac narrow canal arising from the area of the saccule that is part of the membranous labyrinth, and which ends in a flattened sac located in the subarachnoid space lining the brain tissues within the temporal bone; thought to control the buildup of endolymph; may be compromised in Ménière disease

endolymphatic hydrops excessive buildup of endolymph in the scala media and vestibular labyrinth; associated with Ménière disease, which is characterized by episodes of vertigo, fluctuating hearing loss, low-pitched tinnitus, and fullness

endolymphatic shunt operation to redirect or relieve the flow of endolymph as a treatment option for Ménière disease

envelope of the traveling wave an outline of the amplitudes associated with the traveling wave along the basilar membrane for a specified frequency

equal loudness contours representations of dB SPL as a function of frequency that are judged to be equal in loudness; expressed as phons, such that 40 phons is equivalent to the loudness of a 40 dB, 1000 Hz pure tone, according to which all other frequencies are judged

equal pitch contours representation of how pitch is affected by changes in intensity for different frequencies

equivalent volume of the ear canal (V_{ec}) the admittance measured with tympanometry at +200 daPa

eustachian tube connects the middle ear to the nasopharynx; comprised mostly of cartilage that is normally closed, and is opened by action of the tensor veli palatini muscle during chewing and swallowing to equalize air pressure in the middle ear to that of the surrounding environment

eustachian tube dysfunction a condition whereby the eustachian tube is unable to equalize middle ear pressure; common cause of middle ear effusion

excitatory phase transduction process in the cochlea associated with bending of stereocilia toward the tallest row of stereocilia (away from the modiolus); increase in the discharge rate of an auditory nerve fiber

exostosis (exostoses) bony outgrowths in the external auditory canal caused by repetitive irritation from cold water; also known as surfer's ear

external auditory canal (EAC) the canal leading from the auricle to the tympanic membrane; part of the outer ear

externship full-time clinical experience at an approved clinical site during the fourth year of an audiology doctoral program

false positive rate the number of times a patient responds in the absence of a presented sound; number of patients who are incorrectly identified as having a disorder

fast Fourier transform (FFT) mathematical relationship showing that any complex sound is a predictable combination of different pure tones; FFT instruments are available that will produce the spectrum of any complex sound

feedback a whistling-type sound produced by hearing aids due to the amplification of sounds from the receiver reaching the microphone and being reamplified

filtering a process in which certain frequencies are excluded and certain frequencies are passed through

final masking level the highest level of masking noise used in the non-test ear during clinical masking

footplate part of the stapes that connects to the oval window

foreign objects unnatural items found in the ear canal, e.g., cotton swabs, insects, food

formants concentrations of energy for bands of frequencies of periodic speech sounds, e.g., F1, F2 frequencies

formant transitions dynamic changes (rising or falling) in the frequencies of the formants during connected speech

frequency the number of cycles of a vibration that occur in 1 s, measured in hertz (Hz)

frequency counter electronic instrument used to determine the frequency of pure tones

frequency range of audibility for humans 20–20,000 Hz

frequency selectivity/tuning representation of how different measures of the auditory system respond to frequency by intensity combinations, often represented by tuning curves; description of how well the auditory system can differentiate frequencies

frequency theory theory of frequency coding based on the processing of discharge patterns in the afferent auditory nerve fibers

fricatives noiselike sounds produced by passing air through the oral cavity with turbulence caused by positioning of the articulators

functional hearing loss exaggerated or feigned hearing loss, often for financial or psychological reasons; hearing loss with no organic basis; also called nonorganic hearing loss or malingering

fundamental frequency (f_0) lowest frequency component in a complex periodic vibration

genetic hearing loss hearing loss caused by alterations in the genes during embryological development

glomus jugulare a type of glomus tumor that is associated with the jugular bulb along the floor of the middle ear

glomus tumor benign slow-growing tumor of the middle ear

glomus tympanicum a type of glomus tumor that is associated with nerves coursing through the middle ear, especially near the promontory

gold standard an acceptable test for a disorder in which other tests can be compared in order to judge their validity

graded potential a variable electrical gradient in nerve fibers prior to excitation; dependent on amount of available neurotransmitter substance at neural synapse

habenula perforata regularly spaced holes in the osseous spiral lamina through which the afferent nerve fibers leave the organ of Corti and enter the modiolus

half-wave resonator a condition of resonance whereby the fundamental frequency is equal to a half-wavelength, e.g., for a tube open at both ends

harmonics integer multiples of the fundamental frequency (f_0), e.g., $1f_0$, $2f_0$, $3f_0$, etc.

head shadow attenuation of sound by the head in the ear farther away from the sound source; occurs for sounds whose wavelengths are equal to or less than the size of the head

hearing aid an electronic device for amplifying sounds for patients with hearing loss

hearing aid candidacy process of determining whether a patient would potentially benefit from hearing aids

hearing aid orientation part of the hearing aid fitting process in which the patient is instructed on the use, care, and expectations of new hearing aids

hearing aid programming computer-based adjustments of the settings of a digital hearing aid

hearing conservation program industrial hearing care program that monitors noise levels, educates employees about noise-induced hearing loss, and provides hearing protection devices and strategies

Hearing Handicap Inventory for the Elderly-Screening a self-assessment scale of hearing disability generally used with adult hearing screening

hearing protection devices noise-reduction devices worn over the ear or inside the ear canal in work or recreational settings with high noise levels

helicotrema space at the apex of the coiled bony labyrinth in the cochlea where the scala tympani and scala vestibuli are continuous with each other due to the ending of the scala media

helix ridge of cartilage that runs around the outer border of the auricle

Hensen cells support cells in the organ of Corti that lie on the outer margin of the outer cells

hertz (Hz) unit of measure for frequency that represents cycles per second

Heschl's gyrus ridge along the upper surface of the temporal lobe that is the primary auditory reception area of the cortex

high frequency slope the high frequency part of a tuning curve that shows a steep slope

high-pass filter a type of filter that transmits (passes) all frequencies above its cutoff frequency and attenuates those below the cutoff frequency

high-pass masking a physiological masking paradigm used in auditory brainstem responses recordings to provide more frequency-specific information about the function of the cochlea; the cutoff frequency of a high-pass filtered noise is systematically changed to desynchronize some parts of the cochlea in order to observe responses from other regions

High Risk Register factors known to have a high association with hearing loss; recommendations made periodically by a Joint Committee on Newborn Hearing

HI-PRO (Hearing Instrument Programmer) interface device that connects a hearing aid that is to be programmed to the software application using a serial port and specially designed, manufacturer-specific cables

hydromechanical events cochlear transduction processes, including the vibratory energy in the cochlear fluids, followed by the movements of the basilar membrane and bending of the stereocilia by the tectorial membrane

indentification programs programs designed to screen for hearing loss

idiopathic disorder with an unknown cause

immittance term used to encompass both admittance and impedance

immittance audiometry battery of middle ear measures, including tympanometry and acoustic reflexes

impacted cerumen abnormal buildup of earwax (cerumen) that completely blocks off the ear canal

impedance (Z) total opposition to the flow of

energy in an acoustic/mechanical system; measured in units of ohms.

impedance mismatch situation in which two systems have different impedances so that there is an inefficient transfer of energy, e.g., vibrations in air are not efficiently transferred to fluid

incus second of the three middle ear ossicles; consists of a body, short process, long process, and lenticular process; the body articulates with the malleus, and the lenticular process articulates with the head of the stapes

inferior colliculus (IC) auditory nucleus located in the upper brainstem

inferior/descending vestibular nucleus lower region of the primary vestibular nuclei located in the posterior–lateral part of the upper medulla and lower pontine regions of the brainstem

inhibitory phase transduction process in the cochlea associated with bending of stereocilia away from the tallest row of stereocilia (toward the modiolus); decrease in the discharge rate of an auditory nerve fiber

initial masking level (IML) the masker level first applied to the non-test ear using the plateau method of clinical masking; for air conduction the IML = 10 dB above AC threshold; for bone conduction the IML = 10 dB above AC threshold plus the amount of any occlusion effect

inner hair cells (IHCs) auditory sensory hair cells within the organ of Corti; approximately 3,500 IHCs arranged in a single row

inner pillar cells support cells in the organ of Corti that form the inner "leg" of the triangular-shaped tunnel of Corti; also called inner rods of Corti

inner radial fibers afferent nerve fibers originating from the inner hair cells; approximately 95% of afferent fibers come from inner hair cells

inner support cells cells within the organ of Corti that surround the inner hair cells and provide support

input–output (I/O) function measure of how the output of a system changes as a function of the input, e.g., the discharge rate of an auditory nerve fiber as a function of stimulus intensity

insert earphone an air conduction transducer used in audiology that is placed within the ear canal; electroacoustic diaphragm is housed in a small case, which then sends an acoustic signal through a small tube held in place with a disposable foam cuff; common model, ER-3A

instantaneous phase phase of an individual pure tone or resultant combination of pure tones at any point in time

intensity measure of power distributed over an area in units of watts/cm^2 or watts/m^2 depending on the system of measurement being used (MKS or CGS); also generically used to describe the relative level of a sound

interaural attenuation (IA) the difference in intensity between the stimulus delivered to the test ear and the amount that crosses over (by bone conduction) to the non-test ear; the amount of sound level (dB HL) needed to vibrate the skull for different transducers

interaural intensity differences localization cue that is dependent on the different intensities of sounds at the two ears

interaural time differences localization cue that is dependent on the different arrival times of sounds at the two ears

intermittent disorder a pathologic condition that comes and goes or reoccurs often

internal auditory canal opening in the posterior wall of the petrous part of the temporal bone through which the vestibulocochlear (VIII) nerve and facial (VII) nerve exit

interspike intervals (ISIs) time intervals that occur between discharges of an auditory nerve fiber

in-the-canal (ITC) a type of custom hearing aid that has all of the hearing aid components built inside the casing, and which partially fills the lower approximate one-quarter of the concha with the receiver portion extending a short distance into the ear canal

in-the-ear (ITE) a type of custom hearing aid that has all the hearing aid components built inside the casing, and which fills most of the concha with the receiver portion extending a short distance into the ear canal

intra-axial within the brainstem, generally along the midline

intracellular potential electrical potential that is present inside the cochlear hair cells; −40 mV for inner hair cells and −60 mV for outer hair cells

inverse square law decrease in a sound's intensity with distance, expressed by the equation: Intensity (I) = 1/distance^2 or Pressure (P) = 1/distance

ipsilateral acoustic reflex acoustic reflex obtained from ear on the same side as the ear being stimulated; due to the ipsilateral pathway of the bilateral acoustic reflex

kilohertz (kHz) 1000 Hz

kinocilium single large cilium adjacent to the tallest row of stereocilia on each hair cell in the crista; oriented away from the utricle for the anterior and posterior canals, and toward the utricle for the horizontal semicircular canal

labyrinthectomy surgical operation to destroy the vestibular organs

late latency response (LLR) auditory evoked response occurring in the post-stimulus latency range of 100–300 ms reflecting activity of auditory events at the cortical level; later latency than auditory brainstem response and the middle latency response

latency the time it takes for a response to occur relative to the onset of an abrupt auditory stimulus; in auditory evoked responses, latency is measured in milliseconds

latency-intensity function a plot of response latency as a function of stimulus level; often used for interpretation of auditory brainstem responses

late-onset genetic hearing loss hearing loss due to genetic factors that manifests during childhood or adult stages

lateral lemniscus (LL) auditory nucleus of the lower brainstem; prominent nerve fiber bundle formed by ascending auditory fibers

lateral vestibular nucleus lateral region of the primary vestibular nuclei that is located in the posterior–lateral part of the upper medulla and lower pontine regions of the brainstem

lateralization a listening task where the person is asked to judge the location of sound in the head; Weber tuning fork test in which the patient is asked whether he hears the tone in the midline or in one ear or the other

lenticular process slightly enlarged ring at the end of the long process of the incus that articulates with the head of the stapes

lever advantage one of the middle ear mechani-

cal amplification methods that is due to the fact that the manubrium of the malleus is longer than the long process of the incus in the ossicular chain

light reflex reflection of an otoscope's light off the curved tympanic membrane; also called the cone of light

line spectrum amplitude spectrum that plots vertical lines at discrete frequencies present in periodic vibrations

localization ability to determine the direction from which a sound originated

longitudinal fracture temporal bone fracture that runs parallel along the edge of the petrous portion; generally results in conductive loss

longitudinal wave type of wave movement that involves increases and decreases in pressure in the direction of the vibrating object

loop diuretics drugs used to treat edema in patients with heart or lung disease

loudness psychological correlate of intensity

low frequency tail the part of a tuning curve that shows a relatively wide range of lower frequencies at moderate intensities that produce some criterion threshold response

low-pass filter a type of filter that transmits (passes) all frequencies below its cutoff frequency and attenuates those above the cutoff frequency

macula (plural = maculae) sensory organ of the saccule and utricle that is responsive to linear accelerations of the head; also called macula utriculi or macula sacculi

malleus first and largest of the middle ear ossicles, consisting of a manubrium, neck, anterior or lateral process, and head; the manubrium is attached to the tympanic membrane, and the head articulates with the body of the incus

manubrium handle (or long process) of the malleus that is attached to the tympanic membrane; visible through the tympanic membrane with otoscopy

MarkeTrak a publication that serves as a resource on the hearing aid industry from a consumer/patient standpoint

masked thresholds refers to the thresholds obtained in the test ear when masking was used in the non-test ear

masker a noise that is used to elevate or make

inaudible a test signal; noise that is presented in the non-test ear during clinical masking

masking refers to the elevation in threshold of a test signal by the presence of another sound, called the masker

mass susceptance (B_m) the part of the admittance that is related to the mass (inertial) component; mass susceptance is characterized by the force being 90° out of phase with velocity, and 180° out of phase with stiffness susceptance; plotted in the negative direction on a vector plot

mechanical vibrations back-and-forth movements of an object; action of the middle ear ossicles in the transduction process; bone conduction audiometry sets up mechanical vibrations in the skull that stimulate the inner ear

medial geniculate body (MGB) auditory nucleus at the level of the thalamus; receives ascending fibers from the inferior colliculi and sends fibers to the ipsilateral auditory cortex

medial vestibular nucleus medial region of the primary vestibular nuclei located in the posterior–lateral part of the upper medulla and lower pontine regions of the brainstem

mel a unit used to establish a pitch scale; assigns a standard reference value of 1,000 mels to the pitch associated with 1000 Hz (at a loudness of 40 phons), to which other frequencies are judged to be some multiple of 1,000 mels

membranous labyrinth fluid-filled membrane system that is suspended within the bony labyrinth; filled with endolymph; houses the organ of Corti in the cochlea, and the cristae and maculae in the vestibular organs

Ménière disease inner ear disorder related to the excessive buildup of endolymph; characterized by vertigo, fluctuating low frequency sensorineural hearing loss, aural fullness, and low-pitched tinnitus

meningitis inflammation of the meninges (membranous sheets covering the brain)

microtia abnormally small or malformed auricle

middle ear implant (MEI) a hearing aid that is surgically placed in the middle ear and operates using piezoelectric and electromagnetic transduction mechanisms

middle ear reflex (see acoustic reflex)

middle latency response (MLR) auditory evoked response occurring in the post-latency range of 12–80 ms reflecting activity of auditory events at the thalamus and cortical level; later latency than the auditory brainstem response and earlier latency than the late latency response

millimhos (mmhos) unit of measurement for admittance; 1/1000 of a mho

milliseconds (ms) unit of time; one-thousandth of a second (0.001 s)

mini-BTE hearing aids smaller version of the traditional behind the ear (BTE) style, with smaller tubing; can be worn with a more open canal fitting without custom earmold

minimum masking level the lowest level of masker introduced to the non-test ear when using the plateau method of clinical masking that is sufficient to keep the non-test ear from hearing the test tone

mixed hearing loss type of hearing loss in which there is a sensorineural component and a conductive component at a particular frequency; audiogram shows an elevation in bone conduction threshold (BC > 25 dB HL) and air-bone gap greater than 10 dB HL

modiolus porous bony core of the cochlea, where the nerve fibers from the cochlear hair cells come together to form the cochlear portion of the 8th cranial nerve, which then exits the cochlea through the internal auditory canal

monitored live voice method of presenting speech stimuli through the audiometer by speaking into a microphone; to insure proper calibration, the level of the speech is adjusted to peak the VU meter at zero

monomere (monomeric tympanic membrane) healed area of the tympanic membrane that is thinner than the rest of the membrane due to absence of the fibrous tissue layer

morphology the overall shape of an evoked potential waveform

most comfortable loudness level (MCL) dB HL of a tone or speech that is judged to be at a comfortable (preferred) level to listen

motility movement (elongations and contractions) of the outer hair cells that is a normal component of cochlear transduction; responsible for the active process of the cochlea that is necessary for good sensitivity and frequency tuning

mucoid otitis media chronic middle ear disorder in which the fluid in the middle ear becomes thick or pusslike; also called purulent otitis media or glue ear

multiple component tympanometry tympanometric measures that record susceptance (B) and conductance (G) tympanograms using higher frequency probe tones in order to determine relative contributions of stiffness and mass to the middle ear admittance

multiple frequency tympanometry tympanometric measures that record susceptance (B) and conductance (G) tympanograms as a function of probe-tone frequency (226–2000 Hz) to determine the resonant frequency of the middle ear in order to differentiate mass from stiffness disorders

myringotomy a surgical procedure to drain middle ear fluid by making a small incision in the tympanic membrane and extracting the fluid with a needle-type syringe; may be combined with placement of pressure equalization (PE) tubes

narrowband noise band-pass filtered noise concentrated around a center frequency; used in clinical pure-tone masking because it allows efficient masking over a wider intensity range than wideband noise; also called narrowband maskers

nasals speech sounds resulting from opening the velopharyngeal port sending air flow through the nasal cavity

nasopharynx region of the upper throat (above the velum) where the eustachian tube connects from the middle ear

neural synchrony a relatively large number of auditory neurons firing simultaneously

neuromonics a type of tinnitus treatment using sound therapy

neurophysiological basis of tinnitus comprehensive theory of tinnitus and treatment approach established by Pawel Jastreboff and colleagues

NOAH computer software platform that contains programming modules for digital hearing aids of different manufacturers

nodes a property of resonance where two interacting tones cancel each other out

noise aperiodic vibrations that are produced by a combination of many pure tones with random starting phases; unwanted potentials obtained from movement or electrical sources in evoked potential measures

noise floor inherent background signals in electronic equipment or otoacoustic emission measures, which the signal of interest must exceed

noise notch a sensorineural hearing loss in the 3–6 kHz region typical of excessive exposure to high noise levels

noise-induced hearing loss (NIHL) hearing loss resulting from excessive exposure to loud sounds; also called acoustic trauma; see also noise notch

noncompensated tympanogram a way to display a tympanogram whereby the display includes the admittance due to the ear canal (V_{ec} at +200 daPa) and the middle ear (Y_{tm})

nonorganic hearing loss (see functional hearing loss)

notched noise masking a physiological masking paradigm used in auditory brainstem response recordings to provide more frequency-specific information about the function of the cochlea; the noise is notch filtered to desynchronize part of the cochlea in order to observe responses from other regions

nystagmus involuntary horizontal eye movements resulting from neural connections between the vestibular and ocular systems; characterized by a slow (vestibular) component in the opposite direction of perceived head movement and a fast (visual) component that brings eyes back to center; recorded by monitoring the corneoretinal potential during electronystagmography

objective tests measures that do not require patients' subjective judgments or responses, e.g., tympanometry, acoustic reflexes, otoacoustic emissions, evoked potentials; usually independent of age, level of consciousness, and sedation

objective tinnitus relatively rare type of sound in the ear due to some vibratory source in the ear, head, or neck; may be audible to an external listener; often described as whooshing, pulsing, or clicking; usually has an underlying medical condition

occlusion effect (OE) an improvement in the bone conduction thresholds as a result of covering the non-test ear with a supra-aural earphone or wearing some hearing aids; originates from vibrations of the cartilaginous portion of the external auditory canal resulting from bone conducted sounds; greatest OE occurs at 250 Hz and lessens at 500 and 1000 Hz; OE is not significant when there is an air–bone gap in the non-test ear; OE is not significant above 1000 Hz.

octave doubling or halving of frequency

ohm unit of measurement for impedance; also used for electrical resistance

olivocochlear bundle (OCB) band of efferent auditory nerve fibers that originate in the superior olivary complex region and travel to the organ of Corti through the modiolus; approximately 800–1200 crossed (originate on contralateral side of brainstem) and uncrossed (originate on ipsilateral side of brainstem) efferent neurons comprise the OCB

one-third octave band-pass filter that is one-third octave wide at the 3 dB down points; narrowband noises used in clinical masking are one-third octave wide

open canal fitting a type of hearing aid fitting that uses a thin tube that is loosely inserted into the ear canal or held in place by an open ear mold or tip made of a flexible thin material and premade in a variety of sizes; allows more natural sound quality, a more comfortable feel, and no need for a custom earmold; not suitable for all degrees of hearing loss

open-set speech materials in which the patient does not have any prior familiarization or set of choices visually available

organ of Corti sensory organ of hearing that lies within the scala media along the basilar membrane from the base to apex of the cochlea; composed of receptor cells (inner and outer hair cells), support cells, spaces filled with perilymph, and the tectorial membrane

osseous spiral lamina shelf of bone that extends from the modiolus and winds (like threads of a screw) along the cochlea from the base to the apex of the cochlea; serves as the inner attachment of the basilar membrane

ossicles group of three bones of the middle ear—the malleus, incus, and stapes—which articulate with each other to transduce mechanical vibrations from the tympanic membrane to the inner ear; see also ossicular chain

ossicular chain term for the middle ear ossicles, collectively; see also ossicles

ossiculoplasty surgical procedure to repair middle ear ossicles and/or replace with a prosthetic component

osteoma benign single pearl-shaped bony growth in the ear canal

otalgia pain in the ear

otitis externa inflammation of the tissues lining the external auditory canal, usually caused by bacterial infection; also called swimmer's ear

otitis media inflammation or accumulation of fluid in the middle ear; also called otitis media with effusion; can be acute, chronic, intermittent; can be fluid free of bacteria (serous otitis media) or infected with bacteria (purulent)

otoacoustic emissions (OAEs) low-intensity acoustic vibrations measured in the ear canal with a sensitive microphone that originate from energy produced by the motility of the outer hair cells, and reverse transmission of this activity along the basilar membrane and through the middle ear to the ear canal; widely used in newborn hearing screening programs and basic diagnostic tests of auditory function; see also transient otoacoustic emissions and distortion product otoacoustic emissions

otoconia layer of dense calcium carbonate crystals on top of the otolithic membrane in the maculae

otoliths used to refer to the saccule and utricle, saclike sensory organs of the vestibular system; part of the membranous labyrinth located in the vestibule region of the inner ear

otologists appropriately trained and licensed/certified medical physicians specializing in disorders and surgery related to the ears, also called neuro-otologists, otolaryngologists, or ear, noise, and throat (ENT) specialists

otology medical specialty related to the ears, practiced by appropriately trained and certified otologists

otorrhea fluid draining into external auditory canal from the middle ear

otosclerosis caused by outgrowth of bony wall (otospongiosis) around the stapes footplate; commonly causes middle ear conductive hearing loss when stapes is immobilized; less commonly, toxins may invade the cochlea and cause a sensorineural hearing loss; also called otospongiosis

otoscope lighted instrument used to examine external auditory canal and tympanic membrane

otospongiosis (see otosclerosis)

ototoxicity hearing loss due to poisonous side effects from some therapeutic drugs or environmental toxins

outer hair cells (OHCs) auditory sensory hair cells within the organ of Corti; approximately 12,500 OHCs arranged in three rows; have a motoric function (see motility) that is part of the active cochlear process responsible for good hearing sensitivity and frequency

outer spiral fibers afferent nerve fibers that cross the tunnel of Corti and connect to the outer hair cells (less than 5% of afferent neurons are outer spiral fibers)

oval window oval-shaped opening into the cochlea (scala vestibuli) to which the stapes footplate is attached; normal route for transmission of vibrations to the inner ear

overmasking a situation that may arise in clinical masking in which the level of the masker is sufficient to exceed the interaural attenuation and the noise masker crosses over to the test ear and interferes with establishing the true threshold

pars flaccida a small region at the superior margin of the tympanic membrane that is thinner and more flaccid due to the absence of the fibrous tissue layer; also called Shrapnell's membrane

pars tensa major part of the tympanic membrane that is fairly rigid due to the presence of a fibrous tissue layer between the skin lining the external ear canal and the mucous lining of the middle ear space

passive cochlear process the process of cochlear transduction that is related to the physical parameters of the basilar membrane (e.g., narrower and stiffer at the base), which produce the tonotopic traveling waves well documented by Békésy; when measured without the active process of the outer hair cells, the passive process is more broadly tuned and less sensitive

patent open, usually referring to an unoccluded PE tube or abnormally open eustachian tube

PB$_{max}$ the patient's maximum speech recognition score, usually in reference to percent correct of phonemically balanced words used in word recognition score tests; also used as one of the values in the calculation of a rollover ratio from performance intensity functions (PI–PB functions)

PB$_{min}$ the word recognition score at high intensities, beyond PB$_{max}$, that is used in the calculation of the rollover ratio

peak amplitude (A$_p$) amplitude of a waveform as measured from baseline to one of the peaks

peak-to-peak amplitude (A$_{p-p}$) amplitude of a waveform as measured from the most positive peak to the most negative peak

perforation hole in the tympanic membrane

performance-intensity function for PB words (PI–PB function) a method to characterize a patient's word recognition score as a function of presentation level; useful for determining a patient's best word recognition ability (PB$_{max}$) and to calculate a rollover ratio; see PI–PB rollover

perilymph fluid in the bony labyrinth, but outside the membranous labyrinth, that has relatively high sodium (Na$^+$) and low potassium (K$^+$) concentrations

perilymph fistula rupture in the oval window or round window membrane leaking perilymph fluid into the middle ear

period description used to characterize sound waves that refers to the time (seconds or milliseconds) it takes to complete one cycle; reciprocal of frequency

period histogram recording of the firing pattern from a neuron, displayed as a function of the period of the stimulus

periodic vibration sound waves in which the vibratory pattern repeats itself at regular intervals

peripheral auditory (or vestibular) system

refers to auditory and vestibular structures and nerves that are located outside the central nervous system

permanent threshold shifts (PTS) hearing loss due to excessive exposure to noise that does not recover; also called noise-induced hearing loss (NIHL)

petrous part of the temporal bone that is directed medially into the skull and houses the middle ear and inner ear structures

phalangeal process a fingerlike process coming from the Deiter cells, which extends up to the upper surface of an adjacent outer hair cell and fills in what would have been a space between the outer hair cells at the upper surface

phase-locking a characteristic pattern of neural discharges in which they always fire during the same phase of the stimulus

phon a unit used to describe a scale of loudness judgments that are judged equal across frequency; a phon is equal to the dB HL of a 1000 Hz tone, e.g., 40 phons is equal to the loudness associated with a 1000 Hz tone at 40 dB HL; see equal loudness contours

phoneme score a way of analyzing word recognition score performance that counts the number of correctly identified phonemes for each word (each phonemically balanced (PB) word has three phonemes), and reports the score as a percentage of the total available phonemes across the entire list of words (e.g., a 25-item PB word list has 75 phonemes)

phonemically balanced (PB) words lists of single-syllable words in which the consonant-vowel-consonant components occur the same number of times within a list

pillar cells support cells in the organ of Corti that form the tunnel of Corti, which separates the inner hair cells from the outer hair cells

PI–PB rollover performance intensity function for phonemically balanced words, which demonstrates a measured decrease in the word recognition score at high presentation levels; rollover is calculated as $PB_{max} - PB_{min} / PB_{max}$; rollover ratios greater than 0.35 are suggestive of 8th nerve disorder

pitch psychological correlate of frequency

place theory of hearing theory of frequency coding based a tonotopic arrangement along the basilar membrane for sounds of different frequencies

plateau a term used in clinical masking that represents a range of noise increases in the non-test ear that are not accompanied by any change in the threshold in the test ear

plateau method a commonly used masking method, first described by Hood (1960), in which a masking plateau is established; see also plateau

preauricular appendage or tag small skin growth anterior to the tragus due to embryologic alterations

preauricular pit or sinus small dimple just anterior to the tragus due to embryologic alterations

presbycusis hearing loss related to aging

prescriptive fitting method strategy for fitting hearing aids that has been shown to provide the best outcome; uses a mathematical model of selecting gain and output based on the patient's hearing loss

pressure measure of force distributed over an area; units of dynes/cm^2, newton/m^2, or micropascals (μPa) depending on the system of measurement being used

pressure-equalization (PE) tube small polyethylene tube inserted into the tympanic membrane to permit (maintain) ventilation of middle ear; allows equalized air pressure on both sides of tympanic membrane in cases of persistent otitis media and poor eustachian tube function

prevalence an epidemiology term to refer to the number of new and old cases of a disorder present within a specified period of time

primary tones designators of the two externally applied tones (f1 and f2) used to generate the distortion product tone (2f1–f2) during distortion product otoacoustic emission (DPOAE) testing

probe microphone verification (see real-ear measures)

probe tone the tone used in immittance testing that is applied through the probe in the ear canal, and which is used to monitor changes in admittance; standard probe tone is 226 Hz at 85 dB SPL; higher frequency probe tones are sometimes used (see multiple component or multiple frequency tympanometry)

promontory the bony wall on the medial surface of the middle ear that lies between the round window and oval window; used as a site for cochlear stimulation in cochlear implant assessments and transtympanic electrocochleography

propagation the movement of sound waves through some elastic medium

proximal toward the origin or center of a structure or nerve; opposite of distal

psychoacoustics science concerned with how humans perceive sound; study of the psychological correlates of physical properties of sound

pulsatile tinnitus a type of objective tinnitus generally described as a pulsing or whooshing sound; related to the rhythm of blood flow/heartbeat

pure-tone audiometry a basic hearing test that involves finding a patient's thresholds (in dB HL) for different pure tones presented by air conduction and bone conduction; used to describe type and degree of hearing loss

pure-tone average (PTA) the average threshold calculated from the air conduction thresholds at 500, 1000, and 2000 Hz

pure tones simple sound waves that have only one frequency of vibration; also called sinusoids or sine waves

quarter-wave resonator a condition of resonance whereby the fundamental frequency is equal to a quarter wavelength, e.g., for a tube open at one end

rarefaction the phase of a waveform that is associated with a decrease in the density of air molecules, and which corresponds to a decrease in sound pressure

real-ear measures a hearing aid verification step process in which measures are made of the output of the hearing aid at the tympanic membrane of the hearing aid user; requires the placement of a thin silicone tube in the ear canal, which is attached to a measurement microphone, to obtain patient-specific information relative to the ear canal characteristics while it is being worn by the patient

recorded speech materials speech materials that are on some recorded media such as tape or compact disk; used for speech testing

recruitment an abnormal growth of loudness in an ear with a cochlear hearing loss

reference equivalent threshold dB SPL (RET-SPLs) reference levels for pure tones and speech, set by ANSI, that correspond to the average normal thresholds; calibration values used for audiometers for dB hearing level, the most recent of which should appear on the y-axis of an audiogram

reference level for intensity lowest average intensity needed to hear a sound as provided by accepted standards (ANSI); current standard is 1.0×10^{-12} w/m^2

reference level for pressure lowest average pressure needed to hear a sound as provided by accepted standards (ANSI); current standard is 20 μPa

reflex eliciting tones the stimulus tones (500, 1000, and 2000 Hz) used to test for acoustic reflexes; may be presented ipsilaterally or contralaterally

Reissner's membrane the surface of the membranous labyrinth (scala media) in the cochlea that separates scala media from scala vestibuli

rejection rate (see attenuation rate)

reliability a description of a test's ability to obtain the same results when repeated across sessions or multiple testers

reproducibility value correlation between two channels of otoacoustic emission recordings; calculated for different frequency components and displayed as a percentage for each frequency band

resonance the property of a cavity that produces a maximum vibratory response at a particular frequency that is dependent on its size and shape

reticular lamina upper surface of the organ of Corti, formed by the tight mosaic of the tops of all the cells, including the phalangeal processes, tops of the pillars, and the cuticular plates of the hair cells; boundary between endolymph above the reticular lamina and perilymph below the reticular lamina (in the spaces of the organ of Corti)

retraction pocket an abnormal condition of the tympanic membrane in which the pars flaccida region of the tympanic membrane is drawn into the middle ear due to the negative middle ear pressure; early sign of eustachian tube dysfunction

retrocochlear pertaining to the 8th cranial nerve and cerebellar-pontine angle

Rinne test a tuning fork test in which the tuning fork is alternately placed first on the mastoid (bone conducted tone) and then in front of the ear canal (air conducted tone) and the patient is asked to compare the loudness of the two placements or whether the air conducted sound is heard after the bone conducted sound is no longer audible

rollover ratio the ratio of the greatest amount of decline (PB_{min}) of word recognition score that occurs at intensities higher than the PB_{max}: rollover ratio = $(PB_{max} - PB_{min})/PB_{max}$; rollover ratio greater than 0.35 suggests retrocochlear disorder

root-mean-square (RMS) amplitude (A_{rms}) average amplitude (dB SPL) of a waveform integrated over a period of time; obtained by squaring each of the instantaneous amplitudes, averaging the squared values, and taking the square root of the average; equivalent to 0.707 times the peak amplitude for pure tones; measured with sound level meters

Rosenthal's canal channel that coils from the base to the apex located in the bony core of the cochlea just prior to the osseous spiral lamina; location of the spiral ganglia

round window a membrane-covered round-shaped opening between the middle ear and the cochlea (scala tympani); allows for vibrations to enter the fluid-filled cochlea through reciprocal action with the oval window

saccule one of the sensory organs (otoliths) of the vestibular system, located in the vestibule of the inner ear; houses the macula which responds to linear accelerations of the head and orientation relative to gravity; see also utricle

salicylates group of anti-inflammatory drugs, such as aspirin; can cause temporary sensorineural hearing loss

sawtooth waveform complex periodic waveform that is composed of a fundamental frequency and its harmonics; produces a buzzing type of tonal sound

scala media membranous labyrinth within the cochlea; filled mostly with endolymph and houses the organ of Corti; divides the bony labyrinth of the cochlea into its three chambers (scala media, scala vestibuli, and scale tympani); one edge of the scala media is called the basilar membrane and the other edge is called Reissner's membrane

scala tympani lowermost section of the bony labyrinth next to the basilar membrane of the scala media; filled with perilymph; joins the scala vestibuli at the helicotrema

scala vestibuli uppermost section of the bony labyrinth next to Reissner's membrane of the scala media; filled with perilymph; joins the scala tympani at the helicotrema

Scarpa's ganglion (see vestibular ganglion)

scope of practice documents developed (separately) by the American Academy of Audiology (AAA) the American Speech-Language-Hearing Association (ASHA) that describe the services that are considered appropriate for audiologists

screening audiometer a small portable device that only uses pure tones to assess hearing

Self-Assessment for Communication a self-assessment of hearing disability generally used with adult hearing screenings

semicircular canals three orthogonally oriented canals of the vestibular system that respond to angular accelerations of the head

sensitivity the ability of a test to correctly identify those who have a specific disorder or condition

sensorineural hearing loss type of hearing loss described from pure-tone audiometric results that is caused by disorders in the inner ear or neural pathways; characterized by elevation of both bone conduction and air conduction thresholds, with air–bone gaps less than or equal to 10 dB

serous otitis media fluid in the middle ear is clear and not infected

shape of hearing loss one of the parameters used in describing audiograms; refers to the amount configuration of the thresholds across frequency, e.g., sloping, flat, notched, rising

sharply tuned tuning curves with a relatively

narrow (sharp) tip region, as occurs with normal hearing

Shrapnell's membrane (see pars flaccida)

signal-averaging computer a specialized computer that averages synchronous neural responses; typically used in measurement of evoked potentials; response is time-locked to the onset of the stimulus to enhance the response of interest and reduce the random noise signals (improves the signal-to-noise ratio)

signal-to-noise-ratio (S/N ratio) relationship between the level of a sound or evoked potential and a background noise, that is either purposefully presented or is inherent in the evoked response recording

simple vibration sound wave with simple harmonic motion as a function of time; also called pure tone, sine wave, or sinusoid

sine waves (see simple vibration)

sinusoids (see simple vibration)

sone a loudness scale where one sone is defined as the loudness of a 1000 Hz tone at 40 dB SPL (or 40 phons)

sound-field testing presentation of test materials using loudspeakers; also called free-field testing

spaces of Nuel spaces surrounding the outer hair cells of the organ of Corti; filled with perilymph

speaker (or loudspeaker) an electroacoustic transducer that converts electrical energy to acoustic energy; used in audiometry during sound-field testing

specificity the ability of a test to correctly identify those who do not have a specific disorder or condition

spectrogram an graphic output of a spectrograph displaying frequencies (y-axis) as function of time (x-axis); intensity can be represented by the darkness of the displayed frequencies

spectrograph an instrument used to measure the spectra of speech sounds

spectrum (plural = spectra) representation of complex vibrations that determines the individual amplitudes as a function of frequency (frequency spectrum) and/or the starting phases as a function of frequency (phase spectrum); see also fast Fourier transform (FFT)

speech audiometry method used in clinic to evaluate how well a patient can hear and understand specific types of speech stimuli

speech banana a representation of how different speech sounds are distributed on the audiogram; term comes from the general outline of the distribution

speech detection threshold (SDT) speech audiometry test that determines the lowest level at which a patient indicates he is aware that a sound was presented, but does not require the patient to repeat the word; also called speech awareness threshold (SAT)

speech intelligibility index (SII) (see articulation index)

speech noise masker a masking noise used in speech audiometry that is filtered to resemble the range of frequencies representative of those in the speech spectrum

speech recognition threshold (SRT) a speech audiometry test that determines the lowest level at which a patient can correctly identify words at least 50% of the time; used to be called speech reception threshold procedure

speech threshold the lowest level at which a patient is able to respond to speech at least 50% of the time; see speech recognition threshold

speech-language pathologist a professional who has the appropriate degree and license in their state to practice speech-language pathology; typically certified by the American Speech-Language-Hearing Association (ASHA)

speed of sound (in air) 343 m/s or 1,126 feet/s

spike nerve impulse or action potential

spiral ganglion (plural = ganglia) collection of cell bodies of the afferent auditory neurons; located in Rosenthal's canal within the modiolus of the cochlea from base to apex

spiral limbus connective tissue cell within the organ of Corti that lies just above the edge of the osseous spiral lamina; serves as the attachment point for the medial end of the tectorial membrane

spondee words two-syllable (compound) words with equal stress on each syllable, used to obtain the speech recognition threshold (SRT)

stapedectomy surgical procedure in which the

stapes is replaced with a prosthetic device; a treatment for otosclerosis

stapedial branch (of the 7th cranial nerve) branch of the facial nerve that innervates the stapedius muscle of the middle ear; involved in the acoustic reflex

stapedial reflex involuntary contraction of the stapedius muscles when the ear is stimulated by loud sounds as part of the acoustic reflex; innervation through the stapedial branch of the 7th cranial nerve; stimulation of either ear results in a bilateral stapedial reflex; also called acoustic reflex

stapedius muscle small middle ear muscle that arises from the medial wall of the middle ear cavity and attaches to the head (neck) of the stapes; the muscle is innervated by the stapedial branch of the 7th cranial nerve

stapedotomy surgical procedure in which a prosthesis is inserted into a hole drilled in the stapes footplate; a treatment for otosclerosis

stapes third and smallest of the middle ear ossicles, consisting of a head (neck), anterior crus, posterior crus, and footplate; the head is attached to the incus at the lenticular process, and the footplate is attached to the oval window at the entrance to the inner ear

stapes fixation bony growth (otospongiosis) in otosclerosis that encapsulates the stapes and prevents its vibration in the oval window

starting phase position in a waveform's cycle where the vibration begins, expressed in degrees relative to the angle around the circle

Stenger test audiometric test for unilateral nonorganic (functional) hearing loss

stenosis (stenotic ear) abnormal narrowing of the external auditory canal

stereocilia bundles of hairlike microvilli that project from the tops of inner and outer hair cells; stereocilia on each hair cell are arranged in three to four rows with increasing heights and joined to each other by tip links and cross links; stereocilia arrangement looks like a "W" on outer hair cells and a crescent on inner hair cells; bending of stereocilia opens ionic channels that alter the ionic flow to the hair cell

stiffness susceptance (B$_s$) the part of the admittance that is related to the stiffness (spring) component; stiffness susceptance is characterized by the force being 90° out of phase with velocity, and 180° out of phase with mass susceptance; plotted in the positive direction on a vector plot

stops parts of speech in which there is a brief period in which airflow is blocked followed by a burst of airflow when articulators are opened; can be voiced or unvoiced

stria vascularis highly vascularized system of cells along the outer wall of the scala media in the cochlea that maintains the ionic charge of the endolymph

subjective tests tests that require the patient to make a judgment; based on one's perceptions; opposite of objective tests

subjective tinnitus perception of sounds in the ear commonly reported with a variety of hearing losses, and which are not audible to others; typically described by patients as a ringing, hissing, or roaring sound; also known as nonvibratory tinnitus

sudden hearing loss hearing loss with a rapid onset (within a few hours)

superior olivary complex (SOC) auditory nucleus located in the lower brainstem

superior vestibular nucleus upper region of the primary vestibular nuclei located in the posterior–lateral part of the upper medulla and lower pontine regions of the brainstem

supra-aural earphone an air conduction transducer that is placed on the auricle; converts electrical energy to acoustic energy; commonly used model, TDH-50

suprathreshold a decibel level that is above the patient's hearing threshold

table of critical differences a table of values based on the binomial distribution for word recognition scores; used to compare two scores to determine when they are significantly different (at the 95% confidence interval) from each other

tactile response pure-tone threshold that occurs due to the patient feeling the vibrations (sense of touch) rather than hearing them; may occur with bone conduction testing at 250 and 500 Hz between 40 and 60 dB HL; also called vibrotactile responses

targeted screening test a screening test applied to a subpopulation more likely to have the disorder

tectorial membrane thin membrane overlying the stereocilia of hair cells in the organ of Corti; attached medially to the spiral limbus and laterally to the Hensen cells; stereocilia of the outer hair cells are embedded in the undersurface of the tectorial membrane, whereas those of the inner hair cells are not embedded

telecoil an alternative input source to a hearing aid that converts the electromagnetic signal from a telephone or assistive listening device and delivers it directly to the amplifier

temporal bone lateral part of the skull in which the auditory and vestibular structures are found; divided into four main parts, squamous, mastoid, tympanic, and petrous (where most of the middle and inner structures are located)

temporal integration the relationship between the threshold of audibility and the duration of a sound; thresholds for a pure tone generally increase as the duration decreases below 200 ms

temporal lobe part of the cortex on the lateral side, above the temporal bone and below the lateral sulcus; location in the cortex of the primary auditory reception area of the cortex (Heschel's gyrus)

temporary threshold shift (TTS) nonpermanent hearing loss that can occur from exposure to high levels of noise, but recovers within several hours after exposure; occurs at noise levels lower than those that can cause permanent threshold shift

tensor tympani muscle small middle ear muscle that arises from the bony wall above the eustachian tube and its tendon attaches to the manubrium of the malleus; innervated by the 5th cranial nerve; may have some involvement in the acoustic reflex, but in humans it does not play much of a role; see stapedius muscle

tensor veli palatini muscle in the nasopharynx that is responsible for opening the eustachian tube; innervated by the 5th cranial nerve

threshold the lowest level of a pure tone that a person reliably responds to at least 50% of the time for a specified number of trials

threshold of audibility curve graphical representation of the average dB SPL for normal hearing human listeners across the frequency range of hearing

time-domain waveform representation of a vibration's amplitude as a function of time; see also waveform

time-locked a term used in signal averaging to indicate that the physiological response of interest is recorded relative to the onset of each stimulus and is enhanced with signal averaging; random noise is not time-locked and is reduced during signal averaging

tinnitus auditory perceptions in the absence of externally presented sounds, commonly reported with a variety of hearing disorders; often called ringing in the ears; see also objective tinnitus and subjective tinnitus

tinnitus maskability audiometric assessment of how much narrowband noise is needed to mask a patient's tinnitus

tinnitus matching audiometric matching of a patient's tinnitus to a pure-tone or narrowband noise

tinnitus retraining therapy (TRT) a sound therapy treatment approach for tinnitus that is based on a neurophysiological/psychological basis of tinnitus made popular by Pawel Jastreboff

tip region of the tuning curve the narrow range of frequencies with the best sensitivities as displayed by a tuning curve; the tip represents the characteristic frequency of the tuning curve

tip links microfilaments that interconnect the tops of stereocilia of each inner and outer hair cell; thought to be the source of the ion channels that open and close with bending of the stereocilia

tone bursts short-duration tonal stimuli, with a relatively rapid onset (rise time), used for evoked potential testing

tragus flap of cartilage on the auricle that protrudes anterior to the entrance of the external auditory canal

transducer an instrument that converts energy from one type to another; an earphone is a transducer that converts electrical energy to acoustic energy, and a microphone is a transducer that converts acoustic energy into electrical energy

transduction the change in sound energy from one form to another

transfer function of the middle ear experimental measurements that document changes in pressure that occur between the tympanic membrane and the oval window membrane

transient evoked otoacoustic emissions (TEOAEs) type of otoacoustic emissions that are evoked by a series of brief clicks (transients) and measured by signal averaging of the acoustic signals generated by the ear and picked up by a sensitive microphone in the ear canal

transients brief acoustic signals with nearly instantaneous onset and offset and broad frequency spectrum; used to achieve neural synchrony in evoked response measures of the auditory system

transverse fracture temporal bone fracture that is perpendicular to the long axis of the petrous portion of the temporal bone; often causes sensorineural hearing loss due to damage to the inner ear

traveling wave displacement pattern along the basilar membrane that is essential in sound processing, characterized by initial displacements near the base and progressing to its maximum displacement (see traveling wave peak) at the location corresponding to its characteristic frequency; peaks of the traveling waves occur tonotopically, in which high frequencies produce peaks at the base and low frequencies produce peaks at the apex

traveling wave peak location where the maximum amplitude (displacement) of the basilar membrane occurs for any given pure tone, represented by the peak of the traveling wave envelope

triangular fossa indentation formed between the antihelix and the helix on the auricle

tuning curve a representation of the frequency selectivity of the auditory system, generated for a variety of physiologic and psychoacoustic measures; shows the different intensity by frequency combinations that produce some criterion threshold response; characterized by a tip region (around the characteristic frequency), a low frequency tail, and a steep high frequency slope

tuning fork a handheld metal instrument (two pronged) designed to produce a tone when struck; used by otologists during hearing exams

tunnel of Corti space in the center of the organ of Corti, formed by the inner and outer pillar cells, which separates the inner and outer hair cells; filled with perilymph

tympanic annulus outer rim of the tympanic membrane which is embedded into an indentation (tympanic sulcus) of the tympanic portion of the temporal bone, to hold the tympanic membrane in place; also called the tympanic ring

tympanic membrane the membrane that separates the ear canal from the middle ear; has a fibrous tissue layer throughout most of the membrane (pars tensa), but is devoid of the fibrous tissue layer in the superior margin (pars flaccida); transduces acoustic vibrations entering the ear canal into mechanical vibrations of the middle ear ossicles

tympanic sulcus indentation in the tympanic portion of the temporal bone where the tympanic annulus of the tympanic membrane is embedded

tympanogram a graph used for tympanometry to display how the admittance in mmhos (y-axis) changes as a function of applied air pressure in daPa (x-axis)

tympanometric peak pressure (TPP) the pressure (in daPa) where the peak admittance of the tympanogram occurs

tympanometric width (TW) a measure (in daPa) to describe the shape of a tympanogram; determined by the absolute difference between the two pressure values (on the x-axis) that are associated with the intersections of a horizontal line across the tympanogram at half of its height

tympanometry a part of the clinical immittance test battery that measures how the admittance changes as a function of applied air pressure (above and below atmospheric pressure), and how this function is affected by different conditions of the middle ear; produces a graph called a tympanogram

type A tympanogram a normal tympanogram, characterized by a peak admittance of the middle ear (Y_{tm}) in the expected normal range, a tympanometric peak pressure (TPP) at 0 daPa, and a normal tympanometric width

type A_d tympanogram an abnormal tympanogram, characterized by a peak admittance of the middle ear (Y_{tm}) that is higher than the expected normal range, a tympanometric peak pressure at 0 daPa, and a normal tympanometric width (if measurable); suggests a highly flaccid tympanic membrane or a disarticulation of the ossicles

type A$_s$ tympanogram an abnormal tympanogram, characterized by a peak admittance of the middle ear (Y_{tm}) that is lower than the expected normal range, a tympanometric peak pressure at 0 daPa, and a normal tympanometric width; suggests a reduced mobility stiffening of the tympanic membrane that is often seen with otosclerosis

type B tympanogram an abnormal tympanogram, characterized by a flat (no change) admittance across the pressure range; seen with middle ear fluid, impacted cerumen, or perforation of the tympanic membrane differentiated by the measured ear canal equivalent volume (V_{ec})

type C tympanogram an abnormal tympanogram, characterized by a peak admittance of the middle ear (Y_{tm}) that occurs with a tympanometric peak pressure that is more negative than normal range; may have normal or reduced peak admittance of the middle ear and normal or abnormally wide tympanometric width; suggests negative middle ear pressure associated with poor eustachian tube function

type of hearing loss one of the parameters used in describing audiograms; type of loss can be either conductive, sensorineural, or mixed for any frequency

ultra-high-frequency earphone a transducer used for air conduction testing in special situations where the frequencies above 8000 Hz are to be evaluated; common model, Sennheiser HDA200

umbo central location on the tympanic membrane where the tip of the manubrium of the malleus is attached

uncomfortable loudness level (UCL) an intensity level where the patient finds speech or tones to cause discomfort; also called loudness discomfort level (LDL)

undermasking the levels used in clinical masking that are not sufficient to eliminate cross-hearing in the non-test ear (not yet on the plateau); initial masking level to where the plateau begins; also called "the chase"

unilateral to one side; hearing loss affecting only one side

unilateral head turn visual reinforcement hearing test procedure that only requires infant to turn head to one side (where he is reinforced) regardless of the direction or ear to which the sound is presented

universal screening test a screening test applied to a large population

up 5, down 10 procedure threshold search procedure used in audiometry; performed by increasing the level in 5 dB steps when the patient does not respond, and decreasing the level in 10 dB steps when the patient responds

utricle one of the sensory organs (otoliths) of the vestibular system, located in the vestibule of the inner ear; houses the macula which responds to linear accelerations of the head and orientation relative to gravity; see also saccule

validation part of the hearing aid fitting process that obtains information, usually through subjective questionnaires, about how well the hearing aid is working for the patient and the benefit he is receiving

validity a reflection of a test's ability to measure what it purports to measure

verification part of the hearing aid fitting process to obtain confirmation through some measure (e.g., real-ear measures) that a hearing aid fitting has maximized the audibility and speech understanding, has good sound quality, and appropriate loudness perceptions, and is "acceptable" to the patient

vertigo type of dizziness that originates in the vestibular organs of the inner ear, generally described as a sensation of "the room is spinning" or "motion sickness"

vestibular compensation ability of the vestibular system to adapt to vestibular disorders through reinterpretation of the abnormal input by the central nervous system; may improve spontaneously or through vestibular rehabilitation

vestibular ganglion cell bodies for the vestibular peripheral neurons; located within the internal auditory canal; also called Scarpa's ganglion

vestibular nerve portion of the 8th cranial nerve consisting of nerve fibers from the semicircular canals, saccule, and utricle

vestibular nerve section surgical procedure in which the vestibular portion of the 8th cranial nerve is cut in order to alleviate vertigo in patients with serious vestibular disorder

vestibular schwannoma (see acoustic neuroma)

vestibule cavity in the bony labyrinth that lies between the semicircular canals and the cochlea; location of the oval window and the otoliths

vestibulocochlear nerve 8th cranial nerve, composed of the vestibular nerve and the cochlear (or auditory) nerve

vestibulo-ocular reflex (VOR) eye movements that are equal and opposite to the direction of head movements, induced through the vestibular neural pathway and its connections with the cranial nerves that control the extraocular muscles of the eyes

vestibulo-spinal reflex (VSR) body-orientating reflexes, induced through the vestibular neural pathway and its connections with reticular formation and spinal tract nerves that control skeletal muscles

vestibulotoxicity vestibular damage/disorder due to poisonous side effects from some therapeutic drugs or environmental toxins

visual reinforcement audiometry (VRA) a technique used to test children 6 months to 2 years of age using visual reinforcements in a conditioning paradigm

vowels complex periodic parts of speech with a tonal quality; generally carry most of the audible energy in speech

voiced sound complex periodic component of speech generated by vocal fold vibration

voiceless sound an aperiodic component of speech in which vocal folds do not vibrate

VU meter (volume unit meter) a monitoring meter to adjust the input level of signals so that the output is set to be in calibration with the audiometer's intensity (dB HL) dial

warble tones a tone in which the frequency is modulated with small rapid changes; used in sound-field testing to reduce standing waves (where two waves come together and reduce the amplitude)

wave I the earliest positive wave in an auditory brainstem response recording; source is the more peripheral (distal) portion of the 8th nerve; occurs with a latency around 1.5–2.0 ms at moderately high stimulus levels

wave V the most prominent positive deflection in an auditory brainstem response recording; occurs with a latency around 5.5–6.0 ms at moderately high stimulus levels; most common wave peak used for assessment of objective auditory thresholds; origin in the contralateral lateral lemniscus/inferior colliculus regions of the brainstem

waveform pattern of movement of a sound wave displayed with amplitude as a function of time; also is used in reference to evoked responses (otoacoustic emissions or evoked electrical potentials) to describe how the response amplitude varies as a function of time; also called time-domain waveform

wavelength (λ) the distance a sound wave travels in one cycle, measured in units of length; the distance between the same points on two successive cycles of a pure tone; $\lambda = c/f$, where c is the speed of sound in air and f is the frequency

Weber test a tuning fork test for unilateral hearing loss in which the tuning fork is placed on the midline of the skull (upper forehead) and the patient is asked to report if the sound lateralizes to one of the ears or not

white noise a noise with an infinite number of frequencies with random phases and equal amplitudes over the entire frequency range

whole word score a method of reporting the word recognition score (WRS) that reflects the percentage of correctly identified words

wideband middle ear power (WMEP) measures the stimulus power that is reflected from the tympanic membrane (not admitted into the middle ear) for a variety of applied frequencies

word recognition score (WRS) the percentage of correctly identified words obtained from suprathreshold word recognition tests

word recognition testing a supra-threshold speech test using single-syllable word lists (e.g., Northwestern University [NU-6]) that are phonemically balanced (PB) words

Index

Note: Page numbers in **bold** reference non-text material

Whole word score, 202
Wide dynamic range compression (WDRC), 323
Wideband middle ear power (WMEP), 243–244, **243**, 254
Wideband reflectometry, 243
Willeford, Jack, 376
Williams-Steiger Occupational Health Act (1971), 378
Wilson-Vlotman, Ann, 380
Wireless connectivity, hearing aids, 326

Word Identification by Picture Identification (WIPI), 215
Word recognition score (WRS), 201–210, 215, 219
Word recognition testing, 201–210

Z

Zwislocki, Jozef, 368, 369, 370
Zygomatic process, 8